The One Best way?

Studies in Childhood and Family in Canada

Studies in Childhood and Family in Canada is a multidisciplinary series devoted to new perspectives on these subjects as they evolve. The series features studies that focus on the intersections of age, class, race, gender, and region as they contribute to a Canadian understanding of childhood and family, both historically and currently.

Series Editor

Cynthia Comacchio
Department of History
Wilfrid Laurier University

Manuscripts to be sent to

Brian Henderson, Director
Wilfrid Laurier University Press
75 University Avenue West
Waterloo, Ontario N2L 3C5
Canada

Tasnim Nathoo
and Aleck Ostry

The One Best way?

Breastfeeding History, Politics, and Policy in Canada

Wilfrid Laurier University Press

[WLU]

This book has been published with the help of a grant from the Canadian Federation for the Humanities and Social Sciences, through the Aid to Scholarly Publications Programme, using funds provided by the Social Sciences and Humanities Research Council of Canada. Wilfrid Laurier University Press acknowledges the financial support of the Government of Canada through its Book Publishing Industry Development Program for its publishing activities.

Library and Archives Canada Cataloguing in Publication

Nathoo, Tasnim, [date]
   The one best way? : breastfeeding history, politics, and policy in Canada / Tasnim Nathoo and Aleck Ostry.

(Studies in childhood and family in Canada)
Includes bibliographical references and index.
ISBN 978-1-55458-147-4

   1. Breastfeeding–Canada–Social aspects. 2. Breastfeeding–Canada–Political aspects.
I. Ostry, Aleck Samuel, [date] II. Title. III. Series.

RJ216.N36 2009   649'.330971   C2008-906595-6

Cover photo iStockphoto/Gansovsky Vlad. Cover and text design by Blakeley Words+Pictures.

Every reasonable effort has been made to acquire permission for copyright material used in this text, and to acknowledge all such indebtedness accurately. Any errors and omissions called to the publisher's attention will be corrected in future printings.

This book is printed on FSC recycled paper and is certified Ecologo. It is made from 100% post-consumer fibre, processed chlorine free, and manufactured using biogas energy.

Printed in Canada

Contents

Illustrations

Figures

Graphs

Tables

Authors' Note

Historically, practical knowledge and lore about breastfeeding generally has been carried across generations by women. During the writing of this book, we were fortunate to hear many, many stories of individuals' experiences with various aspects of breastfeeding. Family, friends, colleagues, and near strangers who innocently asked about our work privileged us with their own experiences and those of their private networks. In this book, we describe how the intimate and everyday practice of breastfeeding has been shaped by political and economic interests and social pressures. While we have attempted to include stories of women's actual experiences, this book is crafted primarily from written history. We hope that this book serves as a foundation for reconsidering and exploring personal experiences and family stories, and for contextualizing the oral history of breastfeeding practices in Canada.

Throughout this project, we received support from an enormous number of individuals and organizations. We have been fortunate to build on the strength of previous scholarly, professional, and lay work that has documented and preserved that history and politics of infant feeding in various forms. We are grateful to all the research assistants, colleagues, mothers, lactivists, friends and family members who have strengthened this book with their insights and creativity as well as maintained a continual wellspring of enthusiasm for this work—it has been a privilege and a pleasure.

Introduction

The One Best Way?

You will be able to nurse the baby. Never think of anything else.
Nursing the baby yourself is the one best way.
–*The Canadian Mother's Book*, published by the Department of Health, 1923

Dr. Helen MacMurchy wrote the above words in Canada's first piece of federal government-sponsored child-care advice literature for mothers. As the newly appointed head of the Division of Child Welfare, one of MacMurchy's central goals during her tenure was to establish breastfeeding as "the Canadian way"–in spite of the already dramatic decline in breastfeeding rates observed across the country.

While most of us are familiar with the refrain "breast is best," few of us have much appreciation for how breastfeeding came to be considered a public policy concern. MacMurchy, as a social reformer and government official, viewed breastfeeding as a solution to the shockingly high rates of infant mortality during the first quarter of the twentieth century. Breastfeeding became a cornerstone of the federal campaign against infant mortality in the 1920s, and it emerged as part of the debates and policies surrounding issues of mothering. MacMurchy suggested that mothers were responsible for the future well-being of the country, and she described breastfeeding as a national duty. While the motivations behind her desire to increase breastfeeding rates are not as relevant in the twenty-first century as they were in the early twentieth century, breastfeeding has remained part of health and social policy debates. And, while the patriotic and moralistic tone of MacMurchy's early messages might make modern-day readers cringe, nuances of her policies continue to linger in current discussions and debates regarding breastfeeding.

Since MacMurchy created and wrote the first editions of *The Canadian Mother's Book* in the 1920s, the federal government, in all its publications directed at mothers, has officially promoted breastfeeding as "the one best way" to feed infants. However, although breastfeeding has consistently been considered the ideal form of infant feeding, this message has varied somewhat over time. For example, a glance at Canadian federal government publications over the past century demonstrates that the ideal length of exclusive breastfeeding has changed dramatically. In the 1920s, exclusive breastfeeding was recommended for nine months; in the 1950s, it was recommended for three months; and, at present, it is recommended for six months.

As a physician, MacMurchy promoted scientific and medical solutions to child and maternal welfare, and she encouraged women to turn to scientific experts for advice on childrearing. Over the past century, breastfeeding guidelines have consistently been backed by both the state and science. Yet, MacMurchy also cautioned women to be wary of physicians who might prematurely or incorrectly advise them to shift from breastfeeding to bottle-feeding. While, on the one hand, educational materials for mothers have consistently promoted breastfeeding, on the other, scientific knowledge, medical and hospital practices, and a lack of attention to the material conditions of women's lives have often undermined women's ability to successfully breastfeed. As well, throughout the twentieth century, the constancy of "the one best way" message has contrasted sharply with changes in actual breastfeeding patterns.

Choices about infant feeding have implications at both the individual level and the societal level. Consequently, over the twentieth century, physicians, nurses, midwives, government officials, social activists, international organizations, commercial formula manufacturers, psychologists, nutritionists, and, especially, mothers have all become involved in shaping breastfeeding policies and influencing trends in breastfeeding practices. Currently, policy on topics as diverse as early childhood development, nutrition and obesity, environmental sustainability, and childbirth practices emphasizes the importance of promoting breastfeeding. Breastfeeding continues to be inextricably linked with mothering and nutrition policy as well as with public health and health care system policy. Furthermore, it intersects with policy-making not only at provincial and federal levels but also at the international level through initiatives put forward by the World Health Organization and the United Nations.

What is often missing from current discussions about breastfeeding is any knowledge of the historical circumstances that have shaped the major debates and policies. In this book, we describe the history of breastfeeding in Canada from the late nineteenth century to the present, outlining trends in breastfeeding initiation and duration. We contextualize these patterns in relation to breastfeeding policies undertaken between the 1850s and 2000s. In our analysis, we synthesize data from a range of primary and secondary sources, including government reports, medical journals, health and social statistics, food and nutrition policy documents, archival sources, and interviews with policy-makers and advocates in the field of infant feeding. Our inquiry draws upon the disciplines of history, women's studies, anthropology, sociology, and health and social policy analysis.

As we will see, federal breastfeeding policy over the past 150 years has included very different strategies, statements, initiatives, and programs, ranging from the publication of advice literature for mothers, to the ratifications of international conventions, to national campaigns to modify hospital birthing practices. However, central to all policy endeavours has been an emphasis on the promotion of breastfeeding through the education of mothers. Yet, as we argue in this book, breastfeeding practices are clearly more than a matter of individual choice. Policies have repeatedly failed to understand, acknowledge, and invest in changing the determinants of women's infant feeding decisions. We argue for greater attention to the structural determinants of women's infant feeding decisions. These include more accessible maternity entitlements and flexible labour market policies, improving the material conditions of women at "high risk" for decreased breastfeeding, more resources to support the development of breast milk banks, constraining infant formula marketing, and modifying hospital practices that inhibit breastfeeding.

Throughout the nineteenth and twentieth centuries, the Canadian government has been an imitator, not an innovator, of breastfeeding promotion. Canada has tended to adopt policies, programs, and practices developed in other industrialized nations. Breastfeeding policies in the twenty-first century would benefit from considering our country's distinct social, economic, and political history. While the distribution of responsibilities and resources between the federal and provincial/territorial governments has historically been a barrier to the strong and consistent implementation of various international codes, health care practices, and other recommendations, this relationship could potentially provide opportunities for developing innovative policies to meet the diverse breastfeeding goals and material needs of mothers in different regions of the country. That said, the absence of federal leadership in recent years has led to the fragmentation of otherwise encouraging initiatives at the provincial and territorial level. Renewed federal leadership could potentially provide an opportunity for the development of innovative policies that increase women's success in meeting their breastfeeding goals.

The One Best Way? traces patterns of breastfeeding in Canada from the late nineteenth century to the present day. It discusses specific topics and incidences in a roughly chronological order and is divided into four sections, each of which mirrors actual breastfeeding trends. Part 1 shows how the enormous transformations in the economic, political, and social organization of life at the end of the nineteenth century began to alter breastfeeding practices. Breastfeeding remained the dominant form of infant feeding in Canada for the first two decades of the twentieth century; however, as in other industrialized countries, breastfeeding rates in Canada began to decline dramatically after 1920. Part 2 describes the context of this decline. Part 3 shows how breastfeeding rates resurged in the late 1970s and 1980s and climbed steadily throughout the last part of the twentieth century. At the beginning of the twenty-first century, breastfeeding rates have shown some growth but have remained relatively stable in comparison to previous decades. Part 4 offers a summary of breastfeeding practices and policies at the turn of the century.

Part 1: Transitions, 1850–1920

In Chapter 1, we explore early breastfeeding practices in English and French Canada. Using late-nineteenth-century Montreal as a case study, we show how breastfeeding practices were tied to childbirth and childrearing practices in the city's three dominant cultural groups. By the early 1900s, breastfeeding practices began to change in response to urbanization, mass immigration, and industrialization. Concerns about public health and welfare on the part of both government and social reformers shifted breastfeeding from the private to the public domain. In Chapter 2, we examine new scientific ideas about infant feeding and the beginnings of paediatrics in Canada. Gradually, paediatricians became known as scientific experts on infant feeding and became influential in introducing new ideas about infant feeding to the general public. This fuelled the development of modern-day breast milk alternatives. Prior to and during the First World War, motherhood became the ideological root of breastfeeding promotion. Concerns about citizenship and nation building within a context of rapid social change drew differential attention to the breastfeeding practices of certain groups of women. In Chapter 3, we examine how breastfeeding became part of debate and public policy on mothering.

Part 2: Decline, 1920–60

In the 1920s, national initiatives to promote maternal and child welfare led to the development of the first federal government advice literature for mothers. Chapter 4 describes how this early advice literature was informed by scientific and medical understandings of infant feeding and how early federal policies linked breastfeeding to patriotism. By the 1930s, mothers in all classes were adopting scientific methods of childrearing, and medical services were growing rapidly across the country. Using examples from the women's magazine *Chatelaine*, Carnation Milk's marketing campaign, and the development of Pablum, Chapter 5 examines changes in the context of childrearing as well as the increasingly intense infant feeding messages that both health care and commercial sources were directing at mothers. By the 1940s, breastfeeding was no longer considered the norm for infant feeding. Breast milk alternatives were thought to be safer, were readily available, and were considered by many authorities to be a perfectly adequate alternative to breastfeeding. Many women were giving birth in hospital settings, where disruptive hospital practices and a lack of support from health care providers made it difficult for those who wanted to breastfeed. Chapter 6 describes how, by the mid-twentieth century, many of the skills and knowledge essential to successful breastfeeding had been "forgotten." Poor women (who could not afford to bottle-feed) and Aboriginal women were the only groups in Canada that primarily continued to breastfeed.

Part 3: Resurgence, 1960–2000

By the early 1970s, breastfeeding rates were increasing in all areas of Canada, particularly among educated women. The return to breastfeeding occurred in the midst of a range of social, cultural, and political movements, including the natural childbirth movement, the women's movement, international efforts to counter the marketing practices of infant formula companies in the developing world, and the rediscovery of the value of breastfeeding by public health and the scientific medical community. In Chapter 7, we examine the context for this resurgence in breastfeeding. Throughout the 1980s, the federal government led efforts to promote breastfeeding across the country. In Chapter 8, we look at how the 1981 WHO/UNICEF Code of Marketing of Breastmilk Substitutes and the strong movement towards family-centred maternity care brought attention to the practices of health professionals and hospitals. By the end of the 1980s, more than three-quarters of Canadian mothers were initiating breastfeeding. In the 1990s, a variety of initiatives to "protect, promote, and support" breastfeeding were developed. Yet, as we describe in Chapter 9, in many ways, Canada remained a "bottle-feeding" culture.

Part 4: At Equilibrium: Into the Twenty-First Century

Changes in breastfeeding practices have been accompanied by profound changes in the daily context within which women make infant feeding decisions. The availability and promotion of breast milk alternatives, the transmission of breastfeeding knowledge and skills, and the individual and societal value placed on breastfeeding and breast milk are all issues that need to be considered. Thus, in Chapter 10, we provide a brief history of breastfeeding trends and policies. In Chapter 11, we suggest that a historical understanding of the relationship between socio-cultural trends and breastfeeding patterns is essential to informing current policy development and advocacy in the area of infant feeding. We examine the context of policy development in the twenty-first century, including the possible challenges presented by international free trade agreements, questions about federal/provincial responsibility for breastfeeding promotion, the relationship between women's productive and reproductive work, and the need to redefine breastfeeding success at a policy level. As we move into the twenty-first century, breastfeeding has continued to be considered an important practice, with health and social implications at both individual and national levels. In many ways, since the development of the earliest policies on breastfeeding, the "choice" to breastfeed has become a moral one. In the Conclusion, we caution against policies that continue to place responsibility for social problems such as the "obesity epidemic" and soaring health care costs on the infant feeding choices of individual women.

Women giving birth at the beginning of the twenty-first century introduce their infants to a world that is vastly different from the one that existed at the beginning of the twentieth century. However, the question of what to feed those infants is not a new one. Our individual and collective ideas and beliefs about breastfeeding have been shaped by over a century of shifting policies and practices as well as by major social and cultural transformations, particularly in the areas of science and medicine, childrearing and family structure, and the relationships between government and citizens. Yet, inexplicably, current discussions about breastfeeding display only a superficial awareness of the socio-historical forces that have shaped debates about breastfeeding. It is our hope that *The One Best Way?* will aid in rectifying this situation and contribute to dialogue on what still may be.

Part 1

Transitions, 1850–1920

Chapter 1

Infant Mortality, Social Reform, and Milk, 1850–1910

Historical records of early breastfeeding practices in Canada are relatively scarce. However, through the use of infant mortality data, it is possible to explore, albeit indirectly, infant feeding practices in colonial and industrializing Canada. While it appears that, for Aboriginal groups and new settlers, exclusive breastfeeding for many months was typical, variations in breastfeeding practices appear in the earliest available records. In particular, data from late-nineteenth-century Montreal demonstrates how breastfeeding practices were related to class, environment, religion, language, and fertility patterns. At the end of the nineteenth century, several movements were contributing to the development of new ideas, beliefs, and values about breastfeeding. Concerns about child welfare and public health led to a range of activities on the part of charities, religious organizations, and municipal governments to address problems resulting from urbanization, mass immigration, and industrialization. The emergence of a strong social reform movement reduced the distance between "public issues" and "private troubles" and led to breastfeeding's shift from private matter to public concern.

Beginnings: Breastfeeding in Colonial Canada

Before the arrival of European settlers in eastern Canada, Aboriginal women often breastfed their infants for two to three years, sometimes even longer (Prentice et al. 1988, 7; Dodgson and Struthers 2003; Siegel 1984).[1] In the 1600s, immigrants from France, and in the 1700s, immigrants from England, brought their own cultures of breastfeeding with them. Overall, long periods of breastfeeding were widely practised in colonial Canada (Sorg and Craig 1983; Nault, Desjardins, and Legare 1990; Siegel 1984; Henripin 1954). Without adequate alternatives for breast milk, infants who were not breastfed rarely survived. One estimate indicates that, on average, at the beginning of the eighteenth century, infants in New France were breastfed for fourteen months

(Henripin 1954). However, different immigrant groups often had different breastfeeding practices. Women in agricultural communities in Quebec are thought to have weaned their infants earlier, a practice they brought with them from France (Light and Parr 1985). Also, rates of breastfeeding in the seventeenth and eighteenth centuries are known to have been lower in the cities of Quebec and Montreal than they were in outlying rural areas (Nault, Desjardins, and Legare 1990).

With regard to wet-nursing (the practice of a woman breastfeeding another woman's infant, often for payment) in Canada, there is very little information available. In seventeenth-century Europe, wet-nursing was most common among the upper classes. Upper-class women often paid wet nurses to care for infants in their homes. Later, wet-nursing became more common across all classes, and women sent their infants to wet nurses in rural areas. Wet-nursing in Europe began to wane in the eighteenth century. France, however, was one of the few countries in which wet-nursing continued to grow (Sussman 1982). Outside of Canada, in the Protestant colonies established by England and the Netherlands, it appears that most infants were breast-fed by their mothers and that wet nurses were only used in emergencies. In the Roman Catholic colonies established by Spain, Portugal, and France, it seems that it was relatively common to employ wet nurses, who were often of "lower" social status (e.g., black and Aboriginal women). Also, colonists from Roman Catholic countries were inclined to establish charitable organizations, such as foundling hospitals, to care for orphaned children. In these institutions, wet nurses were hired to care for infants (Fildes 1988).

Wet-nursing appears to have occurred in colonial Canada to some extent; however, there are no data on how many infants were wet-nursed, how long they were nursed, who the wet nurses might have been, or whether or not wet-nursing was formally organized. It seems that the practice first emerged in New France in the 1700s, with the development of a nobility and a bourgeoisie. This paralleled the growth of wet-nursing in France (Nault, Desjardins, and Legare 1990; Desjardins 1997). Data from parish registers in New France between 1621 and 1730 indicate that more infants died in the first year of life in wealthy families than in less privileged families. This surprising finding is possibly explained by the higher frequency of births in wealthier families. Because breastfeeding suppresses ovulation and has an effect on the length of time between births, the intervals between birth suggest that wet-nursing was often practised among wealthier families in the cities of Quebec and Montreal (Lalou 1997). One eighteenth-century Montreal merchant, Pierre Guy, hired a wet nurse for each of his children. Madame Guy gave birth to fourteen children, and each of them was put out to nurse the day after he or she was born—some of them in parishes as far away as Saint-Leonard, Saint-Michel, and Sault-aux-Recollets. Few of their children survived, but the ones who did stayed with a wet nurse until the age of two (Clio Collective et al. 1987).

In English Canada, it appears that mothers expected to breastfeed their infants, and wet-nursing was only practised in emergencies, when a mother was ill or had died (Siegel 1984). In the mid-1800s, Letitia Hargrave, a woman who had moved from the British Isles to Manitoba, wrote in her diary

> I fear that my trials began with myself for my breasts got so sore that the irritation brought on a feverish attack and we had to get a nurse for a while for he drank so constantly that I could not get them properly treated. The girl had a thriving baby of her own which she left with her sister. I was nervous about it but they assured me there was no danger. After the second day I nursed him at night myself but from having been ill and leaving off had not enough milk and kept her. (quoted in Siegel 1984, 366)

In Quebec, a French Roman Catholic colony, there is a record of numerous charitable institutions. Homes for "fallen women" (i.e., shelters for unmarried mothers), lying-in hospitals, and institutions for foundlings and sick children were organized. In 1772, an ordinance was passed in which the colonial government agreed to pay for the cost of wet nurses for these "enfants trouvés." In Quebec City, these foundlings were admitted to the Hôtel-Dieu Hospital, and arrangements were made for placements in the homes of wet nurses. The circumstances of these women and the payment provided to them are unknown, although it is clear that Aboriginal women were not allowed to breastfeed infants whose care was subsidized by the government (McKendry and Bailey 1990). Throughout the late 1700s and 1800s, foundlings were often cared for in these charitable institutions, which did what they could to find enough wet nurses. However, infant mortality rates in these places were very high, suggesting that wet nurses could not always be found (Thornton and Olson 1991; McKendry and Bailey 1990). For example, in Ottawa, at the House of Bethlehem, which was run by the Grey Nuns, 88 percent of the infants admitted each year died. Although it was widely known by residents that infant survival in these institutions was low, it was not until the city was petitioned for a grant to cover burial expenses that the situation was seriously investigated. The investigators found that most of the infants came from the local lying-in hospital for unwed mothers and that low rates of breastfeeding were likely the cause of the high mortality rate. Mothers were required by law to breastfeed their infants for two weeks, but the babies were later "dry-nursed" or fed a breast milk alternative, and they rarely thrived. In this particular case, the investigators ordered that the institution be closed until another system of feeding the infants was found (Anonymous 1884).

In general, breastfeeding practices from the Old World mingled with the realities of life in Canada's French and English colonies and shaped early breastfeeding patterns in Canada. Wet-nursing appears to have occurred only in a limited form in colonial Canada, and most women breastfed their own infants for long periods of time.

Three Cultures of Breastfeeding: Montreal at the End of the Nineteenth Century

In 1867, Canada moved from being a British colony to being an independent nation-state. The decades following were a period of enormous social and cultural change. Cities in eastern Canada were beginning to industrialize, and science and technology were emerging as dominant forces. The populations of cities in southern Ontario and Quebec began to increase dramatically as families moved from rural to urban areas. Patterns of family, work, and childbearing began to differ from those of previous generations, and breastfeeding practices began to be affected by various socio-cultural changes. The rich data on infant mortality gathered from parish and population records in nineteenth-century Montreal particularly provide insight into how breastfeeding practices were affected by urbanization. They also reveal that patterns of breastfeeding were clearly related to class, environment, religion, language, and fertility (Thornton and Olson 1991, 1997, 2001).

In 1860, Montreal was the largest and most important city in British North America, with a population of 90,000. The city was rapidly expanding and becoming ever more densely populated as immigrants poured in from rural Quebec and from overseas. Three groups formed the core of industrial Montreal: French Canadian Catholics, Irish Catholics, and British Protestants. Close to half the population was French Canadian Catholic, 30 percent was Irish Catholic, and 20 percent was British Protestant; other groups accounted for less than 2 percent of the population. These communities were divided by language, religion, and geography, and all of them were highly stratified by social class. Irish Catholics shared a language with Protestants from Scotland, Ireland, and Britain, but they shared a religion with French Canadians. British Protestants and Irish Catholics tended to live in different parts of the city, while French Canadian Catholics lived in most neighbourhoods (although a few neighbourhoods were exclusively French Canadian) (Thornton and Olson 1991).

As the city industrialized, women began to take positions in the formal work economy. By 1871, women and children comprised 42 percent of the industrial workforce in Montreal (Ames 1897). While a number of provincial statutes were introduced to increase worker safety and to reduce the length of the workweek, these often excluded employed women and, especially, domestic servants (Ursel 1992). The challenging social and economic circumstances experienced by most of the city's citizens also translated into poor health for women. One study of infant birth weight at Montreal's University Lying-in Hospital, where approximately 2 percent of the city's children were born, showed that mean birth weight fell steadily between 1851 and 1905, suggesting that the quality of women's diet deteriorated quite dramatically, particularly after 1880 (Ward and Ward 1984).

In an era before the enactment of provincial and municipal public health legislation and the establishment of effective urban sanitation, cities presented numerous hazards and ill health for citizens of all ages, particularly infants (Ostry 2006). And, Montreal was less healthy than most other mid-nineteenth-century European and North American cities. Infant mortality rates, measuring the number of children who did not live past their first birthday, were staggering—even by nineteenth-century standards. In 1860, nearly one in three infants born in Montreal died within the first year of life and these rates were much higher than rates in rural Quebec (Thornton and Olson 1991).

Differences in infant mortality rates in Montreal provide some insight into the relationship between infant feeding practices and infant mortality as well as into how breastfeeding practices began to change between 1860 and 1900. The high rate of infant mortality was not consistent throughout the year and across the different cultural groups living in Montreal. Summer posed the most danger. During the 1860s, approximately one-third to one-half of infant deaths were attributable to "weanling diarrhea," or gastrointestinal problems, and these were concentrated in June, July, August, and September. The seasonality of infant deaths was a common pattern across North America, but the poverty and poor infrastructure that defined the living conditions of Montreal intensified the possibility of "summer complaint," or "infant cholera." When the temperatures rose, the city's inadequate housing and its insufficient drainage and sanitation were severely tested. Water and milk were more likely to be contaminated as there was little rain to wash away the dirt of the streets, wells were polluted, and the heat and humidity allowed disease to flourish and thrive. As breastfeeding provided a degree of protection against these threats, infants of mothers who avoided weaning or supplementing their breast milk with cow's milk or water during the summer months likely had better outcomes. In 1860, over half of all infant deaths occurred in the summer. Infants born to Irish Catholic and French Canadian mothers were the most vulnerable as they lived in the poorest, most densely populated areas of the city. However, during the rest of the year, there were no distinct patterns of infant mortality according to neighbourhood (Thornton and Olson 1991).

Another pattern in infant mortality reveals how breastfeeding practices began to shift at the end of the nineteenth century. In 1860, infant mortality rates were much higher in the French Canadian community (28 percent) than they were in the Irish Catholic community (19 percent). Interestingly, two-thirds of the fathers of French Canadian infants were skilled or semi-skilled tradesmen, while half of Irish Catholic fathers were unskilled labourers. Protestants comprised only one-fifth of the population, yet they accounted for over half of the "bourgeoisie," "petite bourgeoisie," and white-collar workers in the city. As Irish Catholics appear to have occupied the lowest position on Montreal's socio-economic ladder and were likely exposed to the poorest sanitary conditions, it is somewhat surprising that their infant mortality rates were considerably lower than were those of the French Canadians. It is unlikely, given their shared religious background, that these differences can be attributed to differences in fertility patterns. They could, however, potentially be explained by changes in infant feeding practices. Overall, estimates based on analyses of birth intervals in Montreal for this time period indicate that approximately 12 percent of mothers either did not breastfeed, supplemented their breast milk, or breastfed for a short period of time (Thornton and Olson 1997).

By 1880, the population of Montreal had doubled. Industrial activity had increased dramatically, and the city had become more densely populated. While more distinct areas of wealth and poverty had emerged, class differences between Irish and French Canadian Catholics, on the one hand, and between Irish and French Canadian Catholics and Protestants of British descent, on the other, remained firmly entrenched. Infant mortality rates in 1880 were virtually the same as they had been twenty years earlier. Among French Canadians, these rates remained much higher than they did among Irish Catholics, and among Irish Catholics they remained higher than they did among British Protestants (Thornton and Olson 1997). Birth interval data indicate that the number of women choosing not to breastfeed, or to breastfeed exclusively for only a short period of time, doubled between 1860 and 1880 to 25 percent. And French Canadian mothers were leading this trend (Thornton and Olson 1997).

By 1900, it was apparent that more women were weaning earlier, supplementing their breast milk, or deciding not to breastfeed. Clear cultural differences emerged in the duration of breastfeeding. At least one-third of French Canadian mothers and one-fifth of mothers from other cultural groups were moving away from long periods of exclusive breastfeeding. Birth interval data indicate, on average, that Protestant women breastfed for two months longer than did Irish Catholic women and for four months longer than did French Canadian women (Thornton and Olson 2001).

The reasons for this trend away from breastfeeding in the last half of the nineteenth century in Montreal are unknown, although it is possible that women's increasing participation in the urban labour force was partly responsible. Some evidence suggests that married French Canadian women were more likely to work than were other women in nineteenth-century Montreal (Cross 1977). Several charities and religious organizations set up facilities to care for young children in French Canadian communities. The lack of daycare facilities in other areas of the city suggests that English-speaking mothers did not work as much as did French-speaking mothers. Perhaps more French Canadian than Protestant or Irish Catholic mothers provided the main source of income for their families. Or perhaps they had larger families, which resulted in the need for two working parents. Poor women may have been motivated to reduce breastfeeding due to the need to work outside the home, while middle-class women may have been so motivated for other reasons, such as an affinity for new scientific methods of infant feeding. Or perhaps traditional weaning practices varied among the different groups. Regardless, the differential rates of breastfeeding in each community suggest that, at the end of the nineteenth century, there were different cultures of breastfeeding in Montreal.

The higher rates of infant mortality in the French Canadian community were not unique to Montreal (McInnis 1997). English Canada and French Canada had very different rates of infant mortality, and this fact persisted into the twentieth century. Also, it is clear that Montreal was not the only city in which French-Canadian women breastfed for a shorter time than did other women. For example, in Ottawa in 1901, French Canadian mothers breastfed their infants for a shorter period than did English Canadian mothers, and this pattern existed regardless of social class (Mercier and Boone 2002). While it may not be possible to fully explain differences in infant mortality between French Canada and English Canada, it is clear that breastfeeding practices, intertwined with fertility patterns and cultural identity, were an important contributor to these differences (Copp 1981).

Social Reform and Domesticity

The changes associated with urbanization, mass immigration, and industrialization contributed to the intensification and increased awareness of social problems. Beginning in the nineteenth century, numerous groups began to mobilize and attempt to ameliorate the slum conditions, poverty, and disease found in urban centres. Towards the end of the century, a diverse and powerful reform movement had emerged. Religious groups, educators, physicians, women's groups, and the trade union movement were all interested in social reform. In particular, women's efforts were recognized as one of the strongest elements of the reform movement, and this drew attention to the importance of women in the family and society. As well, the concepts of public health and child welfare entered public consciousness. Government became increasingly involved in matters of public health and child welfare, and it began to take an interest in what had formerly been thought of as "private" matters. The growth of scientific knowledge, especially in the area of disease prevention, equipped social reformers with new knowledge and the tools with which to address their concerns. Breastfeeding, with its key relationship to infant mortality, became an important focus of public health and child welfare reform efforts.

Initially, social reform efforts were organized by voluntary groups. Voluntary organizations had always been part of community life; however, during the nineteenth century, these local groups began to organize and seek to effect change at both provincial and national levels. Voluntary organizations contributed to the development of a public health movement. In 1875, a citizen's public health association was created in Montreal. Later, organizations such as the Canadian Red Cross, the Canadian Public Health Association, the Canadian Tuberculosis Association, and the Health League of Canada were formed. The Public Health Act, passed in Ontario in 1882, was the beginning of boards and departments of public health in Canada (Ostry 2006). Between 1880 and 1920, various levels of government enacted broadly similar public health legislation (Ostry 1994, 1995a, 1995b). Government involvement with respect to the health of citizens expanded enormously during this period—from a few physicians and volunteers to extensive bureaucracies. For example, in Toronto in the 1880s, there was one full-time employee in public health; by the end of the First World War, the municipal government employed over 500 people in public health (Arnup 1994).

Public health movements gained powerful insights from the new germ theory of disease, which became widely accepted in the 1870s (Tomes 1999). Germ theory holds that living micro-organisms (e.g., bacteria, viruses) caused disease. As understanding about the cause and spread of infectious disease grew, this knowledge was used to develop solutions to diseases such as tuberculosis, typhoid, and influenza. Clean air, water, milk, and food could prevent disease. Germ theory spurred the development of interest in hygiene and cleanliness. In addition to providing the foundation for large-scale public sanitation measures, germ theory brought attention to activities in the home. Domestic activities, such as food preparation, household sanitation, and caregiving practices, were of great interest to public health reformers. Public health efforts to clean up and purify the milk and water supply would be ineffective unless household practices followed suit.

Early public health efforts encouraged mothers to breastfeed, especially during the summer months. Montreal physician Séverin Lachapelle wrote numerous articles and books and, from 1880 onwards, gave lectures about the importance of breastfeeding in reducing infant mortality (Copp 1981). In La mère et l'enfant, he wrote, "Le biberon, voilà la vraie cause de la mortalité excessive de nouveau-né pendant les grandes chaleurs. Le vrai remède, l'unique remède, c'est l'allaitement maternel"[2] (Lachapelle 1888, 10). Other reformers provided advice to mothers on how to keep cow's milk clean:

> To keep milk sweet, get it from a milkmen [sic] whose cart, cans, and horses look clean. If you know where his cows are kept, look at the cows and look at his stable, and see if they are clean ... Get your milk in a pail with a cover, that you keep for the purpose. See that the pail is well washed, scalded, and turned upside down when not in use. Always keep the cover on the pail, when it contains milk. Always keep milk covered

up. Keep the milk in a cool place, or it will grow sour and make the child sick. If you have no ice, wrap a cloth wrung out of cold water around the pail. The water, as it evaporates, will keep the milk cool, but if you possibly can keep your milk directly on ice or in ice water. (Montreal Health Bureau 1914, 3)

In parallel with these public health activities, concerns about childhood moved into public life and the concept of child welfare emerged. In 1887, Ontario passed legislation that permitted municipal councils to set up foster homes and to monitor and inspect them. In 1893, the Children's Protection Act was passed, giving the Children's Aid Society the authority to protect the welfare of the child. Gradually, as Canada continued to grow, these initiatives spread across the country. Child welfare activities slowly expanded from supervision of foundlings fostered in private homes to supervision of daycare centres and institutions for dependent children, supervision and control of medicines, medical inspection and the examination of school children, vaccinations, and the education of mothers.

At the end of the nineteenth century, women reformers were one of the strongest elements of the reform movement. Women's groups, especially those comprised of middle-class women, began to organize around common concerns and issues. Women's role in society was beginning to change, and women were increasingly gaining access to universities and gaining positions in health, education, business, and industry. As a result, women were beginning to recognize the range of social issues confronting the rapidly changing and growing country of Canada. Women's organizations expanded the scope and range of their activities, and these groups took many forms: missionary societies, more secular organizations such as the Women's Christian Temperance Union and the Young Women's Christian Association (YWCA), cultural societies (supporting the arts and literature), and women's rights associations. Most of these organizations emphasized the importance of family life in the Dominion of Canada, and many believed that various features of modern life were weakening the family. As a result of this, there was much concern in the women's movement about moral purity and "race" degeneration. Regardless of their motivation, many of these groups gave guidance and support to working-class girls and women by providing not only education but also services to alleviate harsh living and working conditions. Such initiatives included sheltering immigrant girls, adult education classes, recreation programs, and sick funds (Strong-Boag 1977).

By the 1890s, women's groups were organizing at a national level. Motivated by their own interests and a lack of government involvement, women were taking concrete steps to accomplish their goals. The National Council of Women, an umbrella organization for local women's groups, was formed in 1893. Its mandate was to support the preservation of the family and the state.

In Quebec, a Catholic francophone organization formed for the purpose of linking francophone women's groups. In 1907, the Fédération nationale Saint-Jean-Baptiste was formed. In response to the unique needs of women living in rural communities, branches of the Women's Institute began to appear. These institutes worked to improve rural schools, introduced preventive health for children, and taught hygiene, nutrition, cooking, home nursing, and sewing to women in rural areas. By 1903, the Women's Institute had fifty-three branches (Strong-Boag 1977).

Between 1890 and 1914, women's organizations were primarily concerned with providing education and charity to the poor and with encouraging the government to take a more active role in providing social services, particularly to children. As these initiatives grew, public health boards and departments participated and contributed to expanding the early work of social reformers. In 1895, the National Council of Women became involved in efforts to reduce infant mortality. Two years later, in 1897, it formed the Victorian Order of Nurses (VON). These nurses visited new mothers in their homes and provided education on infant care and feeding. By 1900, there were thirty-two nurses working in rural and urban areas across the country. The National Council of Women also set up well baby clinics, milk depots, baby contests, campaigns for mother's allowances, improved housing, and tuberculosis control. In 1900, the Imperial Order Daughters of the Empire began to establish well baby clinics and nursing services in rural areas. In Quebec, Les Cercles de Fermières and a variety of other women's organizations initiated numerous child welfare activities. Across Canada, branches of the Women's Institute played an important role in child welfare work, especially in rural areas, through the establishment of health services, the provision of school lunches, and the distribution of health literature (Arnup 1994).

All of these reform efforts highlighted the importance of women and the family. In many ways, the differences rather than the similarities between women and men were emphasized. Women were attributed with the virtues of kindness, love, duty, and respect. This being the case, women's reform efforts emphasized women's role as guardians of the family and focused on improving the conditions of mothering. Many believed that, through reform, women could extend their womanly qualities of nurturance and domesticity beyond the home to society at large. Instead of only being carers in the family, women could be carers in society, taking positions as charity organizers, nurses, teachers, and social workers. Even suffragette organizations that were working to get women the vote often used arguments based on the belief in masculine immorality and feminine purity (following which, allowing women the vote would improve the entire community). Thus, by the turn of the century, issues such as working girls, household sanitation, cultural improvement, social purity, and daycare were seen as belonging to the domain of female reformers (Strong-Boag 1977). With increasing attention being drawn to mothering practices and to the role of women in society, breastfeeding was slowly becoming a matter of public concern. By the end of the nineteenth century, breastfeeding was one of the main concerns of a new and powerful social reform movement.

Milk and Infant Mortality

For mothers who were choosing not to breastfeed, who were weaning, or who were supplementing their breast milk, public health and child welfare advocates supported the use of cow's milk. While breastfeeding was encouraged, reformers were aware of the daily realities facing many women and often provided practical advice on how to prepare cow's milk safely. At the end of the nineteenth century, germ theory, which brought with it the idea that bacteria in the milk supply was a source of diarrheal disease in infants, led to a variety of activities to create a safe milk supply, especially in immigrant and working-class neighbourhoods. An awareness that mortality was preventable led to initiatives to clean up cities by purifying milk supplies, building sewage systems, inspecting food, and educating individuals about food, air, and exercise. It also led to the development of milk depots and *gouttes de lait,* one of the reform movement's earliest efforts to exclusively address infant mortality.

Initially, the infant mortality and pure milk campaigns overlapped. During the late 1800s to early 1900s, the relationship between milk and diseases such as scarlet fever, tuberculosis, diphtheria, typhoid, and cholera infantum (weanling diarrhea) became clear. Contaminated milk could be a lethal carrier of disease. In cities, the chances of infants and young children being fed impure milk were significantly greater than they were in the country. Milk was generally collected at dairy farms in rural areas and then transported to the city by horse-drawn carts. By the time the milk arrived in the city, it had travelled long distances without refrigeration and was often sold contaminated with dirt and tuberculosis bacilli. It was also often adulterated with contaminated water, salicylic acid, and yellow dye (MacDougall 1990; Dormandy 2000). Municipal governments were the first to attempt to clean up the milk supply. In the 1880s, Toronto passed laws to regulate dairy barns within the city (MacDougall 1990). In 1893, Quebec City adopted regulations on milk distribution and sales and, one year later, appointed a milk inspector. In 1899, public health authorities suggested inoculating cows with tuberculin, but this did not become mandatory until 1907. In 1908, Ottawa passed legislation requiring the inspection of all cattle supplying milk to the city (Hollingsworth 1925).

Gradually, a system of inspections developed that ensured that cattle were fed hay rather than distillery slops and were contained in sanitary conditions rather than in filthy, cramped barns. Other strategies to improve the milk supply included "certified milk" and pasteurization. Certified milk was "raw" milk that had met stringent hygiene requirements. This milk came from healthy cows raised in sanitary conditions, was kept cool during transportation, and was distributed unadulterated. As conditions for certified milk could be difficult to find and maintain, this product was available in limited supply and, thus, was more expensive than ordinary milk. Dentonia Dairy, located northeast of Toronto, provided certified milk to that city's well-to-do: "The aim at Dentonia is not to make dirty milk palatable, or to kill the germs in it by sterilization, but the whole effort is at keeping the dirt out" (*Globe* 1900). Interestingly, over one-fifth of Dentonia's patrons were physicians. Over time, initiatives to purify the milk supply expanded from the municipal to the provincial level. In 1911, Ontario passed the Milk Act, which mandated the inspection of herds and dairy facilities across the province. In 1914, the Toronto City Council instituted the compulsory pasteurization of all milk sold in the city (MacDougall 1990). In 1914, a water purification plant was opened in Montreal; however, only 25 percent of milk was pasteurized and it took until 1926 for widespread pasteurization to occur (Clio Collective et al. 1987). For a variety of reasons, including debates about nutritive value and taste, pasteurized milk was resisted by both consumers and dairy farmers, and the development of a system that would ensure milk safety across the nation took several more decades.

The milk depot was one of the earliest efforts to exclusively address infant mortality. While certified milk and pasteurization were important in ensuring a pure milk supply and in combating cholera infantum, especially in the summer months, new research was revealing that numerous infant deaths were attributable to diarrhea resulting from bottle-feeding. One influential study, published in Britain by Dr. Arthur Newsholme in 1899, affected efforts to reduce infant mortality across the globe. It examined patterns of infant mortality and emphasized that the majority of deaths were due to diarrheal disease. Diarrhea was caused by improper feeding and hygiene and, thus, was considered to be entirely preventable. Further, rather than simply examining the milk supply, it was also necessary to pay attention to the practices of infant feeding (M. Lewis 1980).

Models for milk depots were borrowed from both Britain and France. At the turn of the century in Britain, child welfare advocates established "pure milk" depots in poor urban neighbourhoods. The purpose of these depots was not only to supply working-class mothers with clean cow's milk, either certified or pasteurized, but also to promote breastfeeding. The milk depot attempted to address two of the perceived barriers to reducing infant mortality rates: (1) mothers who were poor and malnourished and thus unable to breastfeed and (2) mothers who needed to work and so could not breastfeed. Milk was intended to nourish mothers so that they would be able to continue nursing their infants. Gradually, these milk depots began to acquire an educational and supervisory component, and mothers were visited by volunteers or nurses following the birth of their infants.

Similarly, in France, strategies to address infant mortality included the organization of *consultations de nourrissons* and *gouttes de lait*. In 1892, Pierre Budin, chef de service at the Charité Hospital in Paris, organized the first formally structured *consultation de nourrisons*. Women attended an outpatient clinic (the *consultation*) every Friday morning. Infants were weighed and examined, and breastfeeding was emphasized. If it was not possible for mothers to breastfeed, they were given sterilized cow's milk. Budin's methods were so successful in decreasing morbidity and mortality rates that the number of the *consultations* spread rapidly. Parallel to this initiative, Dr. Leon Dufour opened an infant welfare clinic at Fecamp in Normandy in 1894. This was unattached to a hospital and was supported by private donations, and he referred to it as a *goutte de lait*. These initiatives became the model for child welfare work in Canada for the first half of the twentieth century (Comacchio 1993). Although there were several distinctions between these programs in terms of their funding, their connection to various institutions, and their organization, they all encouraged breastfeeding, supplied good quality milk, and provided medical care and supervision during the early years of an infant's life (Dwork 1987).

In 1901, the Montreal Local Council of Women (composed of francophone and anglophone groups), the Foundling Hospital, and several local doctors established two pure milk depots (Baillargeon 1998). Soon after, the Pure Milk League in Toronto established two milk depots that provided certified milk. In addition to providing free milk for those unable to pay, these depots gave lectures, distributed pamphlets, and provided free smallpox vaccinations (Arnup 1994). In Montreal, by 1910, three milk distribution centres were set up permanently. Over the next few years, twenty more depots were set up, the majority of them associated with French Catholic parishes in the poorest areas of the city (Baillargeon 1996, 1998; Copp 1981). Milk depots began to spread to other cities, and they appeared successful in reducing infant mortality rates. In 1914, 3,101 infants were registered at the twenty-seven depots in Montreal, and the Department of Health noticed that infant death rates among registered infants was 50 out of 1,000, less than one-quarter of the overall infant mortality (Copp 1981). Similar successes were recorded in other cities. In the infant clinics in the settlements of Toronto in 1913, there were 364 clinics held, with an overall attendance of 3,926. By 1914, there were 830 clinics with 10,809 infants. This increased dramatically by 1917 to twenty-two centres, 1,033 clinics, and 16,849 infants. Over this four-year period, infant mortality declined from 115 per 1,000 live births to 80 per 1,000 live births, while deaths due to cholera infantum decreased from 637 to 172 (Comacchio 1993). At the milk depot in Hamilton, one member of the VON commented, "Ninety per cent of the deaths among infants were of bottle-fed babies, and it was a pertinent saying that we should not declare 'the Lord giveth, the Lord hath taken away, blessed be the name of the Lord' until we had examined our milk cans" (*Globe* 1912a, 11).

"Pure" Milk and "Perfect" Foods

Public health and child welfare reformers advocated the use of certified or pasteurized cow's milk as a safe alternative to breast milk. However, at the end of the nineteenth century, mothers were also beginning to be exposed to advice about infant feeding from other sources. Beginning in the 1880s, commercial foods for infants became available in Canada. By the turn of the century, there were a variety of cow's-milk products and patent, or proprietary, foods commercially available.

The technology to produce canned milk developed in the 1800s. Condensed milk, developed in 1856 by businessman and inventor Gail Borden, was made by boiling milk, evaporating it to one-quarter of its original volume, and then adding sugar as a preservative; evaporated milk, developed in 1885, was similarly produced but was preserved without the sugar. Both types of milk were intended to be diluted before use. Canned cow's milk quickly became popular for a wide range of uses, as it was easy to transport and store. As these milk products became widely used in the household, they also started to be used in infant feeding. Infants were fed condensed milk, or skimmed condensed milk, diluted with water. By 1911, more than one hundred varieties of machine-skimmed and forty brands of full-cream condensed milk had been marketed (Baumslag and Michels 1995). The development and early production of these products occurred outside of Canada. Some of the earliest products available in Canada included St. Charles Unsweetened Evaporated Cream and Borden's Eagle Brand Condensed Milk (see Figure 1.1).

Patent infant foods became available on the market at the same time as did canned milks. The first commercially marketed patent food for infants was developed by Justus von Liebig in Germany in 1867. His "perfect" food for infants contained cow's milk, wheat flour, malt flour, and potassium bicarbonate. It was originally sold as a liquid and later as a powder. The ingredients of patent infant foods varied enormously and included barley, eggs, oats, wheat, sugar, phosphate of lime, bicarbonate of potassium, and cow's milk. Most of these products were intended to be mixed with water or milk. Gradually, they became available in the Canadian market. Nestlé created a powdered infant food in 1868, which was sold in Switzerland, Germany, France, and England. In 1887, Nestlé products imported from Europe were available in Canada (Nestlé Canada 2005). Some of the earliest products advertised in Canada included Nestlé's Food, Lactated Food, and Eskay's Albumenized Food.

In many ways, the early advertisements for these products reflected public health and child welfare concerns. For example, these products effectively addressed concerns about the relationship between urban conditions and seasonal infant mortality, as they were prepared "away from the city's

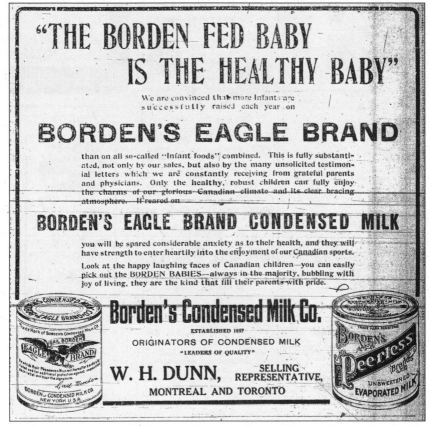

Figure 1.1   Advertisement for Borden's Eagle Brand Condensed Milk. *Globe*, 18 February 1911, 17.

withering heat." Carnation Milk was a sterilized, evaporated milk that came from "contented cows." It was ideal for infant feeding because it was "uniform in richness" and "absolutely pure": "This rich milk is collected every morning from Ontario's fine dairy farms." After being sealed and sterilized, the milk travelled "safely to your home," where it would be opened only when needed (*Globe*, 20 March 1920, 15).

Some products claimed to be the "perfect food" for infants, with the same composition as breast milk (e.g., *Globe*, 24 August 1900, 9). Testimonials from mothers were often used to support these claims. Other ads emphasized the use of their product in the nursery of the Russian Imperial Family (see Figure 1.2) or at the British Ministry of Food (e.g., *Globe*, 22 May 1919, 10). Mothers were often invited to write in to receive instructions for preparing bottles or for samples. Other ads did not claim that their products were superior to breastfeeding but did insist that they should be used to ensure that mothers had the strength to continue breastfeeding. Amazingly enough, these products were also presented as useful should breastfeeding fail for any reason. Glaxo's

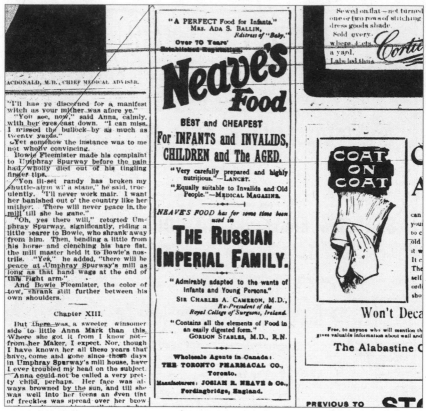

Figure 1.2   Neave's "perfect" food for infants. *Globe*, 13 January 1900, 8.

slogan was "A Happy Baby Makes a Happy Mother." It was claimed that, when a mother drank it two to three times a day before and after birth, Glaxo milk enriched the flow of breast milk: "Should the breast milk fail from any cause, or not nourish Baby satisfactorily, Glaxo can be given to the baby in turn with the breast or as the sole food from birth, for it contains everything to nourish Baby and nothing to cause him harm" (e.g., *Globe*, 15 September 1920, 10).

Although these products were purportedly beneficial for mothers and infants, most public health and child welfare advocates were strongly opposed to their use. Condensed and evaporated milk were rarely produced under sterile conditions. And, once the can had been opened for other household purposes, the purity of the milk could be compromised. Patent foods were too expensive for most families. Indeed, they were more expensive than milk, and many families could not afford milk, particularly certified milk. As well, infants often did not thrive on patent foods, as many of these were composed of predigested cereal and some did not contain any fat, protein, or vitamins. These foods were also intended to be mixed with milk or water, and this, once again, exposed infants to possible contamination.

Conclusion

Breastfeeding practices from the Old World mingled with the realities of life in Canada's French and English colonies and shaped early breastfeeding patterns in this country. Breastfeeding for long periods of time was typical in colonial Canada. By the 1880s, based on infant mortality data from Montreal, it appears that women were beginning to move away from breastfeeding. Mothers may have been choosing not to breastfeed, to wean their infants at an earlier age, or to supplement breast milk with breast milk alternatives. By 1900, it appears that one-third of French Canadian mothers and one-fifth of Irish Catholic and Protestant mothers were moving away from long periods of exclusive breastfeeding (Thornton and Olson 2001). While the reasons for this trend are difficult to determine, social and cultural transformations associated with urbanization and industrialization, such as the extent to which women with young children worked outside the home, were likely important contributors. The shift away from breastfeeding seemed to occur at varying rates in different communities, suggesting that breastfeeding was closely linked to specific cultural childbirth and childrearing practices, fertility patterns, class, and religious traditions.

Reform efforts aimed at reducing social problems associated with rapid urbanization and industrialization, including high rates of infant mortality, were influential in drawing attention to and reshaping breastfeeding practices. Partly in response to the realities of urban life and the trend away from breastfeeding, public health and child welfare advocates began to encourage breastfeeding while simultaneously working towards ensuring safe alternatives to it, including clean water as well as certified and pasteurized milk. Milk depots, a concept borrowed from abroad, began to appear in Canada at the turn of the century and were effective in reducing infant mortality due to diarrhea (Food Controller for Canada 1917). Canned cow's milk and patent foods also began to appear on the market at the end of the nineteenth century. While breastfeeding practices began to alter between 1850 and 1920, at the turn of the twentieth century, breastfeeding remained the dominant form of infant feeding in Canada.

Chapter 2

Theory and Formulas: Scientific Medicine and Breastfeeding, 1900–1920

In the last half of the nineteenth century, physicians began to experiment with developing alternatives to breast milk, primarily for humanitarian reasons. The twentieth century marked the beginning of physicians' becoming increasingly aware of social problems and becoming actively involved in addressing them. Among these social problems was infant mortality. Initially, physicians were eager to apply scientific principles to infant feeding in order to address the problem of infants dying in foundling institutions. Since the mid-1880s, scientists in Europe, the United States, and other parts of the world had begun to develop alternatives to breast milk for infants. At the end of the nineteenth century, Canadian scientists and medical professionals increasingly became part of these discussions, began to apply this new scientific knowledge in their practices, and began to engage in debates about theories of infant feeding. And, at the beginning of the twentieth century, the application of scientific principles to problems of infant feeding became the focus of paediatrics, a new medical specialty. Gradually, paediatricians became known as scientific experts on infant feeding, and they developed a range of modified cow's-milk and customized formulas for infants. While scientific medicine acknowledged the superiority of breastfeeding, many of the new theories and practices indirectly questioned the properties of breast milk and the ability of mothers to successfully breastfeed.

Early Paediatrics in Canada

Although paediatrics was a well-established field in the United States by the turn of the century (the American Pediatric Society was formed in 1888), paediatrics in Canada was much less formalized. During the 1800s, hospitals and medical faculties began to be concerned with the development and care of the child, but it was not until the turn of the century that the first clinical and faculty positions dedicated exclusively to paediatrics were established. The Montreal General Hospital, established in 1822, was one of the first hospitals to focus on the development and care of children, and Dr. A.D. Blackader was the physician "put in charge of the children's services" (McKendry and Bailey 1990) at the hospital. Although he was a lecturer in paediatrics at McGill University and had served as president of the American Pediatric Society from 1892 to 1893, it was not until 1912 that he became professor of paediatrics in McGill's Faculty of Medicine. The Faculty of Medicine at Laval University in Quebec City was founded in 1852. Although it offered some education on the care of infants up to the age of six months, it did not offer a formal clinical teaching course until 1879. In 1895, Dr. René Fortier received the first chair of paediatrics in Canada and became professor of paediatrics at Laval. Parallel to the development of formal positions in paediatrics, the first large children's hospitals were established. Toronto's Hospital for Sick Children was founded in 1875, Montreal's Children's Hospital in 1902 and L'hôpital Ste-Justine pour les enfants in 1907, Winnipeg's Children's Hospital in 1909, and the Children's Hospital in Halifax in 1910.

Although departments of paediatrics existed prior to 1920, individual physicians were usually self-taught and were involved in the treatment of children due to personal interest. In the 1900s, a new generation of physicians went abroad to gain formal training in the field of paediatrics. Individuals went to major centres in the United States and western Europe, including New York, Boston, London, Munich, and Berlin, to learn the science of infant feeding. Alan Brown (1887–1959) was the first Canadian physician to go abroad for formal training in paediatrics; he was later followed by Alton Goldbloom (1890–1968). Brown became the chief of paediatrics at the Hospital for Sick Children in Toronto (a position that he held for thirty-two years), while Goldbloom became the physician-in-chief at Children's Memorial Hospital and professor of paediatrics in Montreal. The students of these two individuals became part of a new generation of paediatricians, all of whom had formal scientific training in infant feeding (Kingsmill 1995). Although the number of paediatricians in Canada was small during the first part of the twentieth century, the influence of this first generation of formally trained paediatricians on the evolution of paediatrics was enormous. At the time of Alan Brown's retirement in 1951, 75 percent of practising paediatricians in Canada had received part or all of their training under his leadership (Kingsmill 1995). And, as infant feeding was the central concern of this specialty, paediatricians were influential in introducing new ideas about the qualities of breast milk, breast milk alternatives, and the practice of breastfeeding to the growing efforts to increase the number of women who breastfed.

Humanizing Milk

Throughout human history, individuals and societies have developed strategies, systems, and alternatives to feed infants when mothers were unable or unwilling to breastfeed. When an infant was unable to receive breast milk (i.e., by being breastfed by a woman other than its mother), various gruels, paps, and animal milks were used, usually with limited success. The first involvement of paediatrics in infant feeding began in the 1800s. Technological advances had resulted in new tools and knowledge regarding the composition of foods. Work in the 1890s on the composition of breast milk and cow's milk led to new interest in developing scientific substitutes for breast milk. The aim of virtually all schools of infant feeding was to develop a substitute for breast milk that matched as closely as possible its chemical and physical properties. In other words, early efforts to develop alternatives to breast milk focused on "humanizing" milk. Scientists worked to modify cow's milk to resemble human milk through a variety of dilutions and additions. Formulas were created from a combination of milk, water, and sugar. Sugar took the form of dextri-maltose or malt sugar, lactose or milk sugar, cane sugar or white sugar, or corn syrup. Milk could be raw, boiled, pasteurized, or certified. Other additions to formulas included acids, in the form of lactic acid, citric acid, vinegar, hydrochloric acid, or lemon juice; cream, barley water, lime water, sodium bicarbonate, and starch were also frequent additions.

The test of the success of these concoctions was whether or not they were digested adequately by the infant. Close examination of the stools of both formula-fed and breastfed infants became a key characteristic of paediatric consultations: "Careful study of the stools is necessary. Normally they are yellow and pasty in consistency, but when upsets occur certain characteristic changes occur" (Spohn 1920, 373), One of the culprits that was often believed to impair the digestibility of formulas was casein, the protein found in cow's milk. As cow's milk was digested, casein produced curds, which were then later "found unchanged in the faecal discharges. It is therefore a constant source of irritation and often gives rise to diarrhea and entero-colitis" (Atkinson 1889, 139). Particular masses in stools were evidence of intolerance of fat, sugar, salt, or some other component of the formula. In response, paediatricians would modify the components of the formula or add agents that would increase the formula's digestibility.

"Divination by stool," or "coprophyllic fetishism" (Goldbloom 1945), became a widespread technique for determining the cause of an infant's ills. For example, infants with hard, grey, and crumbly stools resulting from a high fat content were treated with a low-fat cow's-milk formula with added malt sugar, while infants with green frothy stools were thought to benefit from a simple cow's-milk formula without any sugar added. At Toronto's Hospital for Sick Children, Brown would take his residents on rounds each morning:

> The dirty diaper would be placed at the foot of each cot to await the arrival of Brown and his entourage. The odour, the appearance and the shape of the stools were essential clues to diagnosis. "Stools can tell you everything about a baby—except its name" was one of his favourite

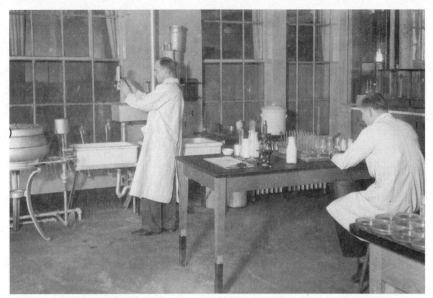

Figure 2.1   Milk laboratory at a dairy, Toronto, ca. 1920. Archives of Ontario. Series RG 2-71. Ontario Legislative Library print collection.

aphorisms. When a fresh specimen of a particular condition could not be obtained he would pull from his pocket an imitation stool he had brought back from Germany for teaching, or one he had requested the hospital's pathology department to make for him. (Kingsmill 1995, 72)

Routine stool analysis and milk composition analysis became the infant feeding tools of paediatric practice. Cow's milk was the favoured alternative because of its supposed resemblance to breast milk and its ready availability:

> Now in cow's milk we have a food containing all the elements found in the natural nourishment for a baby, though the cream, proteid, sugar and inorganic salts are present in percentages differing from mother's milk. However, knowing the percentage of these elements in both the mother's and cow's milk, and knowing, by examining the stools, which of the elements is being perfectly digested and which is not, it is not difficult to alter their relative proportions so that all may be digested. (Rorke 1916, 68)

Cosmopolitan Ideas

Numerous scientific ideas about infant feeding existed at the beginning of the twentieth century. One of the most popular ideas from about 1890 to 1910 was the percentage feeding method developed by Thomas Morgan Rotch (1848–1914) at Harvard Medical School in Boston. Rotch's percentage method was often referred to as "the American method" because it was so widely used in the eastern United States. The percentage feeding method was based on the idea that the digestive capacity of each infant varied and that formulas had to be adapted to the individual and to different stages of growth. Formulas were prepared by diluting cow's milk (in order to lower the percentage of the protein to more closely resemble breast milk) and then by adding sugar and cream to increase the sugar and fat content. Rotch and his followers argued that even slight changes in the relative proportions of fat, protein, and sugar in a formula could have profound effects on an infant's growth and development. For example, if the examination of stool stains discovered the presence of excessive fat, the formula would be decreased by 0.25 percent to 0.50 percent of fat, and then the protein and sugar components would be adjusted accordingly. Often, the protein in milk would be split into casein and whey so that the proportions of these two proteins could be altered. Doctors wrote instructions for preparing infant formulas, specifying nutrient concentrations to 0.1 percent. These prescriptions were based on complex mathematical formulas (this, in fact, is the origin of the term "formula," as in "baby formula") outlining the appropriate percentages for individual infants (Apple 1987; Wolf 2001).

Rotch's percentage feeding method was time-consuming and difficult, and it often required a degree of precision that was not possible in the average kitchen (or even hospital lab). In 1891, Rotch established the Walker-Gordon Laboratory in Boston, the first milk modification lab. By 1903, these laboratories could be found across the United States, Europe, and in Montreal, Ottawa, and Toronto (Apple 1980). At the Walker-Gordon Laboratory located at Dentonia Dairy just northeast of Toronto, orders for modified milk for invalids and infants required a prescription. Once prepared, orders could be shipped express to distant places and used on journeys. Although these prescriptions for modified milk were intended for sick infants, "the chief use of the laboratories [was] in the regular feeding of healthy infants from birth." (*Globe* 1900, 4). Rotch's percentage method declined in popularity after 1910 due to the expense of laboratory milk (only a select few had access to and could afford milk prepared in a laboratory) and the degree of sophistication required to calculate formulas. However, his general principles for milk modification continued to be used into the 1920s.

New York was another popular destination for paediatricians who wanted to learn modern methods of infant feeding. Abraham Jacobi (1830–1919) was considered the "father of American paediatrics" and held the first chair of paediatrics in the United States. Jacobi was considered to be the first to recognize the importance of boiling milk. When Alan Brown arrived in New York City at the Babies' Hospital in 1910 to begin a three-year residency, Jacobi had recently (in 1901) been succeeded by Luther Emmett Holt (1855–1924). Holt was an important figure in American paediatrics. In 1894, he wrote *The Care and Feeding of Children: A Catechism for the Use of Mothers and*

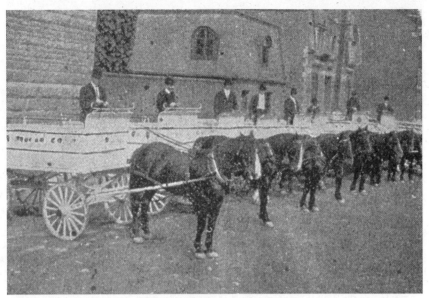

Figure 2.2   Modified milk produced at the Walker-Gordon Laboratory in Montreal was delivered to the homes of consumers by these delivery teams (date unknown). Image courtesy of the Bibliothèque et Archives nationales du Québec, Walker-Gordon Laboratory Co. – Équipes de livraison, rue de la Montagne, MAS 3-112-c.

Children's Nurses. This book was full of advice for middle-class mothers, and it encapsulated his ideas about childrearing. Parents were not permitted to embrace, soothe, play with, or kiss a crying infant as these acts could be harmful: "An infant should not be allowed to sleep on the breasts of the nurse, nor with the nipple of the bottle in his mouth. Other devices for putting infants to sleep, such as allowing the child to suck a rubber nipple or anything else, are positively injurious" (quoted in Colon 1999, 227). This advice manual went through twelve revisions and seventy-five printings. Holt's later book, *The Diseases of Infancy and Childhood*, published in 1897, was a medical textbook. It went through eleven editions in his lifetime and was translated into Spanish, French, German, and Italian. It eventually evolved into the present-day *Rudolph's Pediatrics*, which has the distinction of being the longest continuously printed pediatric textbook (the twenty-first edition was published in 2002). Over the first quarter of the twentieth century, Holt, who was also a supporter of Rotch's percentage feeding method (Colon 1999), was enormously influential in paediatric thinking around the world. Interestingly, the superintendent of the Babies' Hospital in New York was a Toronto graduate by the name of Mary Agnes Smith. As Smith was the director of nursing and intern staff, Holt consulted with her regarding residency posts. Her influence resulted in every chief male resident of the Babies' Hospital from 1912 to 1920 being a Canadian (Kingsmill 1995).

Paediatricians working in Europe also proposed solutions to infant diarrhea and other gastrointestinal disturbances (Levinson 1943; Hill 1967). Adalbert Czerny proposed "Butter-flour mixture" for infants intolerant of fat. Heinrich Finkelstein and Ludwig Ferdinand Meyer developed Eiweissmilch, or "protein milk," in 1910. Protein milk was a low-fat, low-carbohydrate, high-protein mixture designed to counteract the harmful effects of carbohydrates in the intestines, and it was not easy to make. Brown described its preparation in the milk laboratory in Toronto:

> A quart of certified raw milk is taken; two teaspoonfuls of essence of pepsin are added. Warm mixture to 140°F. Keep at this temperature ten minutes. (Too great heat will cause the curd to become tough.) Then let it stand at room temperature for half an hour. The curd is then separated from the whey and placed in a cheese-cloth bag and allowed to drip in the refrigerator or any cool place. This takes from two to four hours and in large amounts may be allowed to drip over night. The curd is then worked through a fine sieve (thirty-six wires to the inch) at the same time adding one pint of a low acid buttermilk, and one pint of water or water to one quart. To every quart of finished protein milk, add one grain saccharin. (Brown, Spohn, and MacLachlan 1918, 512)

By the 1920s, although time-consuming and difficult to prepare, protein milk was popular in Canada. It was widely used by paediatricians, children's hospitals, and baby clinics (Mullen 1915; Brown 1919a). And, unlike Czerny's butter-flour mixture, it was commercially marketed. Physicians located in rural areas or away from a feeding laboratory were advised to use Protein Milk Powder as prepared by the Canadian Milk Products Company, although it was considered somewhat inferior to Finklestein and Meyer's product as it was higher in sugar and fat (MacGregor 1923).

Theory Runs Riot: Controversies in Infant Feeding

Early theories of infant feeding were not without controversy. The rapid succession of new ideas and approaches to infant feeding often left paediatricians with a muddle of concerns and untested solutions. Robert Rudolf, a professor at the University of Toronto, commented that "infant feeding theory has run riot" and that "the proteins, the fat, and the sugar of cow's milk have each in turn been blamed" for difficulties of digestion in infants (1912, 176). Alton Goldbloom remarked, "And so the pendulum has swung. Ten years ago we were adding alkalis to milk as the only and proper way to feed infants ... Now we are adding acid to milk in order to neutralize buffer substances." (1924, 710). In response, many paediatricians concluded that digestive disturbances in infants could be caused by a range of factors: "For many years, physicians working on the problem of artificial nourishment of infants have endeavored to ascertain the reason for the difference in tolerance for cow's and mother's milk. All the constituents of the milk have been blamed at various times for the bad results, and it is probably true that the misfeeding of any one element may cause trouble" (Brown, Spohn, and MacLachlan 1918, 510).

Overall, by the early 1900s, there were two major schools of infant feeding in the United States: the Boston school (percentage feeding method) and the Chicago school (the caloric method) (Apple 1987). The Boston school emphasized precise calculations to determine the appropriate dilutions required to modify cow's milk, while the Chicago school focused on simpler methods of diluting cow's milk and emphasized the heat units, or calories, required for infant growth. Within Canada, these methods were often debated and, in fact, were often combined.

The popularity of the percentage feeding method began to decline after 1910, with physicians opting for simpler milk modification methods and with new solutions to the problems of infant feeding being proposed. As Robert Rudolf observed at a meeting of the Pediatric Section of the Toronto Academy of Medicine, "Percentage feeding is chiefly of American growth and, theoretically sound as it appears to be, it has not found extensive favour on the other side of the Atlantic ... Before recommending the use of laboratory milk we should like to see some more evidence of the necessity for it in this country, and some more unanimity of opinion as to its advantages in America" (1912, 174). Many commented on how Rotch's system was so complicated that it virtually required a degree in higher mathematics. The famous justice Oliver Wendell Holmes joked, "A pair of substantial mammary glands has the advantage over the two hemispheres of the most learned professor's brain in the art of compounding a nutritious fluid for infants" (Holmes 1911, 60).

Gradually, the caloric method began to replace the popularity of the percentage feeding method. Howard Spohn (1880–1973), a pediatric pioneer in Vancouver who had studied in Toronto, New York, and Vienna, was a proponent of the Chicago school of infant feeding. He described the human body as "a steam engine" that converts fuel (i.e., food) into energy and heat (Spohn 1920, 368). The amount of fuel required by the body could be calculated using the concept of a "calory," or the amount of heat necessary to raise one cubic centimetre of water one degree Celsius. Paediatricians preparing infant formulas had to consider the caloric requirements of the infant. One ounce of breast milk or whole milk contained twenty calories, while one ounce of 7 percent milk contained twenty-seven calories. One also needed to consider the differences in carbohydrate and protein content of breast milk and cow's milk. After considering the child's weight and age and the amount of milk, sugar, and water, Spohn concluded that a milk formula composed of one-third milk to one-half water plus 3 percent to 5 percent sugar was a good rule of thumb for a one-month-old infant.

Others argued that it did not matter whether an infant received a cow's-milk formula, buttermilk, patent foods, or milk mixtures as long as it received enough calories within a twenty-four-hour period. Rudolf (1912) stated that an infant requires 90 to 100 calories per kilo when receiving breast milk and 110 to 120 calories when receiving a breast milk alternative. Enough fat, protein, and carbohydrates were required, of course, but the proportion in which they were present didn't really matter: an infant's body would select what it needed. Based on this concept, it was better to overfeed an infant than to underfeed it: "In the former case, the infant will probably reject the excess; but in the latter it has no redress and must fail" (177). Mothers who diluted cow's milk too much would starve their infants: "Either the infant is placed upon a starvation diet, or else must drink far more at each feeding than its stomach is meant to contain" (178). Rudolf concluded that, as long as an infant seemed well and was gaining weight, "we may ignore the presence of 'curds' and mucus in the stools and other so-called signs of indigestion" (178).

By 1920, a new generation of paediatricians well versed in scientific methods of infant feeding could be found in most major urban centres across Canada. Incorporating ideas from a range of institutions and practitioners, and having been exposed to ongoing developments and scientific endeavours abroad, these individuals adapted what they had learned to their own practices and began to develop a distinctively Canadian approach to infant feeding. Brown (1920, 207) commented on the intellectual environment at Toronto's Hospital for Sick Children in 1920: "These men, who came to the hospital already trained by pediatricians of different institutions, bring with them the ideas of their teachers, thus making it possible for the hospital to embody within itself well trained men from various clinics. In this way it cannot help but have a broad mind and lends naturally to the development of what one might term a cosmopolitan clinic, but at the same time endeavoring to develop very definite Canadian methods."

Breast Is Best ... Whenever Possible

In spite of the controversies and debates over various methods of bottle-feeding, physicians in the early part of the twentieth century were very clear about the superiority of breast milk. In addition to the difficulties of providing safe milk and sterile equipment for bottle-feeding, breast milk was believed to contain "some little known substances" that protected infants from a variety of infections (Rorke 1916, 67). However, over time, there were an increasing number of questions raised about the quality of breast milk, about the ability of women to provide sufficient milk for their infants, and about a growing number of circumstances in which mixed feedings were not only acceptable but even recommended.

As paediatrics developed, infant feeding evolved into a science and an art, the mastery of which required several years of training. Most theories of infant feeding promoted the notion that individual infants had unique needs. Indeed, Rotch's percentage method suggested that a variation of even 0.1 percent of a given ingredient was enough to make the difference between an ill-fed and a well-fed baby. Paediatricians, as specialists in infant feeding, increasingly provided prescriptions or were consulted regarding appropriate home-milk modifications. Mothers were no longer seen as the experts on the best nutrition for their infants. Further, mothers' attempts at devising a formula could often be disastrous: "The necessary skill and intelligence required to insure uniformity of result for the extemporaneous peptonizing [or partial predigestion] of milk is rarely to be found in the household, and where this process is adopted, the experiment often turns out to be unfortunate and injurious to the child" (Atkinson 1889, 140).

Breastfeeding was "the ideal which we should always strive to attain" (Rorke 1916, 70). Yet, many paediatricians were suspicious of the quality of mother's milk. Analyses of breast milk composition found a rather surprising amount of variability. A mother's diet and emotional state was believed to affect the quality of her milk. Poorly treated cows could produce milk that was fatal to an infant: "Undoubtedly, many in this audience can substantiate the claim that it is most usually the pet cow, from which the milk is obtained which is put by for the sick baby; that receives all the banging, hurrying, and pelting, and as we all know, is thus likely to yield a milk which may actually be poisonous in its nature" (Atkinson 1889, 138). Similarly, diarrhea was commonly found in infants breastfed by "neurotic" mothers or mothers experiencing disturbances due to menstruation or stress. At the Ontario Medical Association meeting in 1922, MacGregor (1923, 180) stated:

> A type of diarrhea with a passage of eight or ten green frothy stools daily is seen sometimes in breast fed infants with neurotic mothers. This is believed to be due to some temporary change in the breast milk and is not an uncommon thing in this high tensioned age. It may occur during the period of menstruation or at any time the mother is worried, fatigued or otherwise upset. It is further aggravated when the symptoms appear to be induced by the fear that she is not going to be able to nurse her infant.

If this occurred, MacGregor advocated supplementing each breastfeeding with protein milk or a simple formula of cow's milk, with sugar deleted, until the problem resolved itself. Similarly, at the Babies' Dispensary in Hamilton, breastfeeding mothers with infants suffering from diarrhea were provided with advice on how to improve their diet and exercise (Cody 1915).

The discovery of vitamins in the early 1910s also raised questions about the quality of mother's milk. Although vitamins were not fully understood at that time, and although their actual content in breast milk and transmission to infants was unknown, questions were raised about the possibility of a relationship between a mother's diet and circumstances and the adequacy of her breast milk: "Under normal conditions, there is no doubt that mother's milk is an ideal infant's food, but in these days the force of circumstances or numerous other factors ... may so change the composition of the mother's milk that it ceases to be a complete food. This failure ... cannot so far be demonstrated in the laboratory by the ordinary chemical analysis, an analysis to which so many practitioners have attached so much importance" (Brown 1917b, 912). Although conclusive evidence was lacking, it was believed that breastfeeding mothers who did not have sufficient nutrients in their diet could cause illness in their infants, particularly scurvy and rickets.

Whether women were capable of producing enough breast milk for their infants was also an increasing concern. Throughout the early 1900s, many people commented that, compared to twenty to thirty years ago, young women had developed a decreased ability to nurse their infants. The numbers of women providing "insufficient milk" as a reason for turning to the bottle seemed to be on the increase. This was a puzzling trend, and a considerable amount of time was spent speculating on this worrisome issue. Dr. R.F. Rorke, the head of paediatrics at Winnipeg's Children's Hospital, stated, "The reason of the failure on the maternal part may be due to anemia, over-work, bad hygienic surroundings, and particularly a lack of fresh air, insufficient or unsuitable food, or some acute illness ... There is also a number, and a not inconsiderable number, of women who do not seem to respond at all well to the stimulus of the nursing infant" (Rorke 1916, 68). Many suspected that "the unquestioned deteriorating influence of civilization" was responsible for lessening the human milk supply (Hollingsworth 1925, 225). Urbanization was so stressful that it was just possible that mothers' bodies were no longer able to produce enough milk. It was even suggested that the disappearance of women's ability to breastfeed was just the next step in human evolution.

In 1917, Brown published an article in the *Canadian Medical Association Journal* entitled "The Ability of Mothers to Nurse Their Infants." In it, he asked whether women's failure to breastfeed was an actual inability or an apparent one. He concluded that many aspects of modern life could explain the decrease in the number of mothers who were breastfeeding. He suggested that working-class women likely avoided breastfeeding because they had to work and/or lacked adequate nourishment, which could lead to lactation failure. However, upper-class women seemed to be breastfeeding less than were lower-class women. Here, it seemed that the physiology of upper-class women made them more susceptible to the stresses of the city: "In the upper classes, there is undoubtedly often seen an inability to nurse dependent on the more highly organized and hence more easily disturbed nervous organization of the mother. Here, too, is the influence of early mental forcing, early enjoyment of social life, with late hours and the like. Faulty methods of dressing have doubtless in the past been the cause of many hopelessly depressed nipples" (Brown 1917a, 246). Nonetheless, Brown eventually concluded that, overall, "the numerous contra-indications to nursing are more fancied than real" and that "the failure to nurse is to be sought rather in the unwillingness of the mother instigated or abetted often by the advice of nurses and physicians" (Brown 1917a, 246).

Physicians recognized that breastfeeding increased an infant's chances of survival. However, they gradually became more amenable to "mixed feedings"—a combination of breast and bottle-feeding. According to Rudolf (1912, 173), "All are agreed that whenever it is possible, and it generally is possible, an infant should be nourished from the breast. In a few cases, it becomes necessary to wean an ailing child, but this should not be done without grave thought." He suggested that, when a mother could not breastfeed and a wet nurse could not be obtained, the wisest course was to resort to a mixed feeding, where the mother breastfed as often as possible and used a supplement when she could not. However, Brown commented that many physicians suggested weaning far too easily. After only a brief trial period, physicians would conclude that a mother was unable to breastfeed or that an infant was failing to thrive: "The fault lies with the physician, since they are, as a rule, far too ready to abandon their efforts. The mother is perhaps clamorous for weaning, and it is easy to move in the path of least resistance" (Brown 1917a, 247). Reasons for mixed feedings or early weaning varied, depending on the circumstances of the mother and the views of the physician. Breastfed infants suffering diarrhea could benefit from a formula supplement (MacGregor 1923). Others suggested giving the infant a bottle once a day very soon after birth so that, should the mother became temporarily ill, the child would already know how to use the bottle (Rudolf 1912). Spohn (1920) suggested using a supplement if breast milk was scanty, and he emphasized that even a small quantity of breast milk per day could raise an infant's resistance to infection. However, even in normal situations, it was often deemed advisable to provide the infant with one bottle-feeding a day. Holt, in his influential *The Care and Feeding of Children*, suggested bottle-feeding infants during the night so that mothers would be able to rest. In general, while breastfeeding was superior, mixed feeding was no longer out of the question—particularly for mothers who wanted a respite or who worried that they did not have enough milk.

Although opinions on the supplemental use of formula varied from physician to physician, paediatricians were unanimous in their opposition to patent, or proprietary, foods. For one thing, patent foods did not cater to the individual child: "The usual patent foods on the market are unsuitable and undesirable from the pediatric's point of view. All of them are put up for any child and, therefore, make no allowance for the particular digestive ability of the individual infant" (Rorke 1916, 68). Physicians reported cases where infants were introduced to a particular brand of patent food. When the infant failed to thrive, the parents would try brand after brand in rapid succession. Infants fed on Condensed Milk, Horlick's Milk, Mellin's Food, or Allenbury's Food did not thrive when switched to a cow's-milk mixture. Spohn (1920) commented that practically all infants admitted to Toronto's Hospital for Sick Children had a history of being fed patent foods. Patent foods were considered to be "dead foods" as they lacked adequate nutrients, had a tendency to cause rickets and scurvy and to lead to fat babies, and were very expensive.

Knowledge about the properties of breast milk dramatically increased at the beginning of the twentieth century. Although paediatricians were small in number and were primarily accessible through private practices, they were increasingly involved in public discussions about breastfeeding. As well, paediatricians clearly carved out their dominance as the scientific experts in the realm of infant feeding. And, although many alternatives to breast milk had been explored, science had not yet found a superior method of infant feeding: "Whatever we may have learned in recent years concerning the artificial feeding of infants, has detracted nothing from the paramount importance of keeping them at the breast for as long as possible. This is in a sense an admission of defeat, but it is better so, than to begin to feel that science is able now to adequately nourish all infants by artificial means, and that breast feeding can be dispensed with entirely" (Goldbloom 1924, 709).

Conclusion

At the beginning of the twentieth century, Canadians physicians became involved in developing breast milk alternatives. Physicians, particularly paediatricians, grew in prominence. These people began to set up private practices that focused on infant feeding, to take up new positions in paediatrics in hospitals and universities, and to join child welfare efforts at the policy and clinic levels. Although paediatricians viewed breastfeeding as superior, not all physicians were equally trained in both breastfeeding and bottle-feeding, and many increasingly began to prescribe infant formulas to their patients. Dr. Alan Brown (Brown 1918a, 161) commented on "the absolute disregard of modern teachings relative to the feeding and handling of infants by the medical practitioners. In many instances both pacifiers, and the so-called patented foods were highly recommended." Physicians were used to diagnosing and prescribing. Without formal training in paediatrics (and even with it), they had little knowledge of healthy infants and little experience with infants in a clinic setting and/or at various stages of development. Some did not even know how to prepare simple cow's-milk formulas: "In extreme cases some physicians have been reduced to the expediency of ordering condensed milk and instructing mothers to read the labels on the cans" (Brown 1918b, 299).

Physicians often differed on the issue of breastfeeding. Public health and child welfare activists, on the forefront of the infant mortality campaign, saw breastfeeding as a way of preventing infant diarrhea. Physicians in private practice were not so committed to breastfeeding, and they increasingly began to suggest mixed feeding and earlier weaning: "The great importance of breast feeding has long been known, but so far the subject has failed to secure its proper share of attention. Advertisements of infant foods and an abundance of medical literature on scientific feeding have lulled both mothers and physicians into a false sense of security in the practice of artificial feeding. The fearful loss of infant life is so spread over the entire country that the individual physician does not appreciate his own responsibility, though a conservative estimate attributes a full third of all infants' deaths to unnecessary bottle feeding" (Brown 1918a, 150). While some believed that unknown substances in breast milk led to better outcomes in breastfed infants, others believed that bacterial infection was the main cause of poor outcomes in formula-fed infants. Scientific and medical approaches to breastfeeding initiated a divide in breastfeeding discussions: the substance of breast milk became separated from the practice of breastfeeding. These discussions also introduced a contradiction into breastfeeding beliefs: human milk is ideal for infants but it is also vulnerable. Emotions could "pollute" breast milk, and, for unknown reasons, lactation failure was on the rise. Views that breastfeeding was challenging and difficult suggested to some women that they should not breastfeed as they would only fail anyway.

Chapter 3

Nation, Race, and Motherhood: The Political Ideology of Breastfeeding, 1910–20

Social and cultural transformations that had begun in the nineteenth century continued into the twentieth century. By the end of the second decade of the latter, awareness of, and initiatives to address, infant mortality had grown from local efforts to provincial and national efforts. For the next two decades, the intellectual and ideological roots of breastfeeding promotion came from the late-nineteenth-century women's movement. These merged with broader concerns about citizenship and nation building, along with the growing involvement of scientific medicine in social issues, including the campaign against infant mortality. Motherhood was the issue at the root of the ideology of breastfeeding promotion as it emerged prior to and during the First World War.

By the 1910s, reform efforts had shifted from dispensing milk to instructing mothers on infant feeding and hygiene. As the milk supply continued to improve in cities, the child welfare movement began to shift its concern with infant mortality to a broader interest in child development. By 1920, breastfeeding was clearly declining across Canada. In a 1912 newspaper article describing a baby show in Toronto, the reporter commented that there appeared to be "no alarming symptoms of race suicide" and that the best babies came from Earlscourt. This was attributed to the "fresh air of the district and the fact that the good, old-fashioned method of breast-feeding has generally been adhered to" (*Globe* 1912b, 8). Breastfeeding, although favourably viewed, became only one of several different kinds of infant feeding options.

The Future of the Nation

Most industrializing nations at the end of the nineteenth century initiated a "fight against infant mortality" (Rollet 1997; Davin 1978). The campaign against infant mortality gradually emerged out of other urban reform initiatives and paralleled a new social awareness of infant deaths and the recognition of infants as discrete and separate entities (Armstrong 1986). Strategies to combat infant mortality were debated and discussed at an international level. In Canada, as in other nations, addressing infant mortality was perceived as the solution to a variety of social problems. The infant mortality situation was particularly grave in Canada at the turn of the twentieth century. Infants in Canadian cities were more likely to die than were infants in cities in the United States and other areas of the British Empire. In 1901, in the Dominion of Canada, 128 girls and 157 boys out of every thousand born did not make it past their first year–approximately one in four infants (Light and Parr 1983). The infant welfare campaign in Canada followed a similar pattern to those in the United States and western Europe. Ideas for solving the infant mortality problem and other child welfare concerns were primarily borrowed from Britain, France, and the United States (Comacchio 1993). Virtually all of these strategies brought attention to questions of infant feeding and mothering practices. Breastfeeding gradually became the central concern of infant mortality reformers.

In Canada, interest in infant mortality at provincial and national levels began around 1910. Saving the lives of infants became vital as the need for workers in an industrializing society became apparent. The birth rate of Anglo-Canadians and French Canadians began to decline, and the new science of eugenics fuelled debate about "race" degeneration. In the United Kingdom, the advent of the First World War had created a panic over the belief that the "best" of the nation's young men were being lost to the killing fields of France, and this opened international eyes to the need for healthy infants to come to the future defence of their respective nations. In Canada, worries about the future of the nation turned to a concern with "safeguarding the young." In English Canada, which wanted to expand the nation and make it the star of the British Empire, it was feared that the "white" nation was being subsumed by waves of immigrants. The Anglo-Saxon birth rate was declining not only in Canada but also in Britain and the United States. However, in Canada, this decline was aggravated by a concern with the high fertility of French Canadians and non-British immigrants. The Canadian population as a whole grew from 4.3 million in 1881 to 8.5 million in 1920. In 1871, 60 percent of the population was of British origin and 31 percent was of French origin. By 1921, 55 percent was of British origin and 28 percent was of French origin (Prentice et al. 1988). In French Canada the infant mortality campaign was also part of nationalist discussions. However, these discussions were not about the survival of the British Empire but about the "survival of the race."

In 1901, the foreign-born population in the whole country was 3 percent. However, immigration was especially felt in the West, an area that was just beginning to be settled, as many immigrants were attracted by offers of free homestead land west of Ontario. In 1901, the foreign-born population in British Columbia, the Northwest Territories, and Manitoba was 26 percent, 30 percent, and 15 percent, respectively (Prentice et al. 1988). Although small in comparison to the British and French populations in eastern Canada, the immigrant population was transforming society, and some believed that it was creating threatening social problems:

> This is a comparatively young country. The population is still thinly spread over an immense area, except in a few of the larger city centres. It is not possible, therefore, for the people of this country to absorb so many of these foreign-born people.
>
> When these foreigners come to this country they remain in colonies. This is a most dangerous state of affairs. It tends to spread crime, disease, and ignorance.
>
> ... In the vast majority of instances the country would be better off without these people. Take better care of our own people and let them increase in the normal manner. There is no need for the heavy infant death rate we have in this country, nor is there any excuse for the fact that some 8,000 die annually of tuberculosis. The standard of our people socially, morally and physically is of far more importance than their numbers ...
>
> Defective, degenerate, and ignorant immigrants will fill our asylums with insane inmates, our jails and prisons with culprits of all sorts, will leave their trail over the country in a record of murders and crimes, and will give rise to low and degenerate offspring. (Immigrants Coming to Canada 1908, 140)

Reported increases in tuberculosis, alcoholism, divorce, and labour unrest were supposedly due to the erosion of traditional values (McLaren 1990). Fears of race degeneration and race suicide spurred concern with infant mortality.

The sources of contamination in Canadian society, and part of the infant mortality problem, were considered by many to be the masses of immigrants that were pouring into the country. Many programs to address immigration, education, and child welfare were developed by individuals who supported the theories of eugenics. Individuals and groups, such as the Canadian National Committee on Mental Hygiene (which later became the Canadian Mental Health Association), interested in improving society through race betterment, supported a huge range of activities, from improving environmental issues to breeding out hereditary weakness (Dodd 1991). Some believed that hereditary weakness was the cause of anti-social behaviour, crime, and poverty. Supporters of hereditarian genetics advocated for immigration restrictions, marriage restrictions, and sterilization. Other supporters of the principles of eugenics were known as "environmental eugenicists." These people believed that infant mortality, criminality, and other forms of deviance were not solely determined by genetics: they were also determined by social conditions. For this reason, social reform was crucial. The heredity/environment eugenics debate was active throughout the first three decades of the twentieth century, and the reform efforts of environmental eugenicists, in particular, once again shifted attention to mothering and childrearing practices. Infant mortality was not just a question of survival of the fittest: society had a responsibility to ensure that every child was made fit (Dodd 1991). Gradually, mothers came to be perceived as the pillar of the infant mortality campaign in both French and English Canada, and the issue became the survival of the "race" (Baillargeon 2002).

The Infant Mortality Reports

By 1910, infant mortality was no longer solely the concern of lay reformers. Physicians were quickly gaining authority in the new scientific era, and, as government began to expand at all levels, there were increasing opportunities for them to get involved in guiding and reforming society. Their role was beginning to extend beyond clinics into citizenship and nation building. Physicians became increasingly involved in the infant mortality campaign, with the result that infant mortality began to become a medical issue.

One of the first physicians involved in infant mortality discussions was Helen MacMurchy. MacMurchy, part of the second generation of women to attend medical school in Canada, graduated from the University of Toronto with her medical degree in 1901. She was the first woman appointed to the resident staff of the Toronto General Hospital, with a position in the Department of Obstetrics and Gynaecology and a cross-appointment as a lecturer at the University of Toronto. After practising briefly in Toronto, she began a career as a civil servant, first with the provincial government (1906–19) and later with the federal government (1920–34). Among other things, she served as a medical inspector for Toronto schools (1911) and was the first editor for the journal *The Canadian Nurse* (1905–10) (McConnachie 1983). As a public health reformer and supporter of the principles of eugenics, MacMurchy was involved in a wide range of issues, including infant and maternal mortality and feeblemindedness.

In 1910, MacMurchy produced a series of three reports for the Ontario government on the issue of infant mortality (MacMurchy 1910, 1911, 1912). These reports were highly influential in Ontario as well as in the rest of Canada, and they also received international attention. In all the reports (each subsequent one 50 percent longer than its predecessor), MacMurchy provided an analysis of the multitude of factors that influenced infant mortality. Using statistics collected from New York, Boston, Chicago, Philadelphia, and abroad; descriptions of strategies for addressing infant mortality in countries around the world; anecdotes and letters of interest and support; and metaphors from the Bible, the reports highlighted factors such as breastfeeding, urban overcrowding and sanitation (including the problem of getting clean milk), poverty, and women's work.

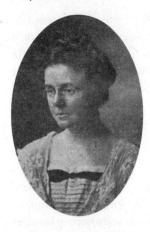

Figure 3.1   Portrait of Dr. Helen MacMurchy, taken from the *Globe*, 28 April 1914. Photo of H. MacMurchy in the University of Toronto Archives, Department of Graduate Records, A1973-0026/293 [67].

MacMurchy (1910) argued that up to 80 percent of all infant deaths could be prevented. The loss of these lives was a social tragedy: "We are only now discovering that Empires and States are built up of babies" (3). MacMurchy emphasized the importance of each individual Ontario child: "Every year nearly Ten Thousand Children in Ontario, under the age of five years go to their graves. We would think ten thousand emigrants a great addition to our population. It is a question if ten thousand emigrants from anywhere would equal in value to us, these ten thousand little Canadians of Ontario, whose lives are sacrificed to our carelessness, ignorance, stupidity" (MacMurchy 1910, 3). In many ways, MacMurchy's reports seemed more concerned with the implications of infant mortality for the "white Imperial nation" than for the individual.

Motherhood was at the core of MacMurchy's concept of public health, and, for her, women's maternal and domestic roles were central to preventing infant mortality. The decline in breastfeeding rates was blamed primarily on women. Mothers failed to breastfeed because they were ignorant ("most mothers think cow's milk is just as good"), because they accepted advice from neighbours or other meddling busybodies ("we must give [them] skilled medical advice"), and because they needed to work ("[this] should not be allowed to happen") (MacMurchy 1910, 30). Breastfeeding was central to reducing infant mortality rates: "The Most Important Thing: One thing we know about Infant Mortality. If the baby is nursed by its mother the chances are that it will live. If the baby is fed in any other way the chances are great that it will die" (MacMurchy 1910, 5).

She posited Jewish infant feeding practices as an example from which all could learn: "It is well known that Hebrew mothers almost invariably nurse their children" (MacMurchy 1910, 10). And, indeed, in Montreal, infant mortality rates were lower in the Jewish population, although as new immigrants Jewish people were primarily among the poorer classes. In 1910, the infant mortality rate for Anglo-Protestants was 163 per 1,000, compared to a rate of 224 per 1,000 for Franco-Catholics, 207 per 1,000 for Catholics of other origins, and 94 per 1,000 among the Jewish population (Baillargeon 1998; Copp 1981). Repeatedly, MacMurchy (1910, 36) stated that the baby represented the future of the nation and that nothing should be allowed to prevent all mothers from breastfeeding: "Our goodly heritage will go to the sons of strangers, unless we put our hands and minds in earnest to the work of rearing an Imperial race. The Jews have discovered the secret of National Immortality ... 'Take care of your children.'"

MacMurchy was vehemently opposed to working mothers. She fervently believed that "the destruction of the poor is their poverty. The rich baby lives, the poor baby dies" (MacMurchy 1911, 5). She described breast milk as the baby's "natural" food and envisioned a country in which all fathers, regardless of their occupation, were paid enough to support a family. Mothers belonged in the home with their children. A society in which mothers needed to work had failed to save the child: "Where the mother works, the baby dies. Nothing can replace maternal care" (MacMurchy 1910, 17).

The *Infant Mortality* reports are filled with strategies for solving infant mortality, including the establishment of infant welfare clinics in poor neighbourhoods, campaigns for clean milk legislation, and the provision of state pensions and nursing allowances for breastfeeding mothers. MacMurchy also believed that mothers should receive greater supervision and care from physicians and nurses, and, as a physician, she evinced suspicion at the attendance of midwives at births. She suggested that information about birth attendants and infant feeding, among other things, be collected when an infant was registered. Although midwives were licensed in Great Britain, MacMurchy (1912) was opposed to their being licensed in Canada.

MacMurchy emphasized the need for better birth registration systems so that infant mortality rates could be calculated and child welfare activities could reach the infants most in need. As birth registration was not enforced, the rate of infant mortality could only be estimated. In 1918, it was thought that 15 percent of infants were not registered (Brown 1918a). However, if the state was careless in tracking births, manufacturers of patent foods were not. MacMurchy (1910, 34) described how the "Baby Exterminators," or patent food manufacturers, sent congratulations, advice, and pictures to mothers following birth announcements in the newspaper. She disapproved of food advertisements that described patent foods as a "perfect substitute for mother's milk." She advocated forcing patent food manufacturers to list the contents of their products on their labels. She was especially critical of "soothing" medicines for infants that contained opium, heroin, morphine, codeine, and other dangerous drugs. The labels of products such as "Mrs. Winslow's Soothing Syrup," "Koepp's Baby Friend," and "Dr. Moffett's Teethina Teething Powders" did not provide contents lists.

While MacMurchy (1910, 30) advocated for collective action to counter the infant mortality problem, she also emphasized maternal responsibility: "It is evident and it must be made known and thoroughly taught and impressed upon everyone, that the great and most effectual means of lessening infant mortality is that the baby should be nursed by the mother." In spite of the dazzling array of alternative strategies described in her reports, MacMurchy chose to focus on education rather than on structural change as the solution to infant mortality. Breastfeeding was prioritized over other possibilities: "It is the mother that we should do something for. She is the one, and the only one, who can save the baby" (MacMurchy 1911, 5).

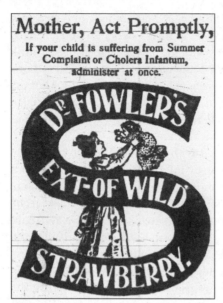

Mother, Act Promptly,

If your child is suffering from Summer
Complaint or Cholera Infantum,
administer at once.

DR **FOWLER'S**

EXT-OF WILD

STRAWBERRY.

Figure 3.2   Dr. Fowler's Strawberry and
Peppermint Mixture contained morphine. *Globe*,
25 June 1900.

Selfish Mothers and Ignorant Mothers

MacMurchy's *Infant Mortality* reports emphasized that the key to solving infant mortality was to "concentrate on the mother" and to "glorify, dignify, and purify motherhood by every means in our power."[1] (MacMurchy 1918, 315) Mothering practices, particularly breastfeeding, were thought to be the solution to the infant mortality problem. Throughout society, increasing attention was paid to the actions of mothers of all classes and from all backgrounds. In policy documents, newspapers and magazines, and pamphlets containing health advice, mothers who chose not to breastfeed were depicted as either ignorant or selfish, sometimes both. Public health and child welfare authorities repeatedly informed mothers that their ignorance was responsible for the loss of the lives of their infants and that their actions were jeopardizing the future of the nation. At the Child Welfare Exhibition held in October of 1911 in Montreal, one exhibit consisted of a screen that flashed a light every ten seconds, "showing that somewhere in the world a baby was paying with its life, the price of ignorance" (Anonymous 1912, 210).

In her 1910 report, MacMurchy (1910, 31) commented, "We expect the ideal mother to know everything by instinct." Mothering was neither instinctual nor natural: it required careful consideration, study, expert knowledge, and intervention. While all mothers needed to be educated about hygiene and breastfeeding, immigrant women were particular targets of intervention:

> To-day we have pouring into this great country of ours thousands of the poor, the ignorant, the superstitious, the down-trodden, from all parts of the old world. The duty falls upon the people of Canada to help these people to become good citizens, to teach them that their prosperity depends, to a large extent upon the care they take of their homes and surroundings. Unfortunately, they are mostly ignorant and careless of the first principles of sanitary protection, and they look upon the health officials as their natural enemies, whose aim and desire is to interfere and make life unpleasant for them. (Laurie 1913, 455)

Graph 3.1

Percentage of breastfeeding durations in Canadian-born mothers, American-born mothers and foreign-born mothers, Toronto, 1915–17

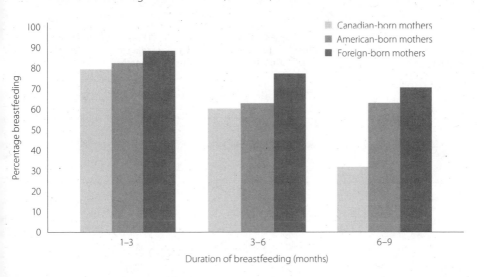

Reformers, often middle-class men and women, were often surprised at the resistance they received from new immigrants. Reformers' efforts, which were motivated by the desire to solve the infant mortality problem, often did not coincide with the practical and material concerns of new immigrants.

Reformers suggested that immigrant women were the least likely to breastfeed. However, an infant feeding survey of 2,079 women in Toronto revealed some surprising results with regard to breastfeeding practices in Canadian-born mothers, "foreign"-born mothers, and mothers from different social classes (Brown 1917a). Between 1915 and 1917, patients from infant clinics (representing the poor) and patients from a paediatrician's private practice (representing the middle and upper classes) were surveyed regarding their breastfeeding practices. Additionally, students and nurses were asked whether or not they had been breastfed, and, if so, for how long. These cases were meant to estimate breastfeeding rates of approximately twenty years before. A look at the clinic cases by country of birth shows differences between Canadian, American, and foreign-born mothers. At three different time intervals over the first nine months of the infant's life, Canadian-born mothers appeared to be breastfeeding less often than did American-born and foreign-born mothers. Foreign-born mothers (i.e., immigrants from outside North America) had the highest breastfeeding rates. Canadian mothers seemed to be "shirking" their "maternal duty" (*Globe* 1917).

Table 3.1

Breastfeeding initiation and duration (three, six, and nine months) in 1900 and 1917 (upper/middle-class and poor mothers) in Toronto

Population	Number of cases	% Bottle fed	% Breast-feeding from birth	% Breast-feeding at 3 months	% Breast-feeding at 6 months	% Breast-feeding over 9 months
Overall 1900	137	12.4	87.6	84.7	76.6	29.9
Upper and middle classes 1917	633	24.0	76.3	46.7	30.4	9.8
"Poor" 1917	946	16.53	79.65	60.51	31.88	—

Note: Reasons for weaning in upper- and middle-class patients: 250 of the cases were weaned in private practice; 32 percent were weaned because of signs of excessive feeding (i.e., vomiting and green stools). The rest were apparently weaned because of insufficient milk (Brown 1917a).

The survey also found that breastfeeding rates had changed since the turn of the twentieth century. Whereas in 1900, approximately 75 percent of women had breastfed until their baby was six months old, by between 1915 and 1917, approximately 30 percent of women were breastfeeding for this length of time, indicating a strong trend towards earlier weaning. By 1917, 10 percent fewer mothers were choosing to breastfeed at birth and, of these, 10 percent fewer were still breastfeeding at three months. Most weaning seemed to occur in the first three months. Further, lower-class mothers were breastfeeding more than were upper-class mothers. The study demonstrated that "well-to-do" mothers, mothers who should have known better, were abandoning breastfeeding. These selfish mothers were neglecting the welfare of the country for their own interests—convenience, more time available to spend with their husbands or on various social activities, or sheer lack of interest in their children. Unlike newly arrived immigrants, who were simply ignorant or poor mothers who often needed to work, these privileged mothers were "choosing" not to breastfeed. Although immigrant mothers and lower-class mothers received a range of advice from public health and child welfare authorities, this was never redirected at the well-to-do mothers who were moving away from breastfeeding in greater numbers.

Working Mothers and Rural Mothers

Industrialization created a divide between women's productive and reproductive work. For the first time, women were leaving the private domain of the home to find employment in the public domain. Women and children were an increasingly important part of the industrial workforce. By 1871, women and children comprised 42 percent of the industrial workforce in Montreal (Ames 1897) and 34 percent of it in Toronto (Kealey 1980). In Canada, women as a percentage of the workforce increased from 20 percent in 1896 to 25 percent in 1931. Women were especially finding employment in urban settings. By 1921, there were 58,000 more women than men in the cities, likely due to employment opportunities in textile mills, factories, retail stores, and domestic service. Often, in these new work environments, women were challenged by harsh conditions, long hours, and inflexible scheduling. However, rather than addressing the actual conditions of women's work, infant mortality reformers chose to focus on poverty in the abstract as the cause of women's failure to breastfeed: "If the mother goes out to work and cannot look after her infant, poverty, by taking the mother out of the home, robs the infant of proper attention and this leads to infantile deaths in the thousands" (*Globe* 1919, 6).

Poverty could influence infant mortality by reducing the chances that an infant would be breastfed, and this was compounded by the environment in which the infant found itself: "Poverty means poor health for the mother, lower intelligence, lack of energy, and general inefficiency, and forces families to live in crowded insanitary surroundings. Poverty forces the mother to work for a living, depriving their babies of breast milk, and, as a consequence, these infants are unable to thrive and develop in the poverty-stricken homes into which they are born" (Brown 1918a, 149).

A 1919 article in the *Globe* commented, "Figures are being given to show that there is conclusive proof of children's deaths, because, by their mothers going out to work, they are deprived of the natural sources of help and have to be kept up on artificial substitutes." The article went on to point out that "it is most impressive to learn that infant mortality decreases during a time of industrial depression, and that a drop in the death rate invariably follows a strike, when women are thrown out of employment and forced to return to the home" (*Globe* 1919; MacMurchy 1910). Although this was a rather expansive claim, studies from abroad did suggest that mothers who worked outside the home (e.g., doing factory work) experienced higher rates of infant mortality than did mothers who worked for pay in the home (e.g., taking in boarders, doing laundry). It is entirely possible that the latter rates were lower because mothers in the home were able to continue to breastfeed (Wolf 2001).

While MacMurchy had suggested in her reports that working women who could not adjust their schedules to accommodate breastfeeding should receive a pension so that they would not have to work, this was pretty much an abstract proposition. An initiative by the Toronto Council of Women argued that mothers who were widowed, deserted, or who needed to work because their husbands were ill or in prison should receive state aid, much as did wives and families of soldiers. The principle behind mother's pensions was "that motherhood is a state of service and should have state recognition" (Huetis 1918, 164). In an attempt to demonstrate to the Ontario government that pensions were "more sane and cheaper" than was granting financial aid to institutions, the Toronto Council of Women adopted six mothers and their twenty-two children and paid them a pension for three years. As mothers were leaving their young children alone at home while they worked for $1.25 per day, the council decided to pay them a pension (ten dollars for the mother and ten dollars for each child) instead of finding them daycare services. In exchange, mothers were required to keep their homes clean, to keep their children in school, and to be home after school (Huetis 1918).

It was common knowledge that bottle-fed infants experienced higher infant mortality rates than did breastfed infants, and it was recognized that mothers who worked were not likely to be able to initiate and continue breast-feeding. A Toronto Department of Public Health report stated, "No mother can properly nurse her child if she must at the same time act as a breadwinner" (quoted in Huetis 1918, 165). However, there do not appear to have been any initiatives on the part of municipal, provincial, or national governments in Canada to provide a mother's pension or nursing allowance. Policies to increase breastfeeding by legally protecting mothers in the paid labour force or creating nursing allowances did occur in many European countries at the turn of the century. In Germany, between 1878 and 1927, a series of laws were enacted that resulted in a twelve-week paid maternity leave. Nursing allowances (i.e., payments for breastfeeding) originated in France in 1892 and began in Germany in 1904. In Germany, these became very popular, and, by 1919, a twelve-week nursing allowance was available to all women. Nursing allowances partly covered lost wages, contributed to the nutritional health of mothers, and provided opportunities to link the provision of nursing allowances with visits to child welfare clinics (Kintner 1985).

Unlike working women in the cities, women in rural areas were seen as having few barriers to successful breastfeeding (MacMurchy 1910). One report suggested that approximately 70 percent to 90 percent of women in rural areas were nursing their infants for at least six months in 1918 (Brown 1918b). Mothers in rural areas had higher rates of breastfeeding than did mothers in urban areas, as they worked in the home and were less likely to be influenced by neighbours or physicians who were improperly trained in infant feeding practices. It was suggested that mothers in rural areas were less likely to bottle-feed as they did not have access to iceboxes and certified milk. However, due to their relative isolation, rural mothers did face challenges in infant feeding. Although they were more likely to breastfeed than were urban mothers, they also had less access to public health nurses, teachers, and clinic physicians. This meant that many rural mothers were more likely to feed at irregular intervals, to breastfeed past the infant's first birthday, and to fail to weigh the baby regularly (all of this was contrary to expert advice but may actually have had favourable outcomes). Rural mothers were also vulnerable to receiving information on infant feeding through magazines and other publications instead of through public health literature and child welfare experts. As a result, patent foods were increasingly favoured in rural areas, with the most popular foods being those advertised in the newspapers and magazines. These patent foods were expensive, had alluring ads, came with full directions on use, and did not adequately describe the difference between their nutritional content and that of cow's milk: "The father and mother love desiring the best for their baby, together with their lack of facilities and knowledge of the technique for feeding cow's milk are all factors in promoting the use of patent foods in rural districts" (Brown 1918b, 298). Thus, rural mothers who continued to work inside the home were more likely to breastfeed than were urban working mothers. However, they often did not have access to expert advice and tended to use patent foods instead of modified cow's milk as a breast milk alternative.

"Literature, Instruction, and Assistance"

Many strategies to address infant mortality emerged in the first two decades of the twentieth century. "Literature, instruction, and assistance" was increasingly provided to mothers through charitable organizations, religious groups, and public health departments. In the second decade of the century, one of the new forums for maternal education and supervision was the well baby clinic. Building upon the milk depots established in the first decade of the century, child welfare clinics began to appear across the country. At the milk depots, mothers received pure milk so that they could maintain their health. Gradually, educational and supervisory components were added to the original milk depots, and, eventually, the dispensing of milk was dropped altogether. The institutions established in Toronto, Hamilton, Ottawa, and London prior to the First World War all underwent this transition from milk depot to child welfare clinic. By the end of the war none of these clinics any longer served as milk depots (Comacchio 1993).

Hamilton was one of the first cities to develop a child welfare clinic. Recognizing a need for local efforts to address infant mortality, local individuals, in conjunction with the VON, established the Hamilton Babies' Dispensary in 1909. They found a suitable dairy farm, and nurses were trained to fill bottles with appropriate formulas of certified milk. Milk was sold at a "ridiculously low" price from two depots at various locations in the city. By 1910, there were five depots in the city, providing milk for about 100 to 130 infants per day. In 1910, the services at the Hamilton Babies' Dispensary began to expand. Physicians were available for diagnostic purposes, nurses provided home visits, volunteers helped with the weighing of babies, while classes, short talks, and demonstrations were provided on topics such as Care of the Baby, Personal Hygiene, and Ventilation. In Hamilton, between 1911 and

1915, infant mortality due to gastrointestinal disease decreased from 57 percent to 19 percent (Cody 1915).

At all the clinics, breastfeeding was encouraged. However, if mothers were unable to breastfeed, babies were placed on formula. In Hamilton, the nurses instructed mothers on how to modify milk at home. The use of certified milk was encouraged, but, if it was too expensive, ordinary pasteurized milk was used. The central message concerned absolute cleanliness in the handling of milk. Mothers were taught to prepare all the required feedings for a twenty-four-hour period and to place the milk formula in separate bottles and then store them in a cool place. Milk was diluted and modified with sugar, and the instructions for doing this were simple enough to enable mothers to carry out the appropriate modifications at home. When necessary, certified milk and required bottles and utensils were sold at cost or given to the mother free of charge. Nurses visited the homes of mothers once a week and focused on the cleanliness of food preparation (Cody 1915).

In Hamilton, as in other cities, mothers were often referred to the clinic by physicians. However, many mothers were "recruited" by a mailing sent from the dispensary and based on a birth registry.[2] Attempts were also made to gain the co-operation of local private physicians. The clinics emphasized that their role was purely to educate mothers and to supervise infant health. Infants requiring treatment were referred back to their physicians or sent to hospital. When women began to attend the clinic, physicians were notified by letter. Education and prevention were key aspects of child welfare clinics: baby clinics were "not so much for curative purposes as for those of education. The mothers of the poor need to learn a lot of things to bring children up safely through the perils that surround them through the conditions in which they are forced to live. That's where the clinics shine—in education" (Anonymous 1913, 94). The focus on prevention also led to increasing the provision of pre-natal care. During routine home visits by nurses, mothers received advice on hygiene, diet, exercise, sleep, and proper care of the breasts. Nurses also took blood pressure readings, collected urine samples, and encouraged breastfeeding. They would then report their findings to the physician (Brown 1919b).

As baby clinics continued to evolve, physicians became more heavily involved in clinic work. For the most part, they took responsibility for the medical side of child welfare work, primarily monitoring and prescribing for the feeding of infants. Nurses and various women's groups addressed the social side of the work. They visited mothers in their homes, provided instruction in the preparation of infant formulas, updated medical history cards, provided advice on hygiene and general care, and gave out set milk formulas (Mullen 1915). Physicians also began to work in government divisions of child welfare. Nurses in the city primarily worked with mothers through delivering services and information; however, nurses in rural areas often attended births and offered bedside care.

The increasing involvement of doctors did not always lead to a seamless transition from milk depot to child welfare clinic. In Toronto, by 1918, there were twenty-two child welfare clinics, all of which gradually moved from focusing exclusively on the regulation of infant feeding to considering the health of school-aged children. When the city took over the clinics in 1916, the decision was made to eliminate the milk depots–particularly in light of the fact that city milk was regulated by the Department of Public Health (between 1913 and 1917, deaths due to gastrointestinal causes in Toronto decreased from 130/100,000 to 37/100,000). In Montreal, the transition of milk depots into child welfare clinics was not as smooth as it was in Toronto. In 1914, women's groups began to be involved in transforming fifteen of the milk depots into child welfare clinics (Baillargeon 1996). However, there were continuous questions about who should be in charge of the *gouttes de lait*. Women's groups, physicians, religious elites, and public health authorities had all been involved in the development of the milk depots and child welfare clinics. Each had their own conception of how the fight against infant mortality should be waged. Women's groups saw saving children as part of the privileged domain of volunteer women social reformers; priests and doctors saw the *gouttes de lait* as charitable institutions; and government saw the infant mortality issue as a quest to improve public health. Physicians preferred that the clinic consultations with mothers remain in their control so that the women and their families would not become targets of state supervision. Also, women volunteers, who visited the homes of mothers with the intent of convincing the women to go to the *gouttes de laits*, upset some physicians because it was thought they might also be providing advice on hygiene and infant feeding. Eventually, women's groups were forced to retire from the *gouttes de lait*. The city health department supported the parish-based clinics but also wished to expand their services so that they would reach a broader range of mothers. Rather than expanding the existing clinics, the city sought the approval of the archbishop of Montreal to open new municipal clinics in areas where *gouttes de lait* did not already exist (Baillargeon 1996). In 1919, the municipal government opened fourteen new clinics, which continued to run concurrently with the private clinics located primarily in French Canadian communities. It wasn't until the 1950s that the municipal government absorbed all of the earlier parish-based *gouttes de lait* (Baillargeon 1998).

Choices and Constraints

By 1920, milk depots had evolved from their original purpose of providing mothers with uncontaminated milk to providing education, consultation, and home visits. A survey of ten Canadian cities in 1918 revealed that there were over fifty-eight infant welfare clinics or milk depots (Brown 1918a). Through child welfare clinics, women had access to health professionals who provided ongoing medical consultations. They weighed and measured infants, developed schedules for infant care, and provided advice on infant feeding. However, child welfare and public health activities focused primarily on philanthropy and surveillance rather than on material assistance. Their emphasis on prevention did result in interventions targeted at altering the physical environment (e.g., building sewage systems in urban areas) but rarely challenged or changed the economic positions of those whom they were intended to help. Mothers were given a central role in the infant mortality campaign; however, the focus on maternal education meant that other causes of infant mortality, such as poverty and overcrowded housing, were ignored. While some interventions were extremely effective in reducing infant mortality, others—such as the attempt by middle- and upper-class mothers to extend their vision of mothers as nurturers to immigrant and working-class women—were resisted.

For the most part, child welfare clinics were created for the poor. Because of their overcrowded living conditions, their perceived ignorance, and their material need, it was thought that the poor required advice on health, hygiene, and lifestyle. It was thought that child welfare clinics could assist with improving home conditions and keeping the community well (Brown 1919b). Families who could pay were expected to see a family physician in a private office rather than attend a child welfare clinic. It should be pointed out that physicians attempted to utilize a preventive focus: as diseases of childhood could be more easily prevented than cured, physicians took it upon themselves to monitor the child's diet, hygiene, and clothing rather than simply to treat specific ailments (Brown 1919b).

Breastfeeding promotion became inextricably linked to the home and to women's role in it. Although women's domestic role was cherished in rhetoric, women's realities did not reflect this. Industrialization had separated paid and unpaid work: paid work was now usually done outside the house. Increasingly, women were led to believe that the husband's role was to bring home a "family wage" and that the wife's role was to care for the family and use the money he "gave" her correctly and efficiently. However, the domestic ideal of a woman with a man to protect her was not as widespread as public discussions would have led one to believe. During the late nineteenth century and the early twentieth century, over 50 percent of the working class lived below the poverty line. In Winnipeg, in 1916, over 20 percent of women between twenty-five and sixty-four were single, widowed, or divorced (Prentice et al. 1988). Demands for cheap labour led to the increasing participation of women and children in the workforce, with the result that families became dependent upon their earning power. Between 1900 and 1920, women represented approximately 25 percent of the Canadian workforce in manufacturing and mechanical work (Prentice et al. 1988). In the new industrial society, there were few options for women who wished to breastfeed. In the 1890s, factory work employed one-third of female workers;

however, women received subsistence-level wages only if they maintained a fifty-four-hour workweek (Ursel 1992). Various pieces of legislation were enacted to protect women and children from working long hours in unsafe environments. However, in 1913, women in Ontario and Quebec factories still routinely worked fifty-five to sixty hours a week and up to seventy hours a week in rush seasons (Prentice et al. 1988). Unless women were able to leave work during the day or pay someone to bring their infants to the factory gates, breastfeeding was difficult, if not impossible.

Conclusion

By the 1920s, mothers were moving away from breastfeeding, but the rate and reasons varied according to class. Mothers' choices were clearly related to social position and structural constraints. Women had differential exposure to new beliefs and values about breastfeeding. Upper- and middle-class mothers received infant feeding advice from physicians in private practice and from advice manuals, while immigrant and working-class women were more likely to adhere to traditional practices or to receive information from physicians in child welfare clinics (or through other philanthropic reform activities).

Although breastfeeding was claimed to be the superior method of infant feeding, not all mothers were choosing to do it. Mothers in urban areas were less likely to breastfeed than were mothers in rural areas; immigrant mothers were more likely to breastfeed than were Canadian-born mothers; and upper- and middle-class mothers were less likely to breastfeed than were working-class and immigrant mothers. Mothers in different classes who chose not to breastfeed had different options available to them. Cow's milk was the most popular alternative to breast milk, but others included canned cow's milk and patent foods (i.e., commercial foods) that were mixed with cow's milk or water. Fresh cow's milk could be raw, certified, sterilized, pasteurized, or modified. Upper-class women could purchase "laboratory milk" and have it delivered to their homes. Middle-class women were more likely, based on advice manuals or a prescription from a physician, to feed their infants milk modified with water and sugar. Working-class women could find affordable milk at city milk depots or could use diluted condensed or evaporated milk. By 1920, breastfeeding practices had moved from being associated with the beliefs and practices of various ethnic groups to being associated with class. As breastfeeding rates began to decline in all class groups throughout the twentieth century, regional and ethnic variations in breastfeeding practices began to emerge.

Part 2

Decline, 1920–60

Chapter 4

Professionals and Government, 1920–30

In the 1920s, the campaign against infant mortality moved from local and provincial activities to attempts at a more coordinated approach at the national level. The formation of the federal Department of Health in 1919 signalled the beginning of Canada's first policies on mothering and breast-feeding. Breastfeeding continued to be considered an important method of solving infant mortality; however, in the 1920s, it took on more political signif-icance and was portrayed as a political and moral act symbolizing patriotism and good motherhood. Following the First World War, growing govern-ment support for the use of scientific principles and the expansion of scien-tific medicine increasingly influenced government activities. Scientific and medical understandings of society merged with national goals. The values of strength, freedom and autonomy, industry, and discipline shaped federal policy at all levels and contributed to the development of new expectations and norms of infant feeding. In the post–First World War era, new attitudes and knowledge about breastfeeding soon carried the authority of the state and of science.

The Canadian Mother's Book

Since the turn of the twentieth century, the federal government had been pressured to form a national department of health. Social reformers and organizations such as the National Council of Women and the Canadian Medical Association advocated for federal involvement in addressing the exceedingly high rates of infant and maternal mortality. However, it was not until the end of the First World War that the government recognized the tragic and preventable nature of infant mortality and its relationship to the strength of the nation. For many industrializing nations, the First World War had highlighted the somewhat embarrassing degree of physical fitness of their recruits. During the war, sixty thousand Canadians had died in battle. Overall, there were approximately 230,000 casualties out of a population of eight million. As well, the worldwide flu pandemic of 1918–19 resulted in the loss of an additional fifty thousand Canadians (McGinnis 1981). By 1919, the alarming loss of life made the idea of a federal Department of Health extremely popular (Comacchio 1993).

The Department of Health Act received its first reading in March 1919, and the federal Department of Health was established on 6 June 1919. The political desire to build the strength of the nation led to the formation of the Division of Child Welfare.[1] The aims of the first division in the new department were "(1) To save and preserve Maternal and Child Life (2) To promote and secure Maternal and Child Welfare (3) To maintain and improve the health, strength and well-being of Mothers and Children and (4) To make known to all the Principles of Maternal and Child Welfare, and the supreme Importance of Home life to the individual and the Nation" (quoted in Arnup 1994, 28).

One of the first acts of the new Division of Child Welfare was the development and publication of a series of "Little Blue Books." In May 1920, at one of the early meetings of the Dominion Council of Health, there was a unanimous request for original Canadian publications on maternal and child welfare, including information on infant feeding (Buckley 1977). Council representatives were appreciative of international sources but weary of relying on them. They stated that they would prefer that "Canada should not continue to borrow, but rather exchange" knowledge and advice on child and maternal welfare (quoted in Dodd 1991, 205). Helen MacMurchy was appointed chief of the Division of Child Welfare on 10 April 1920, and she developed and coordinated the writing and distribution of the first federal-government-sponsored child-care advice literature.

All of the sixteen "Little Blue Books" were well received by women's groups, mothers, and public health officials, with topics ranging from childbirth and childrearing to cooking and cleaning. However, the most popular of these publications was *The Canadian Mother's Book*. The first edition of *The Canadian Mother's Book*, written and later revised by MacMurchy, was received from the printer on 3 March 1921, and 150,000 copies were distributed by the end of the year. Nearly one in four mothers received a copy between 1921 and 1932. By the time the Division of Child Welfare was disbanded in 1933, the book had gone through four revisions (1921, 1923, 1927, 1932), it had grown from 50 pages to over 250 pages, and over 800,000 copies had been distributed. Women received copies through women's groups and from public health nurses (they could also receive a copy through the mail). When a woman registered the birth of her child at one of the various district registrars in each province, she received a request card that could be mailed back to the Department of Health free of charge.

Eleven editions of *The Canadian Mother's Book* were published between 1921 and 1991 (see Appendix C). It is not possible to know the extent to which mothers valued or followed the advice contained in these publications. It does appear, however, that the advice manuals were extremely popular and widely distributed. Regardless, the eleven editions of *The Canadian Mother's Book* are important historical documents with regard to exploring the history of breast-feeding in Canada. These volumes chronicle over seventy years of changes in childbirth and childrearing techniques, in the responsibilities of mothers and fathers, and in the role of health care practitioners and institutions. In terms of infant feeding, they clearly record how "the one best way" has changed over time (Lewis and Watson 1991/92); see Appendix F. *The Canadian Mother's Book* encapsulates federal government policy on breastfeeding and, as well, represents Canada's first foray into two different yet linked areas of policy-making: mothering/family policy and nutrition policy.

Feeding the "Infant Soldier"[2]

As chief of the Division of Child Welfare, Helen MacMurchy influenced all of the division's activities until her retirement in 1934. In many ways, MacMurchy was an ideal candidate for chief of the new division. As a physician, she represented medical and scientific interests; as a maternal feminist, she represented many women's groups that sought to draw attention to and gain respect for women's roles as mothers. MacMurchy wrote and developed the Little Blue Books, including *The Canadian Mother's Book*, by drawing upon her own public health experiences, consulting with other professionals and organizations, and reviewing materials from other countries. In these publications, she demonstrates a desire to establish breastfeeding as "the Canadian way." Breast milk was the perfect food and breastfeeding was "the most successful and the right and natural way to bring up a baby." (MacMurchy 1923, 72)

The first editions of *The Canadian Mother's Book* advised mothers to exclusively breastfeed their babies for nine months. MacMurchy emphasized that bottle-fed babies were nine times more likely to die during infancy than were breastfed babies. Breastfeeding was "safer, easier, cheaper, wiser, and more successful" (MacMurchy 1923, 30) than was bottle-feeding, which was considered to be dangerous and unnecessarily complicated. Mothers were encouraged to breastfeed for the well-being of the nation. Only dedicated mothers could make up for the losses suffered during the First World War: "Children are the security of the home and the nation." (MacMurchy 1923, 7). MacMurchy informed mothers that "the Government of Canada, knowing that the nation is made of homes, and that the homes are made by the Father and Mother, recognizes you as one of the Makers of Canada. No National Service is greater or better than the work of the Mother in her own home. The Mother is 'The First Servant of the State'" (MacMurchy 1923, 5). MacMurchy described breastfeeding as a national duty. She "equated breast feeding with patriotism and artificial feeding with treason" (Buckley 1977, 77). As she assumed that all mothers could and would breastfeed their infants until they were nine months

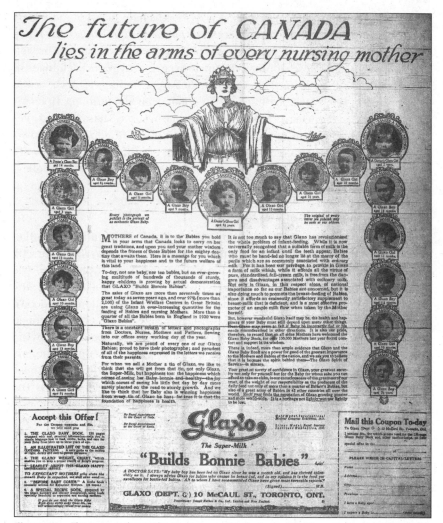

Figure 4.1 The message that mothers were responsible for the health of the nation was also reflected in advertising (including for breast milk alternatives) and other domestic advice literature. *Globe*, 8 July 1921.

old, MacMurchy did not include any information on alternate methods of infant feeding in *The Canadian Mother's Book*: "You can nurse the baby, and you will, for you know it is better for you and better for Canada. It saves the baby's life" (MacMurchy 1923, 31).

Not only was motherhood a national duty, it was also a sacred right. MacMurchy reminded women, "Your greatest happiness is coming to you in the birth of your baby" (MacMurchy 1923, 7). Motherhood was natural and nothing to be afraid of: "Be Brave. This is not some strange thing which is going to happen to you. It is the right, natural and healthy thing for you, just as it was for your own mother when you were born." MacMurchy, single and childless herself, continued: "Too sacred to be spoken, the dearest wish of a true woman is to be a mother" (MacMurchy 1923, 8). Motherhood was described as "sacred" and "natural." Echoing the views she outlined a decade earlier in the Ontario Infant Mortality reports, she stated that breast milk was pure and "specially made by nature for your baby" (MacMurchy 1923, 32). As motherhood was natural and sacred, breastfeeding represented its supreme act. Mothers were selfless, and if they embraced motherhood and approached breastfeeding with the right attitude, they would find any challenges relatively simple to overcome: "Yet, thinking not of herself, she [the mother] gives a supreme proof of her love for her child ... There may be a little difficulty at first in teaching the baby to nurse, but kindness and good sense will win" (MacMurchy 1923, 73).

"Mother's Helpers"

In her desire to promote breastfeeding, MacMurchy quite certainly minimized some of the difficulties that women would encounter. Although she placed ultimate responsibility for breastfeeding decisions on the mother, she also acknowledged the importance of other individuals, who were to support her: "The Mother is the leader, but the Father, the Doctor, the Nurse, the rest of the family and all of us Canadians must help the Mother make Maternal Nursing the Canadian Way" (MacMurchy 1923, 74). MacMurchy's comments regarding these figures in *The Canadian Mother's Book* reflected changes in childbirth and childrearing.

In the past, many mothers turned to their extended families or women in their communities for assistance with childbirth and for advice on childrearing. By the 1920s, urbanization, immigration, life in rural frontiers, and declining fertility meant that many women could no longer draw upon such an extensive network of female advice. As well, the heterosexual nuclear family was being increasingly promoted and viewed as the norm: "Homes are made by the father and mother" (MacMurchy 1923, 7). MacMurchy described fathers as providers, breadwinners, and moral supporters: "Canadian men make good husbands. You must listen to [your husband's advice] even more than usual, for he wants to take care of you, and you need good care now. He can help you" (MacMurchy 1928b, 23). Mothers were given responsibility for the well-being of their babies, the family, and the nation, and fathers were to support mothers in every way possible. They were given responsibility for bringing home a "family wage" and, with respect to childbirth, were to provide understanding and emotional support to their wives during the pre- and postnatal period.

Although motherhood was "natural" and "normal," MacMurchy was quick to advise consulting a physician should there be any problems: "If there is anything wrong with you at all ... ask the Doctor about it at once" (MacMurchy 1923, 11–12). Doctors, and the nurses under their supervision, could provide support with a range of pre- and postnatal concerns: "If there is anything the matter with you, do not say–'O, I suppose it cannot be helped.' It can be helped. Ask the Doctor" (1923, 10). In the unlikely event of any challenges with breastfeeding, doctors could provide practical and emotional support: "There is always something the Doctor can do to make you better. That is what a doctor is for" (11–12). Throughout the pages of *The Canadian Mother's Book*, there is a tension between women being encouraged to follow their instincts and being told to consult a doctor for any problems that might arise.

MacMurchy's advice to seek care from medical authorities reflected the increasing involvement of physicians in pregnancy, childbirth, and childrearing. Paediatrics, the medical specialty focusing on child health, was formalized in Canada in 1922 with the formation of the Canadian Paediatric Society (CPS) (initially called the Canadian Society for the Study of Diseases of Children). In 1923, the first communication by the CPS was a report to the Division of Child Welfare replying to a request to review two publications: *The Canadian Mother's Book* and *Nursing Procedures for Premature Babies* (McKendry and Bailey 1990).

Childbirth was also increasingly supervised by doctors and taking place in hospitals. Many doctors did not consider childbirth a subject worthy of their time and energies; however, other doctors were more "progressive" and argued that childbirth could not be left to "nature." Nurses–private, public health, missionary, and VON–delivered babies for the poor and in communities where there were no doctors. Midwives, who were unlicensed and often viewed negatively by medical and public health authorities, continued to be used, especially in rural and remote areas. However, in urban areas and in the larger provinces, medically supervised hospital births were becoming more common. By 1928, over half of births in British Columbia took place in a hospital (Prentice et al. 1988).

As a physician, MacMurchy promoted medical solutions to child and maternal welfare (Dodd 1991). Supported by the National Council of Women, MacMurchy approved of the move towards more interventionist approaches to childbirth (McLaren 1990). In 1923, MacMurchy produced a report on Canada's maternal mortality rate, which was 20 percent higher than Britain's and twice that of the Scandinavian countries. In the 1920s, twenty-four Canadian mothers died each week (McLaren 1981). This report prompted the Canadian Medical Association to call for an inquiry, the result of which was the report *Maternal Mortality in Canada*, which appeared in 1928. MacMurchy interpreted the data as suggesting that most maternal deaths occurred from a lack of medical care. She recommended increased prenatal care, medical involvement at birth, and improved socio-economic conditions (MacMurchy 1928a). In the following years, government and other child and maternal health agencies focused their energies on the medicalization of childbirth–increasing medical involvement through prenatal clinics, physician attendance at births, and postnatal care–rather than addressing the socio-economic realities of women's lives.

But, while medical involvement was proposed as the solution to infant and maternal welfare, private medical practitioners were creating an ambiguous role for themselves with respect to breastfeeding. MacMurchy cautioned women to distrust any physicians who might suggest alternatives to breastfeeding: "Since the first edition of the Canadian Mother's Book was published, we have received information that, in too many cases, Doctors and Nurses are responsible for the baby being taken from the Mother's breast and fed artificially" (MacMurchy and Department of Health 1923, 74). Many physicians were concerned about the misuse of infant formulas and believed that mothers should not be responsible for making up their own. At one point, the Canadian Public Health Association proposed that "so-called milk substitutes" be controlled by law, the rationale being that, if only physicians could prescribe breast milk alternatives, this would greatly decrease infant mortality (Comacchio 1993, 123). Their desire to have a monopoly on infant formulas and their lack of training in breastfeeding meant that, despite their stated commitment to broader public health goals, many physicians supported the use of breast milk alternatives.

Scientists and *The Normal Child*

In developing the Little Blue Books, MacMurchy drew upon numerous international sources as well as the most recent scientific theories on the care and feeding of children. Several key figures, primarily physicians, soon came to represent scientific authority on childbirth and childrearing in the English-speaking world. L. Emmett Holt in New York was influential in the training of paediatricians in both the United States and Canada. In 1911, F. Truby King became renowned for his role in ensuring that infant and maternal mortality rates in New Zealand were the lowest in the world. His efforts led to the formation of the Royal New Zealand Society for the Health of Women and Children. In 1917, he was invited to set up a centre in London. Soon, centres following his model were formed around the world, including in Canada. King's work focused on the feeding of infants and was widely consulted. For example, in British Columbia, public health nurses distributed publications describing his techniques and procedures for infant feeding (N.L. Lewis 1980).

Canada also had its own scientific authority on childrearing. Alan Brown, head of paediatrics at the University of Toronto, became an internationally known paediatrician. By 1920, Toronto's children's hospital, the centre of the department, was rapidly expanding under Brown's guidance.[3] The hospital was closely involved with all of the city's child welfare work. Toronto's twenty-five child welfare clinics taught medical students how to feed the "normal infant and child" (Brown 1920).

In 1923, Brown published a childrearing manual entitled *The Normal Child*, which *The Canadian Churchman* said was the only Canadian book of its kind containing "just what every mother should know, from the birth of the child–the care and feeding during infancy, etc. and a thousand and one other suggestions" (N.L. Lewis 1980, 63). Brown's book was representative of current scientific advice to mothers, who were told how to establish discipline and routine (prized attributes in an industrial society) through insisting that their children be subject to regimented patterns of sleep, exercise, elimination, and feeding. Although mothers were told to love their children, hugging, kissing, and other signs of affection were thought to spoil them. Inappropriate maternal and infant behaviours were believed to be the cause of problems later in life. The conditioning of children through rigorous scheduling was a North America–wide movement. McGill and Toronto both developed child study centres to investigate the personality of "normal children."

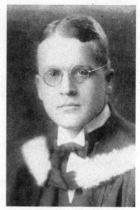

4.2 Graduation photograph of Alan Brown, 1909. Image courtesy of Hospital Archives, The Hospital for Sick Children, Toronto

With respect to infant feeding, breastfeeding was the method of choice for the normal child. Brown was an avid supporter of breastfeeding and believed that the majority of women were capable of it. In *The Normal Child*, he states, "There is no real substitute for mother's milk" (Brown 1923, 106). Although he said that "wet-nursing should be used only as a last resort when a child is extremely ill and all other means have failed" (Brown 1923, 96), he emphasized the value of breast milk to infant health. He believed that women needed to be educated regarding the importance of breastfeeding and that good maternal health was essential: "In fact, with women properly educated and in good physical condition, fully 75 per cent can nurse their infants. One well known authority states that '100 per cent of women, even the flower and fashion of the land, can nurse their children.' Women are better able to breastfeed because they are healthier these days–more exercise and time spent outdoors" (Brown 1923, 73).

Scales and Timetables: Scientific Breastfeeding

Brown applied modern scientific principles to breastfeeding and, like others, emphasized sterility, regulation, and measurement. As with bottle-feeding, sterility was an absolute requirement and mothers needed to cleanse their nipples before and after breastfeeding: "Before and after each nursing, the nipples and adjoining portion of the breast should be cleaned with a solution of boracic acid ... If the nipples are at all sore or tender, the washing should be followed with a sponging with alcohol, and then a little zinc oxide or albolene should be applied" (Brown 1923, 76). MacMurchy, in *The Canadian Mother's Book*, also recommended the cleansing of a mother's nipples with soap, boiled water, and absorbent cotton: "With a tiny soft sponge or some absorbent cotton, having first washed your hands, sponge off the nipples carefully, using cool or tepid water and white Castile or other good soap. Use a soft towel or handkerchief for drying and then rub in a little cold cream or lanoline, or Vaseline, and gently 'draw out' the nipples with the tips of your fingers until the nipple comes out tiny, soft, and round to fit the baby's little mouth by and by" (MacMurchy and Department of Health 1923, 31).

Brown was also an advocate of the new style of parenting, which emphasized regularity and regimentation. He once commented that a child could be trained to be like a "little machine." Fixed times for all activities, including feeding, were vital to ensuring good health. Brown (1923, 78) suggested feeding newborns every four hours: "The baby requires no other food on the first day, except a little warm water with milk sugar, one ounce to twenty ounces of water. Of this he may have from a half-ounce to one ounce between nursings. Six hours after birth the infant should be put to the breast, and then every four hours thereafter." Night feedings were discouraged. *The Canadian Mother's Book* promoted breastfeeding every three hours at 6 a.m., 9 a.m., noon, 3 p.m., 6 p.m., and 10 p.m. Another source commented on night feedings: "From the first, no night feeding should be given—that is from 10 p.m. to 6 a.m. The night was meant for sleeping and baby will soon settle down if he is shown it is expected of him" (Grier 1929, 54).

Strict scheduling was believed to establish proper lactation and to prevent overfeeding: "Always keep strictly to feed times as the regular emptying and stimulating of the breast is essential for the proper establishment of lactation" (Grier 1929, 54). Breasts needed to be emptied at each feeding. The intervals between feeding were important: "By this long interval the breasts are accustomed to become full, and in this way it produces better action and a greater supply of milk" (Brown 1923, 78). Babies were not to be fed early or in between feedings. It was important to distinguish between hunger and thirst, with boiled water being permitted in between feedings. However, straying from the schedule or failing to wake an infant from sleep was thought to lead to overfeeding, which, in turn, was responsible for digestive troubles, especially colic.

Most scientific authorities suggested breastfeeding for no longer than nine months. Brown (1923, 83), too, thought it wise to introduce the infant to the bottle at an early age: "It is always advisable to begin giving a baby one bottle in the twenty-four hours after he is two weeks of age ... There are numerous reasons for this regimen, chief of which are that the mother may be suddenly taken ill or unavoidably absent, or her milk may be temporarily unfit for the baby's use as a result of violent emotion, menstruation, etc. ... Furthermore, it makes weaning much more simple and efficient."

Regularly weighing the infant was an important way of establishing the success of both breastfeeding and bottle-feeding. L. Emmett Holt was one of the first to alert physicians to the importance of infant weight gain. One of the first sets of guidelines on the growth of normal babies was based on one thousand infants during the first four years of life. Weight charts soon became important in treating infant diarrhea. By plotting infant weight gain against standard weight charts, physicians could monitor the progress of illness and treatment. Soon, weighing infants became an established practice in hospitals, clinics, and doctor's offices, and specific forms for recording and comparing infants to standards were developed (Brosco 2002). Holt suggested weighing infants once a week. As for MacMurchy, she advised as follows: "During the first month it is a good plan for the nurse to weigh the baby every day or every other day, perhaps both before and after a nursing at the same hour daily and in the same clothing, so that we know: (1) How much Mother's milk the baby got at that nursing (2) How much he has gained or lost since yesterday" (MacMurchy and Department of Health 1923, 102). As for the importance of monitoring weight: "the loss of a pound in a baby often means as much as if an adult lost fifteen pounds" (MacMurchy and Department of Health 1923, 101). A standard weight chart could be found at the back of *The Canadian Mother's Book.*

Brown (1923, 60) advocated weekly weighings "to make sure growth is going on properly." However, he was more interested in overall trends than he was in how closely infants matched standard tables and charts. He commented that "elaborate algebraic formula" for developing weight charts were still just estimates: "The truth of the matter is that the variation is too considerable to allow of any iron-bound statements regarding it" (Brown 1923, 58). He does mention that bottle-fed babies generally appear to be "less advanced" than do "normal breast-fed babies."

The Sunshine Vitamin

In addition to applying its principles to childrearing, science was also beginning to shed new light on nutrition and health. Beginning in the 1920s, information about vitamins became widespread, and a form of "vitamin-mania" gripped Canadian society. The Canadian government seized nutritional science as a way of addressing endemic nutritional deficiencies such as rickets and scurvy. Knowledge about vitamins, especially vitamin D, was quickly reflected in infant feeding advice and practices.

For the most part, the advice contained in Brown's childrearing manual and in *The Canadian Mother's Book* included the same basic information distributed to mothers in the early social reform period: fresh air, sunshine, rest, cleanliness, good ventilation, and good nutrition. While earlier advice reflected a commonsense approach to nutrition, advice in the 1920s and 1930s began to reflect scientific understandings of vitamins and the caloric content of foods (Dodd 1991). In terms of infant feeding, this was particularly reflected in the advice surrounding vitamin D. In the early 1920s, when *The Canadian Mother's Book* was being developed, the role of vitamins was not fully understood. Early guidelines advised mothers to supplement breast milk with fruit juice–either strained orange, apple, or prune juice–at one month for "health reasons" and to prevent constipation. Rickets and scurvy were two of the diseases associated with childhood that caused health authorities the most concern. Although vitamins were known to be important, their role in the etiology of rickets and scurvy was unclear.

By the late 1920s, it was known that rickets was a "disease of Nutrition caused by lack of Sun and lack of Suitable Food. Rickets may be easily prevented by Sun, Suitable Food and Cod Liver Oil" (MacMurchy and Division of Child Welfare 1929). In the past, cod-liver oil had frequently been given to children to prevent and cure rickets. Initially, scientists were uncertain whether it was something in fish oil generally or cod-liver oil specifically that was responsible for its effect (Goldbloom 1945). Soon, the relationship between cod-liver oil, sunlight, and irradiated substances was more clearly elucidated. "Factor X" was insufficient in cow's milk, so cod-liver oil was a recommended addition to "the diet of all artificially fed and many breast fed infants after the second winter month" (Struthers 1925, 1276).

In 1928, *The Canadian Mother's Book* encouraged all mothers to provide their children with the "sunlight vitamin" through daily doses of cod-liver oil, beginning at two weeks. As scientists had demonstrated a lack of vitamin D in ordinary foods, it was believed that this vitamin must be obtained from sunshine. One study demonstrated that winter sunshine in Toronto was only one-eighth as potent as was summer sunshine; hence, it was thought that the average Canadian received little sunshine for eight months of the year. The *Canadian Mother's Book* suggested that cod-liver oil could be eliminated in the summer, and MacMurchy included a new section on sunbathing: "It is only lately that we have realized that a great part of the sun's influence is in unseen rays" (MacMurchy and Department of Health 1928, 112). She recommended sunbathing for all babies, beginning in the second or third week–indoors during the winter and outdoors during the summer.

In 1929, MacMurchy came out with a special publication entitled *Rickets: Prevention and Cure,* in which she proclaimed that "The Canadian Baby Often Suffers from Rickets" (MacMurchy and Division of Child Welfare 1929). She warned mothers and fathers that rickets was a disease that babies who did not receive sunshine, cod-liver oil, and suitable food were likely to acquire. Rickets "generally means late teething, late standing, late walking, weak bones, bow legs, perhaps a crooked spine or deformed bones" (MacMurchy and Division of Child Welfare 1929, 4). It may not be noticed in childhood, but it could result in harm or even death later in life. The pamphlet stresses the importance of daily sunbathing, and it opens with a picture of a smiling Peace River, Alberta, baby bundled in warm clothing and sitting on a cushion on her snowy doorstep. Suitable food, according to MacMurchy, included maternal nursing, orange or tomato juice, and cod-liver oil: "You may think your Baby is well and strong but unless the Mother eats the right food before and after the Baby is born, and keeps well and strong herself and nurses the Baby at her breast for about nine months and feeds the Baby properly on the right foods, and puts him in the Sun and gives him Cod Liver Oil from two weeks to two years of age, there is danger that your child may have Rickets, and you may not know it. Keep the Canadian Baby Well" (MacMurchy and Division of Child Welfare 1929, 18).

Vitamins aside, mothers had an important role in ensuring the health of their children through good nutrition. Nutrition knowledge soon became a part of scientific childrearing. A study at the Nutritional Clinic at Toronto's Hospital for Sick Children found that 50 percent of malnutrition cases could be attributed to mismanagement and lack of discipline in the home. In particular, "the first evidence of lack of home control is the fact that the child nurses 15 to 18 months. When the parent fails to control a child of that age, what success need one expect in dealing with this same child at 10 years of age?" (Macdougall 1923, 30). The author attributed only 44 of the 370 (12 percent) cases of malnutrition to "improper diet and faulty food habits." In a sense, this report was an indication that breastfeeding was becoming a concern for nutritional science as well as for child welfare.

The New Motherhood: Professionalism, Regulation, and Efficiency

In the post–First World War era, societal beliefs and expectations regarding mothering began to change as tensions between coexisting notions on this subject emerged. Mothering was simultaneously viewed as modern and traditional, professional and instinctive, and scientific and natural. Breastfeeding, a visible and integral part of mothering, was caught between these tensions.

Although women were beginning to seek higher levels of education and were an increasing presence in the workforce, the ideal image of women in films, radio, and magazines continued to be that of the mother. Many middle-class women were urged to obtain a university education. In 1919–20, 13.9 percent of university undergraduates were women; by 1929–30, this number had increased to 23.5 percent. And the number of women and girls over the age of ten represented in the total labour force also increased, from 15.5 percent in 1921 to 17.0 percent in 1931. Women were employed in personal service, clerical, professional, and manufacturing occupations. However, while women were encouraged to achieve a higher education or to find a successful and interesting career, this was understood to be only a temporary phase before they turned their full attention to marriage, housework, and motherhood. Women's employment was not meant to compete with men's, and statistics reveal that 90 percent of women in the formal workforce were single. Middle-class women, especially, were encouraged to seek clean, light jobs that would provide them with skills and knowledge that would make them more capable and self-confident wives and mothers (Vipond 1977).

While the traditional view of women as "primarily mothers of men" (Vipond 1977, 124) remained strong during this period, a new view of mothering also emerged. The growth of science in industry, business, and government was contributing to new notions of "modern mothers." Many women and men, in their efforts to glorify motherhood, argued that mothers were also professionals and that the home could be viewed as a business. Mothers were encouraged to apply scientific management principles to the household. The modern mother was scientific and efficient; she was a household manager and a domestic supervisor. Order, cleanliness, and scheduling would save women time and energy, and they were encouraged to make use of the latest products and equipment to manage their households.

In a political setting, mothers were given enormous responsibility. In an attempt to glorify and professionalize motherhood, MacMurchy emphasized that mothers were responsible for their infants, their family, and their nation. By choosing to breastfeed, mothers could play a vital role in reducing infant mortality and securing the welfare of the nation through providing a stable family life. In her own way, MacMurchy was trying to elevate the status of motherhood in society. On the one hand, MacMurchy's policies could be viewed as empowering; on the other hand, they could be viewed as oppressive. The imperative to breastfeed was all-encompassing: women had a duty to breastfeed and to put aside their own selfish goals and concerns. It was considered an honour and a privilege to support the nation. Breastfeeding became both a patriotic act and a moral act. Mothers were induced to breastfeed for the well-being of the nation, and mothers who did not breastfeed were perceived as killing their infants and placing the country in peril. Breastfeeding became intertwined with good citizenship and good motherhood.

With this switch to new cultural authorities, instinct, intuition, and informal advice were replaced by professional and scientific theories. Rather than paying attention to when the baby seemed hungry or to their own biological cues, women turned to the clock and scales. Rather than trusting their own instincts, women appealed to physicians. And, while it can be argued that women gained much from science, when it came to infant feeding, science undermined their sense of competence. Women benefited from professional scientific advice in many ways, but this meant that they had to relinquish their authority as experts (Apple 1995, 1987; Wolf 2001; Apple 2006).

Unfortunately, the application of scientific principles to infant feeding was disastrous for breastfeeding (Wolf 2001; Hausman 2003; Millard 1990). Clocks and timetables, which were valuable in the worlds of work and school (Strong-Boag 1982), did not work well when applied to breastfeeding. Small and frequent feedings were replaced with scheduled and infrequent feedings, and this inhibited a woman's ability to establish and maintain a supply of breast milk. Nor did breastfeeding fit with scientific ideals such as precision, regularity, and standardization. An obsession with sterility and cleanliness, of utmost importance when bottle-feeding, complicated and created unnecessary obstacles when breastfeeding. The application of scientific principles was intended to save women time so that they could be with their husbands and children; breastfeeding, however, required them to spend more time with their infants. In this scientific era, breastfeeding became modelled on bottle-feeding, and it was the latter that became associated with modern mothering practices.

Advice and Realities

In the view of the federal government, mothers were active, responsible, and rational citizens. With proper education on the scientific evidence supporting breastfeeding, mothers would be able to make choices to support their own best interests and the interests of the nation. However, the advice in the Little Blue Books often failed to match the realities of women's lives. Depending on their class and ethnic background, women often found much of the proffered advice irrelevant, inappropriate, or unrealistic.

The standards advocated for women in *The Canadian Mother's Book* likely made more sense to middle- and upper-class women than they did to lower-class women. MacMurchy described ideal conditions for raising children without paying sufficient attention to economic realities. The fact was, most women did not have enough money to pay private physician fees, did not have the facilities to meet the exacting standards of cleanliness, did not have the time to take prescribed rest periods, and did not have the economic resources to obtain most of the items listed as essential to caring for a newborn. As well, while most childrearing manuals argued that their approaches would, in the long run, save women time, they paid no attention to the great amount of time women would have to spend gathering, reading, and applying this new scientific knowledge.

MacMurchy was not totally unaware of issues for non-privileged, non-urban women. Some Little Blue Books focused on how women could keep a home in a frontier setting (e.g., *How to Make Our Outpost Home in Canada*). However, MacMurchy clearly supported maternity as a primary role for mothers and promoted the relatively new concept of the division of labour between the female homemaker and the male breadwinner. MacMurchy assumed that fathers were present and involved in childbirth and childrearing. The primary role for fathers was to provide practical support to mothers and to have a decent enough job to pay for a doctor. In 1929, 60 percent of Canadian working men and 82 percent of Canadian working women earned less than the minimum necessary to support a family of four (Prentice et al. 1988). The concept of a society based on the heterosexual nuclear family and a family wage was beginning to become a reality for some families but was not a possibility for most.

Rather than focus on culture, geography, and poverty as major influences on infant mortality rates and breastfeeding practices, MacMurchy focused much of the Division's energies on professionalizing child and maternal care. Although motherhood was natural, women still required detailed advice from experts. MacMurchy advised consulting with private physicians and ignoring traditional sources of information. More and more, the medical profession became central to dispensing advice on the care and feeding of children.

There is no doubt that science and medicine had much to offer women (Strong-Boag 1982). Rickets is one example where a scientific solution resolved an old problem. *The Canadian Mother's Book* and other sources of childrearing advice were in huge demand as women required scientific advice in order to fulfill their new roles as professional mothers. As well, the declining fertility rate meant that families were smaller, with the result that women were less able to turn to family and friends for practical support. Between 1921 and 1931, the annual number of births per 1,000 women aged 15 to 19 dropped from 128.1 to 99.5. Moreover, the number of practising midwives continued to decline as they were replaced with physicians and nurses. Women living in frontier areas of the country were often isolated from other women and had limited or no access to health services (Langford 2000).

One of the consequences of placing the health of the family and nation in the hands of mothers was that mothers ended up having a lot of responsibility and very limited support. Mothers had "helpers" in the form of fathers, nurses, and doctors, but they had little in the way of material assistance or consistency of advice. A 1932 letter written by a distraught mother conveys the magnitude of a mother's responsibilities:

> As stated in the Canadian Mother Book: If the baby has three or four stools per day, do not hesitate and call the doctor. This is what I did as soon as I was aware of this fact. Why did my physician assert that this was not serious? and in whom can one place her confidence? Noticing no improvement, I called a second physician who immediately told me a baby suffering from diarrhea should be placed on a diet. This was done, but it was too late. If great are the responsibilities of the mothers (I nursed my child) those of the doctor are of the same degree, although some of them seem to ignore this fact. (Mrs. R. Payne to the National Council of Family and Child Welfare, 21 August 1931, quoted in Buckley 1979)

Any errors or omissions left many mothers feeling guilty and helpless in the face of their perceived responsibilities.

While national survey data on actual infant feeding practices are unavailable, in reality, women appeared to be using a variety of practices depending on their life circumstances and, often, the particular child involved. Florentine Maher, a mother from Montreal, commented in 1926

after the birth of her daughter, "I fed Andrée for eight months, a record!...
This was the first baby that I succeeded in breastfeeding. I tried for the others
but was not successful. This was not a problem. Those mothers who were
able breastfed and the others managed very well with cow's milk" (quoted
in Light and Pierson 1990, 183). Leila Middleton described her decisions
regarding her "succession of daughters." Phyllis Evelyn, born in October 1924
was breastfed for the first two months following her birth and then started
Mellin's Food. Mellin's Food was made up of a malted cereal ingredient and
an alkali which was then mixed with cow's milk. Ruth Eleanor was born in
October 1925: "Used Mellin's food at first and baby is real good." June Patricia
was born in June 1927, and she was followed by Lois Marie in March 1928.
Lois Marie also was fed on Mellin's Food and "she continued to gain and do
well" (quoted in Light and Pierson 1990, 178–79). Ellenor Merriken, living in
a rural community in Alberta in the 1920s, commented on the convenience of
breastfeeding following the birth of her first son:

> He was a fine baby and we took him with us wherever we went.... At six
> months of age, he went with us to the Battle River Stampede and camped
> out for several days. We had no formula to bother with and no bottles to
> sterilize, which eliminated a lot of work and worry and he really thrived
> on mother's milk.... (quoted in Light and Pierson 1990, 197)

Conclusion

The formation of the Division of Child Welfare and the subsequent funding,
support, interest, and activities of the Department of Health represented
the first set of national policies on mothering. The core of these activities
focused on "mothercraft" or teaching women the requisite skills for mothering. Women needed to be educated in scientific and modern methods of
childrearing in order to further national goals. As with the earlier campaign
against infant mortality, breastfeeding was central to these mothering policies, and it took on new political and moral significance. Science was the
new authority on childrearing, and scientific principles applied to infant
feeding blurred the boundaries between breastfeeding and bottle-feeding
practices, putting the emphasis on cleanliness, schedules, and weight gain.
Patterns of breastfeeding were increasingly prescribed by science and the
state. While these new cultural authorities strongly supported breastfeeding,
broader social change and mixed messages from professionals contributed
to a substantially altered culture of breastfeeding. Women's actual practices
and decisions were caught between these political and scientific tensions and
the realities of their daily lives.

Chapter 5

Marketing Infant Feeding, 1930–40

In the 1930s, paediatric services provided by the state, particularly well baby clinics, continued to grow and expand. But these did not spread evenly or have an equal impact on women and children. In some cases, women had to be convinced to adopt new infant care practices. Women were also increasingly exposed to a burgeoning commercial infant feeding culture, of which science and medicine were an intimate part. This is exemplified by the Dionne quintuplets–the face of Carnation Milk. The mid-1930s also represent a turning point in the conceptualization of breastfeeding: breast milk and breastfeeding were two concepts that had been silently diverging. With the advent of the first milk banks, the decline of the need for wet nurses, and the increasing safety of milk formulas made from canned evaporated milk, new images of breastfeeding began to dominate. Women increasingly chose to bottle-feed, influenced in part both by changing ideas about their role in society and by formula advertising. An emphasis on weight gain and ambiguous messages about the value of breastfeeding led to the complicity of scientific experts and professionals in the promotion of bottle-feeding.

The Well Baby Clinic

The 1920s marked a period where the federal government became increasingly involved in matters of infant feeding, particularly through the production and dissemination of advice literature for mothers. In parallel, governments at the local and provincial levels reinforced new scientific infant feeding norms through the provision of services such as child welfare clinics and home visits for mothers. In the 1930s, the distribution of federal child welfare publications proliferated, and the medical supervision of mothers and babies through both public and private services became increasingly routine. Medical services, such as the well baby clinic, checkups in paediatric offices, child development tests, and preventive care, were celebrated in magazines, on the radio, and in government publications. However, services were not equally available to all women across the country, and their reasons for using these services varied enormously. The expansion and popularity of medical services had a dubious effect on breastfeeding practices.

The Canadian Mother's Book remained enormously popular throughout the 1930s, even though the Division of Child Welfare closed down between 1933 and 1937. Helen MacMurchy, in a 1933 radio address, spoke to mothers as follows:

> If any of you has a copy of The Canadian Mother's Book that that you are not using, will you please mail it back tonight, or tomorrow at the latest, to the Division of Child Welfare, Elgin Building, Ottawa ... We have a great many requests every day from mothers for The Canadian Mother's Book—more than we can answer—and if you are not using your copy, perhaps you would mail it back to us and we will send it to some mother who needs it. (Lewis and Watson 1991/92, 13)

In 1934, the Canadian Council on Child and Family Welfare took over the division's work and, among other activities, printed a revised edition of MacMurchy's *The Canadian Mother's Book.* The book continued to be distributed for free and was translated into many languages other than French and English, including Cree, Ukrainian, Japanese, and Chinese (Lewis and Watson 1991/92). By the end of the 1930s, federal child welfare publications were primarily distributed through provincial and local departments of health and other health agencies. Most of these organizations were based in urban areas, and they accounted for 90 percent of the total consumption of these publications. Some of these publications did reach rural areas, as they were often distributed from urban centres by nurses and doctors (Comacchio 1993).

The relative lack of availability of federal government advice literature for mothers in rural areas mirrored the relative lack of availability of medical services in these areas. By the mid-1930s, 28 percent of Canadians were living in the twenty cities that had a population of 30,000 or more. These urban dwellers were served by 45 percent of the nation's physicians, 48 percent of its nurses, and 49 percent of its dentists (Abeele 1988). In Ontario, in 1936, only ten municipalities had a full-time medical officer of health. Out of a population of 3.6 million, only one-third lived in places where public health services were available (Abeele 1988). In rural areas, public health nurses were often the only medical professionals available to provide support and education for mothers. While mothers had unequal access to public health services, depending on their geographical location, services were found in some surprising contexts. A 1936 issue of *Canadian Child and Welfare News* reports on a Sikh well baby clinic at a lumber camp near Lake Cowichan on Vancouver Island. This report provides an interesting commentary on the primacy of infant feeding advice in clinics provided by the state. At this clinic, babies were weighed and the nurse provided instructions on "proper diet," using pictures cut out of magazines. The mother was "told when and what to feed her baby and [was] given a book on infant feeding. Though the majority of mothers know only a few words of English, the fathers can generally speak and read it with ease" (Anonymous 1936, 18). This shows an early focus on the infant feeding practices of various immigrant groups and the gradual displacement of traditional child-care practices by modern, "Canadian," scientific practices.

Mothers were attracted to public health and medical services for a variety of reasons. In some contexts, public health officials found themselves in the position of having to convince mothers to come to various clinics and accept the advice provided. In an exploration of the lives of mothers who attended the Montreal *gouttes de lait* between 1910 and 1965, Baillargeon (1996) documents a shift in the 1930s, with mothers of all classes abandoning traditional childrearing practices and adopting medical advice. When the *gouttes de lait* began in 1910, poorer mothers were the most motivated to attend the clinics as they were able to receive material aid there. The clinics, in an effort to encourage mothers to attend, also held baby contests, and mothers were drawn to the valuable prizes they could win. Efforts by the *gouttes de lait* staff to promote breastfeeding were met with disinterest when placed beside the promise of material aid in the form of cow's milk or a free doctor's exam for a sick infant.

The number of *gouttes de lait* in Montreal grew from three in 1910 to sixty-eight at the beginning of the 1930s. With the wider availability of services targeted at all mothers, by 1930 one-third of infants born in Montreal were being seen in the *gouttes de lait*. Women in the upper classes were rarely seen in the *gouttes de lait*, as they continued to see physicians in private practice. As well, many women in the upper classes had already fully embraced scientific motherhood, including the abandonment of breastfeeding. For other women, the *gouttes de lait* provided a service they would not otherwise have had. For many, the clinics were a place for social encounters and a place to show off their maternal successes. One woman described how all the mothers took extreme care to present their infants at their best. Conversely, the clinics could be a somewhat hostile environment for mothers who were unable to keep up with the comparisons that formed part of a subtle maternal competition. While medical concerns were not a priority for many of the women who attended these clinics, it is clear that poverty and large families functioned as barriers to many women who would have benefited from the medical services provided there.

Bigger Babies Are Better Babies

In a survey of thirty-one women attending the Montreal *gouttes de lait*, the majority reported that they visited the clinics primarily to get their baby weighed. The idea of weight gain as the best indicator of infant health had thoroughly infused public awareness by the 1930s. While regular weighings had always been an important part of paediatric practice, the idea that a fat baby equals a healthy baby became a popular ideal. Weighing the baby became the key event in all well baby clinic encounters, while baby shows and other child welfare events gave out prizes for "ideal weight." Charts describing typical weight gain were widely available in publications for mothers, and mothers could weigh their infants in the baby departments of pharmacies and department stores (N.L. Lewis 1982–83). The pressure for weight gain was soon recognized by public health officials as contributing to more mothers' turning away from breastfeeding.

The paediatric interest in weight gain can be traced back to the late 1880s. Holt is quoted as commenting, "Of what importance is the weight of the child? Nothing else tells us so accurately how well it is thriving" (Holt 1907, "Weight, Growth and Development"). Initially, infants treated for gastroenteritis or diarrhea were monitored by plotting their weight against a standard weight chart to see if the treatment was effective and/or to track the progress of the disease. Weight gain soon became a measure of infant health. As time went on, paediatricians continued to monitor physical growth with more complex weight-height-age charts that were more sensitive to different skeletal types. If infants failed to gain the appropriate amount of weight as indicated by the chart, then they were considered "malnourished" even if they appeared to be perfectly healthy. Deviations from weight gain symbolized "failure to thrive." Often, it was mothers who were blamed for these failures.

By the 1930s, maternal competitiveness had led to a "pounds race." Breast milk alternatives soon became associated with faster weight gain. Images of round babies rapidly gaining weight on products such as Eagle Brand Evaporated Milk permeated the media. Cow's-milk formulas, with their higher caloric content, were seen to result in faster weight gain. Chandler (1929), the director of the Montreal Child Welfare Association, commented on the pounds race in the context of breastfeeding promotion: "The very emphasis we have put on the baby-scale is working to our disadvantage, as the mother knows that her baby should be gaining regularly. She is upset if the neighbor's baby on a bottle's gain is more regular and with far less trouble to her and more sleep to the father" (Chandler 1929, 664). The public association between bottle-feeding and weight gain is interesting in light of research documenting lower weight gain, differential patterns of mental development, and higher susceptibility to illness in bottle-fed babies. In the May 1929 issue of *Child Welfare News*, put out by the Canadian Council on Child Welfare, there is a report of a five-year American study on children between the ages

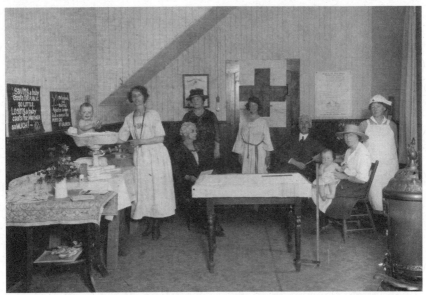

Figure 5.1   Kamloops Well Baby Clinic, sponsored by Red Cross members, was officially opened May 10, 1922. The Clinic was held in Red Cross rooms with Miss Christine Thom, R.N., in attendance and Dr. M.G. Archibald physician-in-charge. At the time of the opening Mrs. D.W. Rowlands was president, Mrs. F.J. Fulton, convener. This photo was taken 25 April 1923, and shows (from left) Mrs. L. Sadlier-Brown, Mrs. D.B. Johnstone (President), Mrs. R.H. Lee, Mrs. R.L. Johnstone, Dr. Archibald, Mrs. D.G. Miller, and Miss Thom. Photograph courtesy of Kamloops Museum & Archives.

of seven and thirteen. The study found that twice as many bottle-fed babies as breastfed babies between four and nine months old were more than 10 percent underweight (Canadian Council on Child Welfare 1929).

Chandler (1929, 669) was aware of the impact of images of mothers successfully bottle-feeding thriving infants on mothers struggling to breastfeed, and he attempted to create separate clinics for mothers who were breastfeeding and bottle-feeding:

> No doubt the mingling of the mothers at the health centre and the apparently excellent results achieved with the bottle-fed baby have an important bearing in discouraging the mother who is having a hard time to feed her baby naturally. To obviate this we established two years ago a separate clinic just for breast-fed babies. It was carefully explained to the mothers that they were on the honor roll as long as they nursed their babies, and would have to go to the general clinic when weaning was necessary. The results from this type of clinic are not at all convincing that the extra expense was justified.

Undoubtedly, many mothers were unable to resist the temptation to switch to bottle-feeding or began to supplement their own milk supply with formula in order to ensure adequate weight gain and, thus, the health of their infants. Alan Brown (1938, 340) commented in a 1938 issue of the *Canadian Public Health Journal* on appropriate situations for the use of formula supplements: "If the baby is not getting enough milk, a fact which would be indicated by stationary weight or slow gain, by waking before the proper feeding time, etc., then the baby should be allowed to nurse for ten minutes from each breast, at each feeding every three hours. If the baby at the end of a few days is still not receiving sufficient food, the required amount should be completed after nursing by a modified milk feeding as prescribed." Concerns about "failure to thrive" resulting from poor weight gain and faulty breastfeeding advice led to more mothers' and paediatricians' choosing to supplement or use formula exclusively.

Placing the Blame: "Fictitious Difficulties" and a Lack of Proper Teaching

By the beginning of the 1930s, many professionals were despairing at their inability to revive and maintain breastfeeding rates and were beginning to reflect on some of the potential reasons for this. For the most part, it was still thought that mothers did not place enough importance on the value of breastfeeding. But, others, especially Chandler and Brown, also commented on changes in the socio-cultural environment and the unintentional effects of the rise in the stature of paediatrics: "Is there any connection with the rise in popularity of pediatrics as a specialty ... and an apparent decline in nursing?" (Chandler 1929, 663).

Many commentators were surprised at the continuing decline in breastfeeding, given the strong rhetoric that supported it. Scientific research was continuing to highlight the benefits of breastfeeding and to document different strategies for managing breastfeeding difficulties and re-establishing a failing milk supply. Brown noted the low rates of gastrointestinal disease in breastfed babies. Of 1,500 infants under one year of age admitted to the Hospital for Sick Children with infections, only 15 percent were breastfed (Brown 1940). According to Brown (1933, 265):

> Most babies are weaned in the first few weeks of life. In some cases, it seems, natural feeding is not attempted. Mothers who succeed in nursing very commonly require help in the nourishment of their infants, and there is recurring familiar difficulty in prolonging function to its term. Every country records a similar experience. Even in child-welfare centres, where breast feeding forms the first article of a universal creed, the percentage of breast-fed babies rarely reaches 100.

Brown suggested that many of the difficulties that women experienced were "fictitious." He also recognized that the majority of mothers who were struggling to breastfeed were not the "poorest mothers," and he questioned whether "there may have been something of a moral change, wide-set in the community, that injures breast feeding nearer its source" (Brown 1933, 266–67).

Chandler, in his report on declining breastfeeding rates in Montreal's health centres, attributed these discouraging findings to a variety of factors, including cultural change (Canadian Council on Child Welfare 1930). He commented on the changing role of mothers, who were seen to be working from an early age and becoming increasingly involved in recreational activities outside the home: "the girl is a pal before marriage and she is carefully taught she must remain so afterwards if she is to retain her husband" (Canadian Council on Child Welfare 1930, 30). He also described the influence of modern urban living: boarding homes and one-room apartments were crowded and detrimental to successful breastfeeding.

And, although difficult to acknowledge, Chandler suggested that scientific medicine, in particular paediatrics, might have to accept part of the blame for declining breastfeeding rates. Nutritional research had led to the universal advice to administer cod-liver oil and orange juice in order to prevent scurvy and rickets in infants: "We can no longer claim that the bottle-fed child is almost sure to develop rickets–in fact, we know that cod liver oil will protect him, even in this climate, from any but the mildest manifestations" (Chandler 1929, 664).

Chandler also placed part of the blame for mothers' unsuccessful attempts to breastfeed on maternity hospitals and private physicians. He believed that many physicians lacked proper instruction on breastfeeding techniques and too quickly moved towards bottle-feeding when difficulties arose. Paediatricians, for their part, had based their specialty on the development of breast milk alternatives:

> When the obstetrician hands the baby over to the podiatrist does he not imply that he is not familiar with modern methods of artificial feeding rather than not being conversant with breast feeding? ... Is not the keen competition in pediatrics having a tendency to make us show our skill in artificial feeding rather than keeping the baby on the breast which is less spectacular and much more difficult? Both the medical student and the graduate interested in children devotes almost his whole time to the artificial feeding of children and little or none to the difficulties of breast feeding. (Chandler 1929, 663)

Chandler called for medical students and paediatricians to be better trained in breastfeeding techniques and to put slightly less emphasis on bottle-feeding. In other words, he recognized a discrepancy between expert advice to mothers (which advocated for breastfeeding) and a lack of practical support on the part of health care professionals. Albeit indirectly, paediatrics and scientific medicine were part of the changes in the socio-cultural environment that were contributing to the decline in breastfeeding.

Scientific Infant Food: Alternatives and Complements

If, in developing safe alternatives to breast milk, paediatrics had unintentionally promoted bottle-feeding, the involvement of paediatricians in the development of commercially produced "scientific" and "nutritional" infant food products made the boundary between the promotion of breastfeeding and the promotion of breast milk alternatives even more blurry. Beginning in the 1930s, Canadian paediatricians followed the international trend of blending nutritional research and commercial enterprise.

In 1910, the first instance of an infant food product being developed by a paediatric researcher and being produced commercially by a private company occurred. The American physician J.S. Leopold returned to New York City following his studies abroad to find that the two sugars commonly used in breast milk alternatives to improve tolerance and digestibility in Germany, dextrin and maltose, were unavailable in the United States. He managed to convince the Mead-Johnson Company to manufacture and distribute the product "Dextri-Maltose" and to have it evaluated at the Babies' Ward of the New York Postgraduate Hospital (Greer 1991).

In the 1930s, researchers at the Hospital for Sick Children ("Sick Kids") in Toronto followed this model. In 1929, Alan Brown appointed Frederick Tisdall and Theodore Drake to direct and expand the hospital's nutritional research laboratories and to develop products to improve children's diets. By early 1930, Tisdall, Drake, and Brown announced their first major product. Sunwheat Biscuits contained whole wheat, wheat germ, milk, butter, yeast, bone meal, iron, and copper and included vitamins A, B_1, B_2, D, and E. Sunwheat Biscuits were marketed by McCormick's Food Company, and all royalties were returned to the Toronto Pediatric Foundation for further research at the Hospital for Sick Children.

Six months later, Tisdall, Drake, and Brown announced the development of the first precooked cereals for infants. In the 1932 edition of *Common Procedures in the Practice of Paediatrics*, Brown and Tisdall described the composition of "Mead's Cereal": wheat meal (53 percent), oatmeal (18 percent), cornmeal (10 percent), wheat germ (15 percent), bone meal (2 percent), dried Brewer's yeast (1 percent), and alfalfa (1 percent). These were all ground, mixed, dried, and precooked to create an infant food high in vitamins A, B, and E, with low fat, protein, and mineral content (Brown and Tisdall 1932). This new cereal product was sold by the Mead Johnson Company in the United States and soon became known as the popular cereal Pablum.[1] The 1939 edition of *Common Procedures in the Practice of Paediatrics* states that Pablum should be introduced into an infant's diet at around three months because nutrition research was showing that infant iron reserves were being used up earlier than had previously been believed: "Pablum should be added to the infant's diet at about three months of age, particularly on account of its iron content. It is perfectly safe to do this, as no untoward effects were noted on addition of pablum to the diet of infants as young as one month of age" (Brown and Tisdall 1939).

Throughout the 1930s, the nutritional research laboratories at Sick Kids were responsible for a variety of innovations in infant feeding. Among other activities, the hospital was involved in convincing dairies and bakeries to add vitamin D to their milk and bread products in order to eliminate the need for daily doses of cod-liver oil in children. Sunwheat Biscuits and Pablum represented the hospital's most successful commercial ventures. In 1935, Tisdall set up the Paediatric Research

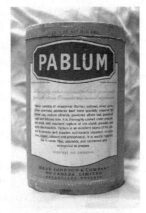

Figure 5.2   An early package of Pablum. Image of Pablum box circa 1934 courtesy of Hospital Archives, The Hospital for Sick Children, Toronto.

Foundation to receive the royalties from Pablum and Sunwheat Biscuits, and this income was used to support laboratory costs. In 1951, the foundation turned over $1,700,000 to the Hospital for Sick Children Research Institute (Kingsmill 1995). In 1977, Berton (1977) comments that Sick Kids had collected more than a million dollars in licence fees from international sales. Aside from the noteworthy commercial success of emerging paediatric nutrition research, the development and marketing of Sunwheat Biscuits and Pablum contributed to the notion of applying scientific principles not just to the infant feeding process but also to actual infant foods: "Food itself became scientific" (Comacchio 1993, 124). It was becoming increasingly common to see scientific nutritional research used to promote commercial infant feeding products.

Advice and Advertising: Chatelaine's Baby Clinic

Public health and paediatrics were not the only sources of information and advice aimed at mothers. Beginning in the 1930s, a new commercial culture aimed at women began to emerge. Although commercial infant feeding products had been available and marketed since the end of the nineteenth century, the marketing campaigns directed at mothers in the 1930s differed in the extent of the advertising; the overlap between commercial marketing, scientific medicine, and public health; and the variety of media formats in which information was dispersed. Following the shortages and costs of the First World War, many women had acquired a new consciousness of the marketplace. In the past, many women purchased goods for their family by shopping from catalogues or bargaining with merchants. A growing cash economy and mass production were contributing to the development of new patterns of shopping. Chain stores and supermarkets were increasingly aware of the role women played in household maintenance and were providing appropriate shopping environments (such as having female customers served by female clerks). Massive marketing campaigns reached women through radio, billboards, store windows, magazines, and books (Strong-Boag 1994). Women were an important part of a newly emerging marketplace, and products and information directed at mothers, including those associated with infant feeding, were one of the key elements of this commercial culture.

The new commercial culture altered the informational environment in which mothering advice was provided and discussion occurred. Advice on mothering was available not only from public health organizations and medical professionals but also from a variety of groups, institutions, and companies ranging from the Royal New Zealand Society for the Health of Women and Children to the Metropolitan Life Insurance Company. Newspapers and magazines carried regular daily, weekly, or monthly advice columns for mothers. Mothers could ask to receive free product samples by mail, and they were provided with free childrearing manuals, product information, and weight charts. Advertisements for mothers reflected the creation and availability of a wide range of products, including condensed milk, prepared infant foods, medicines, clothes, and toys.

An interesting example of shifts in patterns of infant feeding can be seen in a monthly column entitled "The Baby Clinic" that appeared in the women's magazine *Chatelaine*.[2] This column was published from 1933 to 1939 and was edited by John W.S. McCullough, the chief officer of health in Ontario from 1910 to 1935. Every month, McCullough commented on some aspect of childrearing, including immunization, feeding, and habit training, and he responded to letters written by mothers across the country who were seeking expert advice. The column was surrounded with advertisements for a wide variety of baby products. These advertisements were concentrated in this one section of the magazine, and, as the decade progressed, they expanded and became more elaborate. An examination of "The Baby Clinic" demonstrates some of the interesting interactions between scientific childrearing advice, mother's questions and experiences, and commercial pressures.

Like most medical professionals, McCullough stressed the importance of breastfeeding, partly reflecting the public health concern with unsafe milk. The caption for the August 1936 column read, "Fifty to seventy-five per cent of babies dying from intestinal troubles should have their death certificate labeled 'Poisoned by dirty milk'" (McCullough 1936, 42). While he promoted breastfeeding for the first nine months, he also provided mothers with information on how to create formulas appropriate for infants from two weeks to nine months of age: "Breast milk in whole or in part should be the food of the baby for the first nine months. If breast milk requires to be supplemented, modified cow's milk is the best addition" (McCullough 1933a, 66). On the other hand, reflecting an awareness of the unique properties of breast milk, he suggested that premature infants should have wet nurses. In his September 1933 column, he provided instructions on how to choose a good wet nurse (McCullough 1933a).

Letters from mothers requesting advice from McCullough provide insight into changing infant feeding practices. In one column, McCullough commented on the common practice of mothers' giving babies water between meals and letting them fall asleep with a bottle of water. He suggested that this practice interfered with an infant's desire for food and contributed to breastfeeding failure as it was easier for infants to feed from the bottle than from the breast (McCullough 1933b, 64). Many of the responses to mothers' letters reflect a concern with overfeeding and, indeed, most digestive troubles were attributed to this. It is also clear that, as the decade progressed, many mothers who were still choosing to breastfeed were supplementing their breast milk with formula.

The emphasis that McCullough placed on breastfeeding is in conflict with the advertisements that surrounded the column. Ads for baby foods, vitamins, cod-liver oil, and evaporated milk frequently used medical science to make a case for their products. Advertisements made appeals to scientific authorities, using statements such as

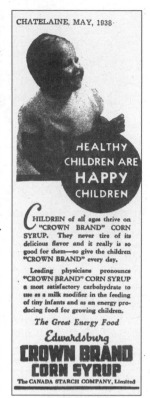

CHATELAINE, MAY, 1938

HEALTHY
CHILDREN ARE
HAPPY
CHILDREN

*C*HILDREN of all ages thrive on "CROWN BRAND" CORN SYRUP. They never tire of its delicious flavor and it really is so good for them—so give the children "CROWN BRAND" every day.

Leading physicians pronounce "CROWN BRAND" CORN SYRUP a most satisfactory carbohydrate to use as a milk modifier in the feeding of tiny infants and as an energy producing food for growing children.

The Great Energy Food

Edwardsburg
**CROWN BRAND
CORN SYRUP**
The CANADA STARCH COMPANY, Limited

Figure 5.3   Advertisement for Crown Brand Corn Syrup. *Chatelaine*, May 1938, 59.

"Physicians and paediatricians know." They also included testimonials from medical professionals. An ad for corn syrup, a common addition to infant formulas, stated, "Leading physicians pronounce Crown Brand Corn Syrup a most satisfactory carbohydrate to use as a milk modifier in the feeding of tiny infants" (see Figure 5.3). Many advertisements described issues related to food safety and nutritional deficiencies–problems that were invisible to the eye and whose solutions required a faith in science: "Scientific tests *prove* that Libby's homogenized Baby Foods are thus easier to digest, and work no hardship on Baby's delicate digestive system" (see Figure 5.4). New infant products designed just for bottle-fed babies were emerging: "Does bottle bother baby?" read the ad for Baby's Own Tablets. Infants that had been successfully bottle-fed used these tablets to aid in digestion and stomach problems known to result from bottle-feeding (Anonymous 1938).

Many of the earlier advertisements reflected a hesitancy on the part of mothers to provide their infants with anything processed or canned. The Montreal paediatrician Goldbloom (1959, 282), in his memoir, commented

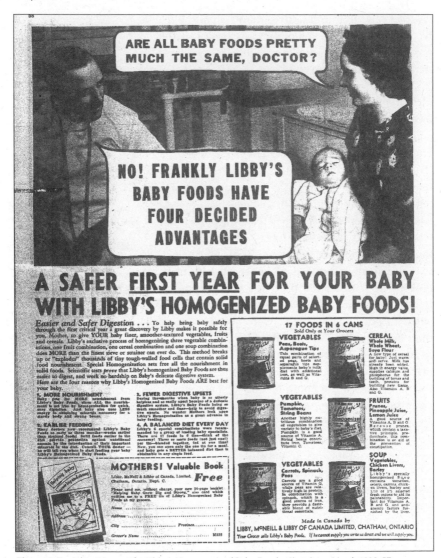

Figure 5.4   Advertisement for Libby's Homogenized Baby Foods. *Chatelaine*, March 1938, 57.

on how many mothers were reluctant to give their infants tomato juice to help prevent scurvy: "Tomato juice was found to be effective, but you could obtain this only by draining off the juice from a tin of canned tomatoes. Many mothers objected to this practice, because they abhorred the idea of giving their precious infants anything out of a can. It required some years to eradicate this prejudice." Similarly, an ad for Carnation evaporated milk started with "Odd, isn't it, how our ideas about 'canned milk' have changed! Mothers used to be doubtful about giving it to babies. They thought it might lack some essential nourishing quality … But today medical science knows,

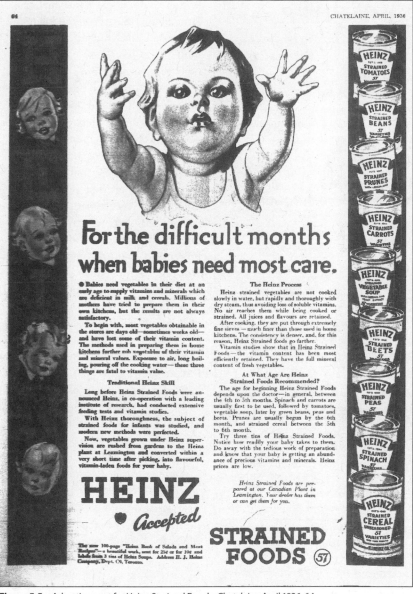

Figure 5.5   Advertisement for Heinz Strained Foods. *Chatelaine*, April 1936, 64.

beyond a doubt, that Carnation Milk is an ideal food for even the tiniest of babies" (Anonymous 1933, 3).

As with the development of Pablum, so with the development of other infant foods: nutritional research was rapidly discovering the importance of minerals and vitamins in the diet and their role in nutritional deficiency diseases. Mothers were being advised to introduce cereals and cooked vegetables into

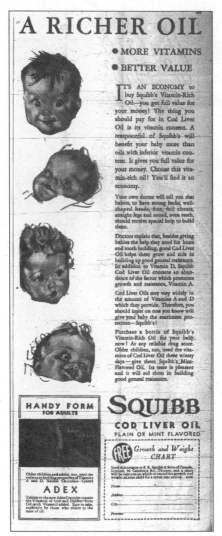

Figure 5.6 Advertisement for Squibb Cod Liver Oil—Plain or Mint Flavored. *Chatelaine*, December 1935, 55.

their infants' diets at an earlier age. One ad for Heinz strained vegetables suggested the introduction of solid foods by at least four or five months (see Figure 5.5). The earlier introduction of solids and the development of commercial baby foods reflected changes in technology. Mothers who prepared cereals at home often had to cook it for four to six hours. Factory-prepared cereals and vegetables were developed that retained nutrient quality, were more digestible, and saved mothers considerable time and energy (Brown 1940). Advertisements for cod-liver oil argued that the oil would provide babies with protection from nutritional deficiencies and increase their overall strength and resistance. As cod-liver oil was renowned for its bad taste and smell, mothers could also buy it in a mint flavour (see Figure 5.6).

By the end of the 1930s, evaporated-milk formulas dominated in terms of alternative infant feeding methods. The most popular evaporated milk on the market was Carnation Milk. The Carnation Milk Products Company started in 1899 in the United States. The first Canadian plants were established in Aylmer and Springfield, Ontario, in 1916. As the two most easterly "condenseries," these plants supplied the growing market for evaporated milk in Canada, Detroit, Cleveland, Buffalo, Pittsburgh, Philadelphia, and Boston (canned milk crossed the border free of charge). Carnation's advertising was tailored to specific regions. Bilingual and Canadian advertising for Carnation Milk included slogans such as "Lait Carnation–de Vaches Bien Nourries"; "Frais, Riche, Toujours à Votre Portée"; "Good Cow's Milk on the Prairie"; "If you spent your childhood on an Ontario farm, you know how wonderfully sweet and rich was the fresh milk from high grade cows well cared for. That's the kind of milk we use for Carnation Milk" (Weaver 1974).

One of the reasons for the popularity of Carnation Milk had to do with an innovation that first appeared in the mid-1930s: irradiated evaporated milk. Irradiation involved exposing milk to ultraviolet rays produced by a quartz mercury lamp, and it could result in milk fortified with vitamin D. For a variety of reasons, many people were opposed to adulterating milk, and evaporated milk was subject to irradiation before regular milk (Harrison 1991). Carnation Milk fortified with vitamin D was a perfect solution for mothers reluctant to give their children daily doses of smelly, poor-tasting cod-liver oil.

Milk Banks and Miracles

While little is known about the history of wet-nursing practices in Canada, it is clear that the 1930s marked the demise of the traditional wet nurse. The increasing use of infant formula in the 1930s and the advent of the first breast milk bank in Canada meant that wet nurses were no longer deemed necessary for infant survival. This event signified an important shift in thinking about the relationship between breast milk and breastfeeding. With wet-nursing, breast milk was a product linked to the practice of breastfeeding. With the availability of bottled breast milk, breast milk became dissociated from women's bodies (Golden 1996): breast milk, with all its valuable properties, could be viewed as a product on its own. In the 1930s, breast milk, rather than the practice of breastfeeding, continued to be valued for its life-saving properties. This was especially true with regard to the birth and survival of the Dionne quintuplets in 1934. Ironically, while their survival is attributed to donations of breast milk, they later became known as the celebrity face of Carnation Milk.

Milk banks appeared in North America in the 1910s in the United States, with the first milk bank opening in Boston in 1910. By 1929, over twenty cities in the United States were providing bottled breast milk to sick and premature infants (Golden 1996). The first "human milk depot" in Canada opened in the mid-1930s at the Royal Victoria Hospital in Montreal. In its 1936 annual report, the hospital described a 50 percent decrease in infant mortality, from ".70 to .38 per cent." Breast milk was frozen and distributed for free. In their first year, the hospital distributed over sixty-seven gallons (*Globe and Mail* 1937).

Golden (1996) reports that, in the United States, mothers were often paid per ounce for breast milk and that women's motives for selling this milk ran the gamut from greed to altruism. Frederick Tisdall (1942, 87), in the 1942 edition of his child advice manual *The Home Care of the Infant and Child*, also commented on the payment that mothers received for their breast milk: "Due to the progress made in the artificial feeding of infants and the fact that breast milk can now be obtained in most cities, it is very seldom necessary to procure the services of a wet nurse. To-day in the children's hospitals of most cities, breast milk is available for use when necessary. It is obtained from mothers throughout the city, who, for one reason or another, are willing to sell it."

Yet, breast milk was not always viewed as a commodity for purchase. In the case of the Dionne quintuplets, mothers from both Canada and the United States were more than willing to donate breast milk to aid in their survival. The Dionne quintuplets were born on 28 May 1934 in Callander, Ontario, a rural northern community. Yvonne, Annette, Cécile, Émilie, and Marie were the first known set of identical quintuplets to survive. As such, they made world headlines and attracted intense curiosity and attention. Soon after their birth, the Ontario government assumed guardianship of the quintuplets. They were placed under the medical care of a local physician, Allan Roy Dafoe, and later became the focus of a research program conducted by psychologist William E. Blatz and the Toronto child study centre (St. George's School of Child Study). In one of the two books he published on the quintuplets, Blatz comments, "For most of us our early childhood is wrapped in oblivion. But for these five children every nook and corner of their lives has been exposed to the gaze of the photographer and the scientist and the layman. Every ounce of mother's milk is recorded and every vitamin tabulated. Even the number of their diapers has been broadcast to the world at large" (1938, 9).

In the first hours after their birth, the quintuplets received only a few drops of warm water. The following morning, Dafoe reportedly gave the quintuplets a cow's-milk formula made up of milk, water, and corn syrup (Berton 1977; Dafoe 1936). In the afternoon, he managed to obtain two ounces of milk from nursing mothers at the North Bay hospital. Offers of donated breast milk then came in from both Canadian and American sources. Dr. Bundeson from Chicago Board of Health called Dafoe on 29 May and offered to send breast milk from Chicago donors. The packages of milk were packed in dry ice, flown by airplane, and then sent by rail to arrive on 30 May. On Thursday, 31 May, the fourth day after their birth, breast milk arrived by rail from the Toronto Hospital for Sick Children. This was the first of 120 shipments. The breast milk was collected by breastfeeding mothers in the Toronto Junior League and taken to the hospital, where it was boiled, bottled, and refrigerated; it was then shipped by rail to Callander. Breast milk also came from the depot at Montreal's Royal Victoria Hospital. In total, the quintuplets received over 8,000 ounces of breast milk (Berton 1977).

Arnup reports that many of the women who provided milk for the quints were patients of Dr. Dafoe. One mother, whose first child was born on 10 June 1934 described her recruitment: "The head nurse came to my bedside and asked if I would be interested in feeding the famous quintuplets ... I thought it was a wonderful contribution I could make but when I found out I was to be paid, I was really excited." She received 10 cents an ounce for her breast milk.

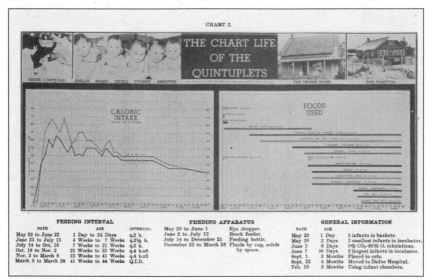

Figure 5.7   Charts describing the Dionne quintuplets' diet. The chart entitled "Foods Used" describes the introduction of various foods, including (in chronological order) breast milk (30 May–26 October), tomato or orange juice (9 July), cod-liver oil (started 28 July), ferrous chloride, prune juice, cow's-milk dilution, dextri-maltose, Pablum (26 October), evaporated milk, bacillus acidophilus, cooked vegetables, egg yolk, and cooked fruit pulp. "Further history of the care and feeding of the Dionne quintuplets" reprinted from *CMAJ* January 1936; 34(1), pages 26–32, by permission of the publisher. © 1936 Canadian Medical Association.

Another mother commented, "I suppose my part in the lives of the quints was minimal but it was a small satisfaction for me—and a fun thing for our family" (quoted in Arnup 1994–1995).

The quintuplets received undiluted, boiled breast milk via medicine dropper for approximately five months. By five months, the quints were collectively consuming a gallon of breast milk a day—more than two major hospitals could provide (Arnup 1994–1995). Louise de Kiriline (1936, 13), the nurse to the quintuplets for the first year of their lives, reports that, at five months, the medical staff were unable to ensure a stable supply of breast milk and the quintuplets then began to receive a cow's-milk formula. Later, she reports that the quintuplets were switched to evaporated milk due to concerns about purity and cleanliness. In keeping with scientific infant feeding practices, the quintuplets also received tomato, orange, and prune juice as well as vitamin D in the form of cod-liver oil. Pablum was the first solid food that was introduced to their diet (Dafoe 1936).

The quintuplets' doctor, Allan Dafoe, became an international hero. He also became a well-paid spokesperson for Carnation Milk. The fame of the quintuplets spawned "The Quintuplet Industry," and the quintuplets were used to sell more than forty products, ranging from Quaker Oats to Musterole Chest Rub to Remington Rand Typewriters. Specific infant feeding products

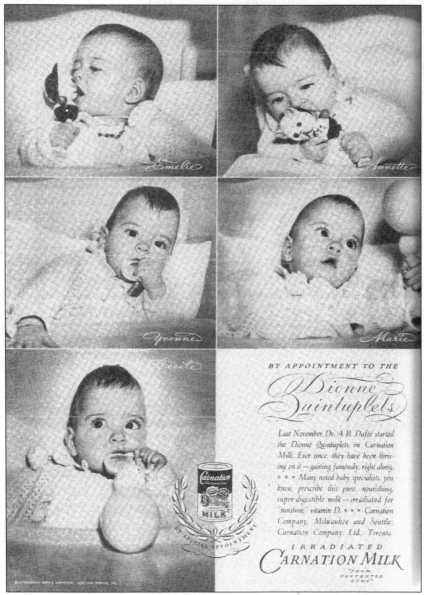

Figure 5.8   Advertisement for Carnation Milk featuring the Dionne quintuplets. *Parents Magazine*, 1935, 10(5): 47.

included Purest Cod Liver Oil, McCormick's Biscuits, and Karo Syrup (Berton 1977).

In the spring of 1934, when Carnation evaporated milk was first enriched with vitamin D, the advertising director at the American-based Carnation Milk Company heard the story of a woman in a small Ontario town who had just given birth to five baby girls. Representatives from Carnation Milk contacted William A. Dafoe, a Toronto obstetrician and brother to the quintuplets' physician, Allan Dafoe, soon after the birth. Reportedly, William Dafoe "courteously, firmly, and almost pleadingly advised against disturbing his brother, who ha[d] been inundated with hundreds of person[s] interested in every conceivable product" (Weaver 1974, 88). Jack Coyle, the "Carnation Man" in Canada, sent a letter in which he wrote: "We understand that the babies are being given breast milk feedings and are gradually gaining. You are certainly to be congratulated upon your success in this most unusual feeding case. We recognize the superiority of breast milk feeding and advocate Carnation Milk feeding only in its absence–this in spite of the enthusiasm for Carnation formulas because of their soft curd and digestibility which are similar to those of breast milk" (Weaver 1974, 88). Eventually, in exchange for exclusive rights to the quintuplets' name and pictures, Carnation made an offer of a free year's supply of evaporated milk, three thousand dollars, and a monetary gift to Allan Dafoe. The deal was made on 26 November 1934, and in April 1935 the quintuplets were used to launch a marketing campaign that was to see Carnation evaporated milk enriched with vitamin D. One advertising department declared it "the greatest publicity campaign we have ever seen" (Weaver 1974, 89). Berton (1977) reports that the quintuplets actually hated Carnation milk and refused to drink it. This in spite of advertisements claiming that the quints had consumed 2,500 tins of Carnation milk in their first eighteen months.

The birth of the quintuplets attracted the attention of mothers of all backgrounds and brought interest and awareness to breast milk and milk banks. McCullough was one of many who attributed their survival to breast milk, and he encouraged mothers to consider their case before abandoning the breast for the bottle. Yet, in a perverse twist of fate, the quintuplets were later used to market Carnation evaporated milk as a safe, scientific, and modern choice in infant feeding.

Conclusion

In the 1930s, commercial, public health, and medical and scientific interests strongly encouraged mothers to modernize their infant feeding practices. All of these groups had different aims and purposes, some explicit, others implicit, ranging from improving maternal and child health to strengthening the position of scientific medicine to selling new products in a growing consumer culture.

It is impossible to know the extent to which mothers followed the recommendations they received from all these sources, particularly as there is so much overlap between commercial, scientific, and public health sources. Undoubtedly, some mothers were eager for, others overwhelmed by, and many put off by the information they were offered. Yet, clearly, mothers of all classes were exposed to more "marketing messages" than ever before.

The messages that mothers received were sometimes ambiguous. Breastfeeding was promoted at the same time as were "safe" alternatives to breast milk. Physicians and medical scientists invested time and energy in the development of breast milk alternatives and infant foods such as Pablum. While their training in "artificial feeding" was extensive, many physicians lacked a basic understanding of the challenges of breastfeeding and ways to overcome possible difficulties. As well, nutrition research on blood and hemoglobin was showing that iron reserves in infants were depleted by six to nine months (Brown 1940; Brown and Tisdall 1939), and mothers were encouraged to introduce supplemental foods into their infant's diet after three months. Ironically, scientific medicine, which purportedly valued breastfeeding, was complicit in its decline.

The promotion of breastfeeding was also likely hampered by challenges in communicating the risks of bottle-feeding. Cow's milk no longer appeared to be dangerous. Electricity was more readily available for refrigeration, and many mothers were aware of the importance of boiling milk and water. Between 1920 and 1939, the number of residential users of electricity doubled. In 1941, 69.1 percent of occupied dwellings had electric lights (Strong-Boag 1994). In 1937, Dr. J. Hershey at the Peace River Health unit reported low levels of dysentery in younger children and attributed this to mothers' practices of boiling milk and water used for feeding children (reported in N.L. Lewis 1982–83). Infant feeding products, especially evaporated milk, were promoted as safe and hygienic. Images of fat, rosy-cheeked babies and anecdotal reports of successful bottle-feeding contributed to diluted messages about the dangers of not breastfeeding.

Ambiguous messages about breastfeeding, the lure of safer breast milk alternatives, and an emphasis on weight gain likely contributed to more and more women choosing to bottle-feed or to "mix feed" by supplementing their breast milk. The sales of commercial milk products as well as anecdotal reports suggested that breastfeeding was continuing to decline. The emergence of milk banks symbolized the end of the traditional wet nurse. The case of the Dionne quintuplets illustrates the widening physical and psychological association between the producers of breast milk and the users of breast milk. A greater heterogeneity of infant feeding practices appears to have proliferated in the 1930s. Mothers were choosing to breastfeed, bottle-feed, or to combine the two. Many mothers who chose to breastfeed were beginning to wean their infants at an earlier age, likely as a prelude to, or consequence of, introducing solids into their infants' diet at an earlier age. Homemade formulas from whole cow's milk, evaporated milk, and a range of "milk modifiers" were increasingly used. Mothers were providing their infants with vitamins in the form of juice, cod-liver oil, and enriched evaporated milk.

Chapter 6

Old-Fashioned, Time-Consuming, and a Little Disgusting, 1940–60

By the 1940s, breastfeeding initiation and duration rates were rapidly declining. An article in *Saturday Night*, a widely circulated national magazine, commented, "The Canadian baby is fast becoming a parasite on the cow, and the female breast (to quote a Toronto paediatrician) fit only for hanging a sweater on" (Howes 1950, 46). Although several scientists, medical researchers, and health professionals continued to recognize and promote the merits of breastfeeding, the value of breastfeeding to individuals in both health settings and the general public was continuing to diminish.

Government publications containing infant feeding information continued to describe the benefits of breastfeeding; however, unlike in the 1920s, breastfeeding was no longer a sign of patriotism or a requirement of good motherhood. As well, directions on bottle-feeding, the earlier introduction of solid foods, and earlier weaning began to appear in these publications. The profound shift in government advice on infant feeding over this twenty-year period was accompanied by a seismic structural change in the delivery of maternity care in Canada. In 1940, approximately 35 percent of Canadian women gave birth in hospitals. By 1960, almost every woman birthed in a hospital. The shift towards hospitalized birth resulted in the increasing influence of physicians and nurses in disseminating infant feeding advice. As well, a range of hospital practices both directly and indirectly affected women's breastfeeding success.

In the two decades following the Second World War, federal government attention shifted from concerns about infant mortality to the persistently high rates of maternal mortality, and no real initiatives to support breastfeeding emerged. More troubling were signs that the practical knowledge and skills required to breastfeed successfully were disappearing. Women who were interested or committed to breastfeeding were unable to find the necessary emotional and practical support either in their own social networks or from health professionals. "Emotional barriers" were the reasons commonly cited by women who chose not to breastfeed. By the 1960s, many women viewed the practice of breastfeeding as burdensome and repulsive, a relic from their grandmothers' time.

"Dr. Couture's Book": *The Canadian Mother and Child* (1940 and 1949)

In 1937, the federal Department of Pensions and National Health announced the formation of the Division of Child and Maternal Hygiene. Ernest Couture, a specialist in obstetrics and gynecology, was appointed the division head and guided its activities between 1937 and 1953. During Couture's years, the division focused on research (particularly on maternal mortality), consulting with provincial health departments, and developing and providing educational materials (Lewis and Watson 1991/92; Burns 1967). Building upon the success of *The Canadian Mother's Book*, Couture developed a new manual for mothers entitled *The Canadian Mother and Child*. This guide to motherhood and child care was often referred to as "Dr. Couture's book." The first edition was published in 1940, and it quickly became a Canadian bestseller, with approximately two million copies distributed in a thirteen-year period. In 1952, the Division of Child and Maternal Hygiene distributed approximately ten thousand copies a month, which closely corresponded to the number of first births in the population (Department of National Health and Welfare 1952).

In *The Canadian Mother and Child*, Couture (1940, 4) described motherhood as "the most glorious achievement in the life of a woman, for, in becoming a mother she fulfills the special purpose of her existence as a woman." Breastfeeding was a "complete realization of motherhood" (Couture 1940, 108). He insisted that a mother's love for her child was the greatest incentive to breastfeed: "The very presence of your baby, and your feeling of love for it, should prove more eloquent than words to persuade you to breast-feed your infant, if you are able to do so. In doing this, you are providing it with the best food that Nature can give" (Couture 1940, 108). In contrast to the earlier *The Canadian Mother's Book*, Couture suggested that not all mothers were necessarily able to breastfeed. However, the increasing number of mothers who were choosing not to breastfeed was the result of a lack of knowledge regarding the importance of breast milk for infants: "The failure to appreciate this fact ... accounts for the widespread tendency to neglect this maternal function" (Couture 1940, 108). Couture was careful to emphasize that "the way a baby is fed during the first year of life, may make a child either strong and healthy, or weak and sickly" (Couture 1940, 120).

Couture described the numerous benefits of breastfeeding, including preventing infant mortality and helping to restore women's "organs of reproduction" following birth. Other topics included instructions on maintaining a cheerful state of mind, the importance of cleaning the nipples with a warm boracic acid solution prior to breastfeeding, and the appropriate

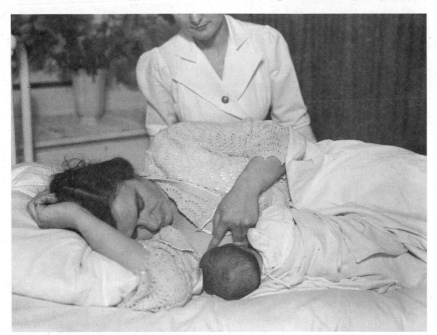

Figure 6.1 "For the first few days the baby may have to be taught how to nurse." *The Canadian Mother and Child*, 1940, 112. Library and Archives Canada, PA-803154.

use of breast pumps and breast shields. Mothers were advised not to use a lead shield as "lead poisoning of babies has been known to result from this type of shield" (Couture 1940, 124). Couture commented on the use of beer and porter to increase milk flow, and he advised women not only to consult with their physician regarding alcohol use but also to find other strategies for increasing their milk supply.

One of the most significant changes in *The Canadian Mother and Child* involved infant feeding schedules. During the 1940s and 1950s, views on child development began to relax, and this influenced infant feeding practices. In the 1920s and the era of the scientific management of children, infants were to be fed according to a strict timetable. Although experts argued over the correct time interval, a four-hour schedule was typically promoted. The 1940 edition of *The Canadian Mother and Child* presented a three-hour schedule as an option if the infant was not thriving as well as it should. In the post–Second World War era, new, less rigid ideas about childrearing emerged. Benjamin Spock's popular *Baby and Child Care* manual was published in 1946 and is likely the most well-known example of these new ideas. Spock encouraged mothers to relax and trust their instincts. Ethel Cooke (1955), in *The Canadian Nurse*, commented, "Feeding, being the great joy of the baby's life, is the first important step of his learning process. Dr. Benjamin Spock has written. 'He gets his ideas about life from the way his feeding goes—and he gets his first ideas about the world of people from the person who feeds him.' So he suggests that mothers should set their clock by the baby–not the baby by the clock."

Self-demand feeding allowed infants to set their own schedule. It was believed that babies would gradually space out their feedings and adopt a more regular schedule. The 1949 *The Canadian Mother and Child* encapsulated these more "permissive" views. It advised the use of a three-hour or four-hour schedule but added the following caveat: "In many instances doctors are recommending that the baby be allowed to establish its own feeding schedule … When the doctor is not available to give guidance in regard to the self-demand method, the schedule indicated above should be followed" (Couture 1949, 110). This method of infant feeding became more frequent in the years following the Second World War. In 1948, Alan Brown commented in the *Lancet* that "the days of rigid schedules are now a thing of the past." Further, "The increased freedom that the mother has in the management of her child produces a less tense mother and a more contented baby. This type of régime is well worth looking into and may provide a means for increasing the incidence of breast-feeding" (Brown 1948, 877). In a complete turnabout from his previously espoused views, Brown added that night feedings were now permissible and that it was no longer necessary to wake an infant who sleeps through its regular feeding time.

For mothers who were unable to breastfeed or who had insufficient milk, Couture provided instructions on the preparation of infant formula. Mothers could prepare the formula themselves, without consulting a doctor. Formulas consisted of varying amounts of cow's milk (pasteurized, certified, evaporated, or powdered) or goat's milk, sugar, and water. All infants were to receive cod-liver or halibut oil and sunshine in order to protect against rickets and tetany, and they were to receive orange or tomato juice to protect against scurvy. He also told all mothers to offer infants water in a bottle three to five times a day, even if the infant refused it. He was particularly concerned about water intake during the summer and provided suggestions on how to encourage the baby to drink by changing the temperature and sweetness of the water. Couture suggested introducing cooked cereal, homemade or store-bought, at two and a half months. During the third month, mothers should start giving their infants a food containing iron. The 1949 edition of *The Canadian Mother and Child* encouraged the introduction of solid foods at ten to twelve weeks of age to augment breast- or formula feeding. Solids contained minerals and vitamins, especially vitamin B_1, and helped to train the infant to accept solid foods of varying colour, taste, and consistency. Mothers could wean their children through the gradual introduction of solid foods.

Other than producing the popular *The Canadian Mother and Child*, the federal government did very little to promote breastfeeding during Couture's years. In the fall of 1940, a special committee of the Division of Child and

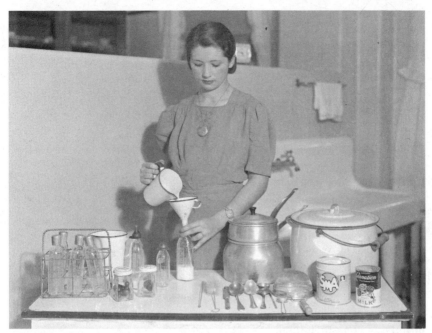

Figure 6.2   "When preparing the formula have everything you require at hand. It is of the utmost attention that every utensil be scrupulously clean. Wash your hands well before preparing the formula." *The Canadian Mother and Child*, 1940, 130. Library and Archives Canada, PA-163732.

Maternal Hygiene was appointed to study, and make recommendations for reducing, maternal and infant mortality. The committee made recommendations regarding nursing services, incubator services, human milk depots, and blood transfusion services. These recommendations were never translated into programs, supposedly due to wartime resource limitations (Burns 1967). In 1948, a national health grant strategy was introduced, whereby the federal government provided money to the provinces for specific health purposes. Some of these annual grants went towards purchasing equipment to ensure safer formula preparation in hospitals (Burns 1967).

In terms of breastfeeding promotion, in 1949 the Division of Child and Maternal Hygiene supported a collaborative project with the Saskatchewan Health Department and other provincial groups. The Mother's Milk Service in Regina was intended to provide breast milk to premature and debilitated babies and to increase interest in the value of breastfeeding. As a demonstration project, it was hoped that it could be used as a model for other similar projects across the country (Burns 1967). Mothers were paid ten cents per ounce for their breast milk, which was collected from their homes and delivered to a plant where it was pooled, pasteurized, and dispensed, with a doctor's prescription, for free. Recognizing that infant feeding decisions were made prior to birth, the milk service also provided consultation for prospective mothers.

Although the demonstration project did not spur the development of other similar projects, it did highlight the declining rates of breastfeeding in one part of the country. One project collaborator commented, "It is estimated that in most areas, not one-half and in certain sections not one-quarter of the number of babies born are breastfed for even a short period" (Tinkiss 1948, 6).

On the surface, during the 1940s support for breastfeeding remained strong in *The Canadian Mother and Child* and in other government initiatives. However, as the length of exclusive breastfeeding was reduced from nine to three months and the earlier introduction of solid foods promoted, state-produced literature was clearly shifting away from breastfeeding. For the first time, advice on bottle-feeding was included in state-produced advice manuals. The emergence of self-demand feeding in the advice literature suggested that infant feeding practices were becoming less rigid, and this may have encouraged more successful breastfeeding in that, through more frequent feedings, a woman's milk supply was able to replenish itself. However, these more permissive breastfeeding guidelines occurred at the same time as did enormous changes in Canadian maternity practices, and it is to these that we now turn.

Birth: From Home to Hospital

Historically, the only women who gave birth in hospitals were the very poor or the unmarried. Throughout the first half of the twentieth century, physicians gradually replaced midwives and traditional birth attendants in the homes of women giving birth. As scientific medicine became more professionalized, middle-class women who could afford to pay physicians were both choosing and encouraged to shift to hospital births. Technological advancements had resulted in a variety of interventions, such as antibiotic therapy and oxygen and incubation for infants. Hospital births were more convenient for physicians than were home births, and they appeared safer and more scientific to mothers. Middle-class mothers demanding the most up-to-date treatments initiated the trend towards hospitalized birth (Mitchinson 1993; Light and Pierson 1990). British Columbia led the other provinces in the move towards hospitalization. Between 1926 and 1940, the hospitalization rate in that province increased from 48 percent to 84 percent of live births (Strong-Boag and McPherson 1990). Nationally, in 1941, fewer than 50 percent of babies were born in hospital, but by 1961, the rate was 97 percent (Prentice et al. 1988). (See Appendix D.)

The shift towards hospitalized birth affected breastfeeding success in a number of ways. First, in the past, physician involvement in breastfeeding generally resulted in dubious effects. Physicians tended to have a merely symbolic commitment to breastfeeding and would switch to bottle-feeding at the first sign of difficulty. Second, in a hospital environment, women had much less control and decision-making ability than they did in the home.

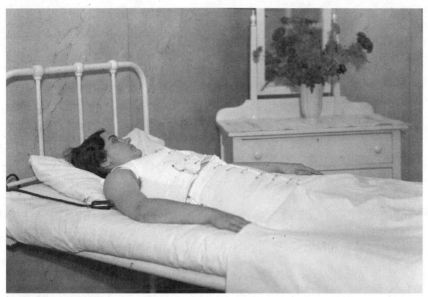

Figure 6.3   "Immediately after the birth, the mother can be made more comfortable by means of carefully applied binders." *The Canadian Mother and Child*, 1940, 63. National Archives of Canada. PA-803153.

Not only did physicians have sole authority, but hospitalization deterred the involvement of grandmothers, mothers, and other women who might possess practical breastfeeding knowledge. The expectation was that delivery and care were to be entirely in the doctor's hands (Strong-Boag and McPherson 1990). Third, various hospital interventions made it extremely challenging for mothers to breastfeed successfully.

Some of the new practices that were increasingly part of the childbirth process included the use of X-rays, anesthetics, the use of piturin to stimulate contractions, the artificial induction of labour, episiotomies, shavings, enemas, Lysol washes, stirrups, arm straps, and the use of forceps. Although some births likely benefited from the appropriate use of some of these practices, "By promoting hospitalized care administrators and specialists brought women into an environment where the staff and the equipment, and thus the opportunity and temptation, for greater intervention were more readily available" (Strong-Boag and McPherson 1990, 81). Many of these interventions affected the physical ability and/or comfort of women attempting to initiate breastfeeding. In 1950, Hilary Bourne (1950, 971), a physician in the Department of Obstetrics and Gynecology at the Royal Victoria Hospital in Montreal, commented: "It should be pointed out that Cesarean section is no contraindication to breast feeding unless of course the mother is having a stormy post-operative recovery."

After the birth, a woman had restricted access to her infant. Early care of the mother following birth included a prolonged period of rest: mothers were supposed to recline in bed for five or six days and were not allowed to leave the hospital for twelve to fourteen days. At Vancouver General Hospital, women were not permitted to attempt breastfeeding until at least six to eight hours after birth. "Standing Orders" recommended feedings at four-hour intervals for fifteen minutes (Strong-Boag and McPherson 1990). Beatrice Whitehair, part of the first generation of women to give birth in hospital in the Prairies, described her experience in Calgary:

> The new General [hospital] was open by the time my twins were born ... But I lost the boy. He was twelve days old but he was dying ... Well I put it down to that they didn't bring him often enough to have nurse. And I told the doctor so. I said "You know Dr. Crawford that baby isn't getting any nourishment. I have to squeeze it into his mouth, he hasn't got the power to, he's getting weaker and weaker." Well he said, "I'll tell them to bring him to you all the time." But they didn't ... (quoted in Langford 2000, 165)

Couture, in *The Canadian Mother and Child*, suggested that women clean their nipples before and after feeding with a saline solution and warm boiled water to prevent bruising and cracking as well as breast abscesses. Mothers were to breastfeed for two to three minutes on each breast eight to ten hours following the birth. Afterwards, the baby was to receive a "dessertspoonful of warm boiled water from a bottle" (Couture 1949, 99). In hospitals, staff were encouraged to provide supplementary bottles of formula to infants in order to allow mothers to rest and to prevent weight loss in the infant. Women also frequently received free samples of formula (Arnup 1994).

Both physicians and nurses lacked adequate training in encouraging successful breastfeeding and often inadvertently made bottle-feeding seem like a more attractive option. A nurse in the Maternity Pavilion of the Vancouver General Hospital commented, "As a rule, on or about the third day a mother's milk comes in with a rush ... Since pediatricians do not always make daily visits, some mothers are left unrelieved if there has not been an order written to express, pump, or to use a nipple shield. Even if these orders are given later to relieve the discomfort, the damage has often been done" (Anderson 1954, 895).

The paediatrician Alan Brown disagreed with many principles of hospital care. He argued that nurses trained especially in breastfeeding should handle the "nursing couple" during the first two weeks following birth. He believed that supplementary feedings in the first few days lessened the chance of a woman establishing an adequate milk supply and suggested that "the use of dilute lactose water is preferable, at least, until it is evident that the maternal milk-supply is inadequate" (Brown 1948, 877). Brown also argued against separating mothers and infants following delivery: "The advantages of having the baby with the mothers has also been investigated … A normal mother can undertake a great deal of care of the baby from the second day on, and having her infant in close proximity seems, in most cases where the mother wishes it, to be helpful to her" (877). "Rooming-in," the practice of having infants stay with mothers for part of the day, also permitted frequent, on-demand feedings, which would stimulate the milk supply.

Accepted, Familiar, and Attractive: Bottle-Feeding in the 1940s and 1950s

Throughout the 1940s and 1950s, bottle-feeding was becoming a more familiar and accepted form of infant feeding. During the Second World War, the federal government acknowledged the number of mothers who utilized evaporated milk for infant feeding and, during wartime conditions, ensured that an adequate supply was available. Interestingly, while the number of women in the labour force increased during and following the war, there did not seem to be any conflict between women's paid work and infant feeding choices. Women's roles following the Second World War seemed to have changed very little, while childrearing norms and the role of men as fathers began to change dramatically. Fathers became more involved in supporting women throughout pregnancy and childbirth and took on new responsibilities with regard to childrearing. Breastfeeding was seen to be an often taxing activity, and bottle-feeding enabled fathers to become more involved in infant care. Furthermore, bottle-feeding was seen as providing many of the same advantages as breastfeeding.

The advent of the Second World War does not seem to have inhibited the decline in breastfeeding either due to women's increased presence in the labour force or to a decreased availability of cow's milk for making infant formulas. In Europe during the war, where conditions were often desperate, there is some evidence of increased breastfeeding as women who were unable to obtain supplies for infant formula reverted to breastfeeding. For example, in wartime France, rates of breastfeeding reportedly increased from 38 percent to 90 percent due to the unavailability of infant formula (Applebaum 1970). The situation was much different in Canada.

During the war, Canada dramatically increased its food exports (including condensed, powdered, and evaporated milk) to meet its wartime commitments as an ally to Britain and the armed forces abroad. Yet the Wartime Prices and Trade Board made special provisions to ensure that all mothers who required evaporated milk for infant formula would be able to obtain it. In January 1943, "Evaporated milk is being distributed by priority in this order: To the British Ministry of Food, the armed forces, areas without a fresh milk supply and mothers with young babies" (*Globe and Mail* 1943, 1). By the end of 1943, evaporated and partly skimmed evaporated milk was restricted to infants and those requiring it for health reasons. Parents were required to apply for evaporated-milk cards at their local ration board, where they would present a medical prescription, a doctor's formula, or a certificate from a physician, a public health nurse, or a recognized health agency (Canadian Press 1943).

During the war, women's participation in the labour force surged. Yet, there does not seem to have been any conflict between this new historical development and breastfeeding practices. In 1944, at the peak of wartime employment, one-third of all women over the age of fifteen were in the paid labour force. However, in 1946, only one-quarter of these women were working for pay. This decrease was attributed not to the withdrawal of women already in the workforce but, rather, to a decline in the number of younger women entering the workforce. In the post–Second World War period, younger women were more likely to prolong their education and to get married and start a family at an earlier age. Although young mothers did not make up a large proportion of women in the paid workforce, the proportion of married women continued to increase (these were women who did not have children or who had older children). In 1941, only slightly more than 10 percent of all employed women were married; during the war, this increased to between 25 percent and 35 percent; by 1961, it increased to nearly half (Prentice et al. 1988).

In spite of their increasing presence in the labour force, attitudes towards women's proper role in society appeared to have changed only minimally in the postwar period. Images of femininity and domesticity dominated, and women were portrayed as homemakers and mothers (Pierson 1977). Interestingly, the economic need, or the desire, for paid work does not seem to have been a major source of conflict for mothers who were making infant feeding decisions. A 1952 national survey found that the major reason married women under the age of forty left their employment was to engage in child-care responsibilities (Krahn and Lowe 2002). In 1955, the Department of Labour conducted a survey of employed married women in eight Canadian cities. Of those who participated in the survey, more than 50 percent had dependent children and 80 percent worked full-time. The high number of married women in the labour force was largely due to the massive wave of immigration after the war: one-third of all workers in the survey were born outside of Canada (Prentice et al. 1988).

While women's proper roles as homemakers and wives did not change substantially following the war, views about parenthood, especially father-hood, continued to evolve. Dr. Jean Webb, a specialist in paediatrics and public health, replaced Couture in the Division of Child and Maternal Hygiene and revised the 1953 and 1957 editions of *The Canadian Mother and Child* (Lewis and Watson 1991/92; Burns 1967). Webb acknowledged that motherhood was not always joyful. In particular, she acknowledged the dif-ficulties of breastfeeding: "Many women get discouraged with their first few attempts to nurse their babies. Both you and your baby have to learn to nurse successfully and it usually takes a little time. The more you nurse your baby,

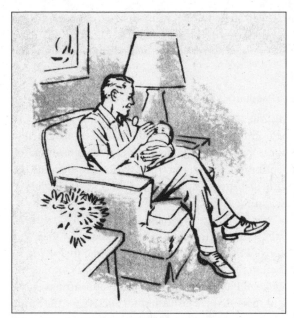

Figure 6.4   Beginning in the 1940s, the content of *The Canadian Mother and Child* began to reflect the gradual involvement of fathers in childrearing practices. The image of a father bottle-feeding a baby was Included in the 1967 edition (edited by Jean Webb). *The Canadian Mother and Child*, 1967, 91.

the more milk you will have, so it pays to persevere" (Webb 1953, 78).

The 1940 edition of *The Canadian Mother and Child* claimed, "Parenthood is a partnership requiring the hearty cooperation of each partner" (Couture 1940, 35). It then went on to devote two pages to describing the role of fathers. Fathers had a responsibility to ensure that mothers received proper prenatal and postnatal care, to be acquainted with the makeup of a woman's constitution and temperament, and to provide their pregnant wives with sympathetic treatment. In the postwar period, the role of fathers in childrearing began to expand. For example, in 1952, the Toronto Department of Health began teaching prenatal classes for first-time fathers. By 1957, joint classes for both women and men were introduced (MacDougall 1990). Webb's manual provided more detail on how to involve fathers in infant care than had earlier advice manuals. Indeed, according to Webb (1953, 80), the "one advantage of bottle-feeding is that it gives Daddy a chance to feed the baby occasionally, and this helps develop a happy relationship between father and baby."

Breastfeeding had often been considered the best way of providing infants with nourishment and comfort. Yet, the new guidelines assured mothers that bottle-fed infants could receive the same quality of attention as did breastfed infants. The more permissive childrearing guidelines, which encouraged self-demand feeding (an idea that was firmly established by 1953), emphasized providing children with love and attention, and breastfeeding was thought to be an ideal way of doing this: "A special advantage is that the breast-fed baby gets the full attention of his mother while he is nursing. It may be hard to realize that a small infant can be aware of these things, but there is no doubt that even the tiniest baby needs that feeling of human touch and security that he gets lying happily in his mother's arms, filling himself with food" (Webb

1953, 76). Mothers who bottle-fed their babies were instructed to give their infants the same attention as they would if they were nursing, thus ensuring that they would not miss out on the comfort and companionship acquired through breastfeeding.

"Ironing Out the Difficulties": Paediatrics Abandons Infant Feeding

The subject of infant feeding was the foundation for the medical specialty of paediatrics. However, by the mid-1940s, the field began to turn its attention to other concerns. As the paediatrician Alton Goldbloom (1945, 284) commented, "We have ironed out most of our difficulties, and we have finally relegated the whole subject of infant feeding to its proper place in pediatrics ... From baby-feeders we are gradually becoming physicians for children–or pediatrists."

By the 1940s, paediatrics was no longer a struggling specialty trying to establish itself as a respected part of the medical profession. In 1922, the Canadian Society for the Study of the Diseases of Children had just 13 members; by 1951, it had 216 members (McKendry and Bailey 1990; Comacchio 1993). In 1939, the Royal College of Physicians and Surgeons became responsible for certifying all medical specialists. The Canadian Society for the Study of the Diseases of Children, originally open to all physicians with an interest in child health, became the more exclusive Canadian Paediatric Society, which had a restricted membership (Comacchio 1993).

In the early years of paediatrics, the development of adequate breast milk alternatives had consumed much of the time and energy of paediatric researchers and practitioners. Aspiring paediatricians spent at least one to two years studying various methods of infant feeding. The intent of all these different methods was to alter cow's milk to resemble human milk. This had led to debates about such things as the caloric properties of various milks and sugars, the addition of acids, and raw milk versus boiled milk. Complex mathematical equations were used to tailor formulas to individual babies, and formulas were developed following detailed stool analysis. The discovery of vitamins in the 1910s had sparked further speculation on necessary vitamin content. By the 1940s, these discussions and trials were part of the distant past: "Present trends in infant feeding are all towards simplicity. Formulas which used to be changed by the doctor about once a week are now hardly changed at all. Spoon feeding with semi-solids, once withheld until the second half of the first year, are now given as early as six or eight weeks, rarely later than three months, and the variety of foods is only limited by the ingenuity and daring of the physician" (Goldbloom 1945, 284).

Simple formulas of cow's milk, water, and sugar were now considered able to meet the needs of most babies, and mothers could prepare these at home. Also, numerous breast milk alternatives were available on the market. Although Canadian data are not available, in the United States, in 1959, there were over 200 brands of evaporated milk, 78 brands of infant foods, and 26 carbohydrate modifiers available on the market (Meyer 1960, cited in Hill 1967). Researchers had never found any problems with deficiencies due to a lack of vitamin B complex or vitamin A, and efforts to educate mothers to dose their children with vitamin D in the form of cod-liver oil or irradiated evaporated milk and vitamin C from orange and tomato juice seemed to have been effective. Brown commented that rickets and scurvy were rarely seen at the Toronto Hospital for Sick Children. In 1947, there were five cases of rickets and five cases of scurvy out of 11,748 hospital admissions and 63,741 outpatient visits (Brown 1948).

Paediatricians seem to have solved most of the major problems of infant feeding, and many of the fears about the purity of cow's milk had disappeared. The second generation of paediatricians in Canada had never witnessed the high rates of infant mortality that were evident in the first part of the twentieth century (see Appendix B for a statistical overview). Goldbloom commented as early as 1930 that "Weaning, either in summer or winter, has lost its terrors and diarrhoeal diseases in summertime are far less frequent than they were" (Goldbloom 1930, 807). However, the fresh milk supply was not as safe as some might have believed. A 1951 survey conducted by the Health League of Canada examined the percentage of each province's milk supply that was pasteurized and came up with some interesting findings. In Nova Scotia, 55 percent to 60 percent of milk consumed was pasteurized; in New Brunswick, 88 percent of milk sold by licensed dealers; in Quebec, 85 percent of commercial milk; in Ontario, 99 percent of all milk sold; in Manitoba, 65 percent to 70 percent of milk consumed; in Saskatchewan, 35 percent of milk consumed; in Alberta, 32 percent of milk consumed; and in British Columbia, 85 percent of milk consumed (Anonymous 1951). Perhaps because of this, evaporated milk, packaged safely in a sterile can, was the most frequently used form of cow's milk in infant formulas (Grewar 1958).

Goldbloom's comment that the variety of solid foods was "only limited by the ingenuity and daring of the physician" was reflected in the medical literature. Beginning in the 1940s, it was increasingly common to see reports of physicians experimenting with the age of introduction and the variety of solid foods fed to infants. Rather than prohibiting most foods for the first year of life, "grown-up" foods were now being introduced in the first few days of life. Reports described infants being fed foods such as sardines, creamed tuna, shrimp, peas, and carrots at one month. Gough summarized six years of experiments in infant feeding. His approach was to begin feeding the infant orange juice, vitamin D, and cereal in the first week after birth. He introduced fruit in the second week and meat and vegetables in the fourth week. He commented on his excellent results: "In general practice, it is not good medicine to subject patients to extra expense merely for experimental purposes. However, the results, in the persons of children, speak for themselves, and the keynote is simplicity" (Gough 1953, 545).

A survey of two thousand paediatricians in the United States in 1954 reported that 66 percent of them recommended feeding solids at six to eight weeks of age or earlier (Butler and Wolman, cited in Fomon 1991).[1] Although medical research did not provide proof of any particular nutritional or psychological benefits to the earlier introduction of solids, there did not appear to be any real harm either. The potentially strong effect of the earlier introduction of solids on breastfeeding initiation rates and the subsequent ability of women to maintain an adequate milk supply were never discussed; rather, it was believed that infants appeared to be remarkably adaptable to whatever they were fed (Hill 1967, 267).

The earlier introduction of solids did raise other questions, though: "The apparent increase in height and weight of today's children in comparison with the normal nineteenth century specimens raises the question whether yesteryear's children were undernourished or whether today's children are overfed and overweight" (Cochrane 1959, 456). Mothers were often believed to overfeed their infants and to become upset when they did not eat enough or gain enough weight (Royer 1962). Cochrane (1959, 454) suggested that perhaps mothers weren't the only ones to blame: "Today mothers are being constantly bombarded with advertising suggesting that bigger babies are better babies. Paediatricians are not altogether free from blame, for many encourage the feeding of solid foods almost before the umbilical cord has been tied." Advertisements for infant feeding products in *Chatelaine* between 1955 and 1964 reveal a new concern with infant growth (Potter, Sheeshka, and Valaitis 2000). Furthermore, over-nutrition and obesity were increasing concerns in adult nutrition and public health. By the late 1950s, questions were being asked regarding whether current infant feeding practices might be contributing to this new trend. However, as yet, there was no evidence to suggest that childhood obesity was harmful or problematic in the long term.

Old-Fashioned, Time-Consuming, and a Little Disgusting

In 1950, Hilary Bourne (1950, 969), a physician in the Department of Obstetrics and Gynecology at the Royal Victoria Hospital in Montreal, commented, "It is a well-known fact that the worst place in the world as regards breast feeding is the United States; Canada runs a close second. It is also well known that the European, and in particular the Scandinavian, countries are best in this regard. The difference, however, is not due to geographical location, or anatomical development, or even physiological insufficiency. The great difference is one of temperament, education, and so-called modern living." By 1960, support for breastfeeding was difficult to find, and, across the country and in all socio-demographic groups, breastfeeding rates were at an all-time low.

Ann Sharkey (Sharkey 1952), in *The Canadian Nurse*, reported on the numerous excuses and objections to breastfeeding that she often encountered.

These ranged from needing to return to work to feeling confined to the house to avoiding getting one's clothes messy. According to Sharkey, "In this modern hustle-and-bustle era there has developed a negative attitude towards breast-feeding, chiefly due to lack of knowledge. Some women retain childish attitudes of prudery or disgust; others may have had inadequate health and sex education; while still others may have insufficient knowledge regarding the value of breastfeeding" (Sharkey 1952, 188–89).

Other, less practical, reasons for not breastfeeding were also increasingly common. Women often described psychological or "emotional barriers" to breastfeeding. Breastfeeding was seen as burdensome or old-fashioned. Many women had never seen a baby breastfed and were further dissuaded from initiating breastfeeding by the advice and example of their friends and family (Bourne 1950). By the 1960s, the sight of a woman breastfeeding in public was as foreign as was the sight of a woman bottle-feeding at the beginning of the century, when "reasons for weaning, once breastfeeding ha[d] been started, were abnormality of the breast or nipple, unwillingness to continue feeding and insufficiency of milk, either actual or fancied" (Grewar 1959, 844). Negative attitudes towards breastfeeding were also reflected in the media, although the extent to which this might have actually influenced behaviour is impossible to untangle. In an analysis of infant feeding messages in *Chatelaine* between 1945 and 1995, Potter, Sheeshka, and Valaitis (2000) found that letters, editorials, and articles about breastfeeding were predominantly negative.[2]

Survey data on actual rates of breastfeeding during this period are unavailable. Howes (1950) reported in a magazine article that only 40 percent of Toronto's babies were breastfed for any length of time. It also appears that the only non-Aboriginal women continuing to breastfeed were poor women who were unable to afford formula. A number of Aboriginal communities retained traditional practices of breastfeeding throughout the 1950s (Dodgson and Struthers 2003). However, an article in the *Canadian Medical Association Journal* commented on shifting infant feeding practices in Aboriginal groups in Manitoba, and Grewar (1958) described how some First Nations groups were continuing with traditional breastfeeding practices while others were adopting "white man's ways" and shifting towards breast milk alternatives and bottle-feeding. He also commented on the increased rates of infantile scurvy between 1954 and 1956, and he attributed this to the bottle-feeding.

A 1951 survey of 297 women who attended prenatal classes held by the Toronto Department of Public Health found that 172 of them were breastfeeding. Of the 125 women who were not breastfeeding, only 19 reported that they had never attempted it. Most women breastfed for a few days to three months. Reasons for not breastfeeding included insufficient milk (63); cracked, small, or inverted nipples (10); breast infection (6); doctor's orders (3); worry (2);

and other (13). Several women in the survey criticized hospital staff because they did not help or encourage them to breastfeed. Others expressed a desire for more information about breastfeeding (cited in Arnup 1994). Grewar deplored the decline of the "natural nurser"–a mother who took it for granted that she would breastfeed and who succeeded with little or no instruction. He contended that physicians frequently lacked both knowledge of and faith in breastfeeding: "A moment's thought will indicate how deplorably little time is devoted to the mechanism and management of breast feeding in the medical student's present curriculum" (Grewar 1959, 845).

Conclusion

By the 1960s, breastfeeding was almost forgotten. Although still promoted in government advice to mothers, guidelines were more permissive and breast milk alternatives were presented as acceptable infant feeding choices. Throughout the 1940s and 1950s, increasing numbers of women were giving birth in hospital. Hospital births, in conjunction with smaller family sizes, meant that often the first birth a woman attended was that of her own child. Scientific medicine, not women's lay knowledge, now guided the birth process. A lack of practical experience, coupled with unsympathetic hospital procedures, made breastfeeding a challenging prospect even for women who wanted to breastfeed. At a two-generation remove from a time when breastfeeding was the norm, many women had lost the skills and knowledge needed to breastfeed. As well, the values, beliefs, and social structure that had once supported breastfeeding had now been replaced.

The field of paediatrics was no longer interested in problems of formula feeding, and infant mortality due to unsafe milk or inadequate formulas was no longer a concern. Physicians heavily promoted the early introduction of solids, which likely had an impact on breastfeeding duration rates. By the 1960s, infant feeding was primarily a matter of personal preference. Indeed, bottle-feeding was attractive in some cases as it provided fathers with an opportunity to participate in child care. Except for women who could not choose to bottle-feed due to economic pressures, and for some Aboriginal communities that retained traditional practices, bottle-feeding was now a familiar and ordinary part of life.

Part 3

Resurgence, 1960–2000

Chapter 7

The Return to Breastfeeding, 1960–80

Throughout the early 1960s, breastfeeding initiation and duration rates remained relatively low, with less than one-quarter of mothers initiating breastfeeding. However, while breastfeeding continued to be abandoned by some groups of women, other groups were increasingly interested in choosing to breastfeed. By the late 1960s and early 1970s, breastfeeding rates began to increase in all regions of Canada. As with the shift away from breastfeeding two generations earlier, so with the shift back: women from higher socio-economic backgrounds led the trend.

The return to breastfeeding occurred in the midst of a range of social, cultural, and political movements. The natural childbirth movement emerged strongly in the late 1960s in conjunction with the women's movement. Women began to re-evaluate their roles in society and in the workplace as well as their relationships to their children and partners. Attitudes towards childbirth and reproductive practices were challenged and altered. The formation of La Leche League, a lay organization supporting breastfeeding, was key to supporting and strengthening the return to breastfeeding in Canada. As well, international efforts to counter the marketing practices of infant formula companies in the developing world found tremendous support among Canadian women in the late 1960s and early 1970s, creating awareness about the potential dangers of infant formula. Finally, by the late 1970s, public health and the scientific community "rediscovered" the value of breastfeeding, and this lent the practice increasing medical authority.

"Fashions" in Infant Feeding: Breastfeeding in the 1960s

A 1964 *Globe and Mail* article commented, "Breastfeeding seems to go in and out of fashion in Canada, depending on the current mythologies, the status of women, and even the geographic area" (*Globe and Mail* 1964, W3). The article reported that breastfeeding rates varied considerably from area to area and from one social group to another. In some places, 50 percent of women were breastfeeding, while in others, only 10 percent were breastfeeding. While overall breastfeeding rates continued to decline in the early 1960s, new "fashions," or patterns, pertaining to infant feeding were beginning to emerge. Two retrospective surveys on breastfeeding practices in the 1960s and 1970s provide the first comprehensive overview of breastfeeding in Canada, and they show how breastfeeding varied according to social class, ethnicity, and province.

New fashions in infant feeding both encouraged and discouraged breast-feeding. Interest in breastfeeding underwent a revival in Newfoundland in the early 1960s following an outbreak of gastroenteritis that took the lives of seventy-two babies. In the mid-1960s, Toronto public health nurses were reporting that many upper-middle-class mothers were initiating breast-feeding (*Globe and Mail* 1964). Many young mothers, especially university graduates, were interested in child development, particularly the concept of maternal-infant bonding (Grant 1968). Beginning with the work of John Bowlby in the 1950s and 1960s, new research was exploring the concept of attachment and the role of breastfeeding in developing a strong and nurtur-ing bond between mother and child. Potter, Sheeshka, and Valaitis (2000) reported that maternal-infant bonding themes became significant in adver-tisements for infant feeding products in *Chatelaine* between 1955 and 1964, which is perhaps one indication of the popularity of this scientific research in public consciousness.

In some groups of women, breastfeeding was still considered the norm. One public health nurse commented on how most mothers in Ottawa who had recently immigrated from Europe breastfed their first infant. However, by their third or fourth child, they often no longer chose to breastfeed as they found it was something they should only do in private. Other women who were interested in or attempted breastfeeding were discouraged by a number of factors. Some mothers complained of meeting overt scorn or disapproval from neighbours and even of having to deal with "the fear of the husband that it will spoil the wife's figure." One prominent female physician railed against the new fad of breastfeeding and called it "some sort of mystical status symbol." In Ottawa, many female civil servants viewed women who chose to breastfeed as "letting down the side" (*Globe and Mail* 1964, W4).

In contrast, many women believed that only poor women breastfed, and they saw bottle-feeding as the "normal" way to feed a baby. In the 1960s, while many affluent women were returning to breastfeeding, poorer women were just beginning to abandon the practice. One article commented on how upper-middle-class mothers who chose not to breastfeed were causing harm not to their infants but, rather, to the infants of poorer mothers who chose to follow their example (Associated Press 1964).

Data collected in the Nutrition Canada survey (1970–72) provide the first comprehensive, national, and representative overview of breastfeeding practices for the years between 1965 and 1971 (see Appendix E for an over-view of national studies of breastfeeding initiation and duration). This study revealed that the breastfeeding initiation rate across Canada was 26 percent, with approximately 2 percent of mothers breastfeeding exclusively. At three months, about 75 percent of these infants were no longer being breastfed. While 2 percent of mothers breastfed exclusively, 24 percent combined breast- and bottle-feeding and 74 percent bottle-fed exclusively. Myres (1979a) also reported that the proportion of breastfeeding mothers was three to four times greater in the highest-income group than in lower-income groups. As well as wide variations in breastfeeding initiation rates according to social class, there was also enormous variation according to region: 11 percent breastfed in Quebec, 15 percent in the Maritimes, 33 percent in Ontario and the Prairies, and 41 percent in British Columbia. This shows a strong east-to-west gradient.

While breastfeeding initiation rates varied according region, interestingly, the pattern for the introduction of solids did not. The median age for the introduction of solids was one to two months (the median age for First Nations infants was three months, and for Inuit infants it was five months). Approximately 50 percent of infants were introduced to solids by one month, and 80 percent to 90 percent were introduced to solids by three months of age. It was clear that there was a relationship between the initial feeding method and the age at which solids were introduced. Mothers who exclusively breastfed their infants tended to introduce solids at a later age (three months) than did mothers who never breastfed (one month) (Myres 1979a).

The national survey also provided information on the types of milk used in infant formula for the years between 1965 and 1971. According to the survey, 98 percent of infants received some form of milk formula. Some formula types were more frequently used than others: 21 percent to 40 percent of bottle-fed infants received a commercially prepared formula, while 4 percent to 40 percent of infants under six months of age were fed home-prepared formulas of evaporated milk, water, and carbohydrates. Evaporated-milk formulas were used more frequently in Atlantic Canada than in other parts of the nation. As an interesting comparison, in the United States, less than 5 percent of infants were fed evaporated-milk formulas (Nutrition Canada 1976).

The national survey showed that, as income increased, the use of unmodified cow's milk decreased and the use of prepared infant formulas and infant cereal increased (Myres 1979a). Further, the survey found that the type of milk consumed was also related to income. Whole milk and evaporated milk were used in the lowest- and low-income groups, while skim milk and 2 percent milk were used in the higher-income groups. Lower-income groups used prepared infant formulas at about one-fifth the rate of the higher-income groups. These differences in milk consumed led to differences in the amount of vitamin C, fat, and iron consumed: lower-income groups had a higher intake of fat and vitamin C and a lower intake of iron than did higher-income groups. However, there were no obvious patterns in nutrient intake with respect to income level, and all income groups consumed nutrients above the levels recommended by the Canadian Dietary Standard.

The national survey found that the proportion of infants initially breast-fed was 46 percent in the Inuit population, 31 percent in the First Nations population, and 26 percent in the general population. Inuit and First Nations women also had the highest rates of exclusive breastfeeding: 8 percent in the First Nations population and 3 percent in the Inuit population as compared with 2 percent in the general population (Myres 1979a). The Maternal and Child Health Survey conducted in 1962 found that 69 percent of First Nations women initiated breastfeeding–a considerably higher percentage than was found in the general population (cited in Stewart and Steckle 1987). These two surveys suggested that rates of breastfeeding initiation were declining among Aboriginal women in the 1960s just as it was increasing among most other women.

Up until the Second World War, Aboriginal people in Canada's North had remained relatively isolated from the rest of the country and had mostly retained a traditional way of life. The Second World War had led to the construction of airports in the North as well as to the construction of the Alaska Highway and the American Distant Early Warning military radar line (known as the DEW line). This led to increased Aboriginal contact with "white culture," with the result that, after 1955, traditional lifestyles were disrupted. One of the consequences of increased contact was escalating rates of tuberculosis, with increasing numbers of individuals being sent to hospitals in the south. At one point, 12 percent of the Inuit population in the north had TB and was taken to southern areas (Kome 1981). It began to be more frequent for Aboriginal women to leave their communities to give birth in northern regional medical centres or in the south, and traditional birthing practices, including beliefs and knowledge about breastfeeding, were adversely affected (O'Neil and Kaufert 1996).

In the mid-1950s, high rates of infant mortality were observed in the North. In particular, Otto Schaefer, a physician who began working in the North in the 1960s and who lived there for thirty-two years, noted the detrimental impact of bottle-feeding on infants. He observed that infants who were not breastfed had high rates of diarrhea, respiratory and ear infections, and anemia. He also noted that breastfed infants were walking, on average, three months earlier than were formula-fed infants. In 1964, he became the first director of the Northern Medical Research Unit. As part of his role, he became an early advocate for a return to traditional Inuit practices of breastfeeding up until the age of 3 (Hankins 2000).

In the 1960s, a variety of social and cultural factors were influencing fashions in infant feeding. The national nutrition survey indicates that breastfeeding rates in the general population were extremely low but that there was enormous variation according to social class and region. In particular, and this is backed by anecdotal evidence, it appears that women in western Canada and women with formal educations were increasingly initiating breastfeeding. As women from higher socio-economic backgrounds were moving towards breastfeeding, Aboriginal women, among whom breastfeeding had been common, began to abandon the practice.

Reclaiming Breastfeeding

In Canada, interest in breastfeeding was rekindled in the 1960s and early 1970s by the emergence of the natural childbirth movement (hallmarks of which included the Lamaze method and La Leche League) and by the "second wave" of feminism. Although each of these movements was distinct, they did overlap in several ways, as each was part of a societal trend to question faith in scientific medicine and technological advancement as well as to emphasize the importance of women's experiences and knowledge. In one way or another, each movement sought to reclaim babies from experts. One of the founding members of La Leche League, Edwina Froehlich, commented, "The babies belonged to the doctors in those days … One of the things we said right from the beginning was, by golly, let's give the baby back to the mother" (quoted in Gorham and Andrews 1990).[1] These movements also re-emphasized the practice of breastfeeding by valuing the process and experience rather than just the desirable properties of breast milk.

By 1965, 99 percent of women were giving birth in a hospital environment. Initially, childbirth in hospital was viewed as safe and comfortable; however, increasingly, some women and physicians were viewing the process as cold, manipulative, and alienating. The use of interventions like forceps and anesthesia was no longer ideal and "modern." Long hospital stays and separate nurseries for infants, which originally had given women respite following birth, now felt like surveillance and meant that mothers returned home strangers to their own babies. The natural childbirth movement was one of the results of mothers' and physicians' questioning hospitalized birth.

The start of the natural childbirth movement is unofficially attributed to Dr. Grantley Dick Read, a British obstetrician who recognized that women often fare better when birthing at home than when birthing in hospital. He suggested that the fear and pain of childbirth that women experience was reinforced by the hospital environment, which provided isolation and pain medication rather than support, touch, and encouragement. In 1944, he published *Childbirth without Fear: The Principles and Practice of Natural Childbirth*. This book was read by many women in Europe and North America who were questioning current obstetrics practices. In 1959, the revised edition was published—the same year that an American woman, Marjorie Karmel, published *Thank You, Dr. Lamaze* (Kroeger 2004).

The early natural childbirth movement spread slowly by word of mouth, popular media, and physicians willing to change their practices in response to the demands of women (Sandelowski 1984). Natural childbirth had many meanings, including conscious childbirth, drug-free childbirth, educated childbirth, and "primitive" childbirth. Generally, these different viewpoints all regarded childbirth as a normal, family-centred event. Breastfeeding and rooming-in were two practices associated with natural childbirth (Sandelowski 1984). In 1949, Howes published an article in *Saturday Night* describing how the practice of rooming-in challenged hospital routines that separated mother and infant. Some of the benefits of rooming-in that she described included the need for fewer staff, less chance of epidemics, happier mothers, more involved fathers, and an opportunity for mothers to learn about their infants (Howes 1949). Articles on rooming-in and the relationship between natural childbirth and breastfeeding began to appear in the scientific and professional literature in the 1950s and early 1960s (e.g., Anderson 1954 and Newton and Newton 1970). Many of these articles recognized the adverse impact of medical interventions, especially complete anesthesia, on initiating breastfeeding.

In Canada, in the mid-1960s, there appeared to be a range of childbirth practices in hospitals. In some hospitals, fathers were permitted to stay with mothers during labour, and a few hospitals were beginning to practise rooming-in. In 1968, the federal government published a document entitled *Recommended Standards for Maternity and Newborn Care.* This guide for Canadian hospitals was developed by a subcommittee of the Maternal and Child Health Advisory Committee, with the support of the Canadian Anesthetists' Society, the Canadian Council on Hospital Accreditation, the Canadian Medical Association, the Canadian Nurses Association, the CPS, and the Society of Obstetricians and Gynaecologists of Canada. Although rather neutral on the subject of breastfeeding, the guide reflects some of the new discussions and shifts in childbirth practices: "The newer philosophy of obstetrical care places emphasis on the emotional as well as the physical aspects of childbirth. More attention is being given to the feelings and reactions of women during labor and at the time of delivery. With the newer approach to preparation of women for labor, fewer women are heavily sedated consequently more are able to participate with conscious effort during the final stages of labor and during delivery" (Child and Maternal Health Division 1968, 33). The standards reflect more awareness of the psychological experience of childbirth and a move away from heavily medicated childbirth. However, some of the standard procedures of care still included enemas, perineal shaves, perineal cleansing with a disinfectant solution every two hours, restricted food intake, and rectal examinations. Mothers were required to give birth in the lithotomy position, lying on their backs with their legs strapped into stirrups.

In terms of breastfeeding, the authors comment, "Encouragement and assistance should be given to the mother who wishes to breastfeed her baby" (Child and Maternal Health Division 1968, 48). This meant following the feeding routine outlined by the doctor, with the first feeding occurring eight to twelve hours after birth. Then, women were provided with the opportunity to breastfeed for two to three minutes every three or four hours, with the feeding time gradually increasing to ten minutes. The authors recognized that rooming-in was helpful to mothers learning to breastfeed. Further, "The mother who does not wish to breast feed her baby or who fails in the attempt because of psychological or physical reasons should not be made to feel guilty. These mothers require encouragement and help as they learn to give an artificial feeding" (Child and Maternal Health Division 1968, 125). The authors comment on one unexpected potential barrier to successful breastfeeding: "One common concern of nursing mothers is the bluish, watery appearance of breast milk. They expect their breasts to secrete milk comparable to cow's milk. They need to have the difference in color explained, before they have decided to discontinue nursing because of the appearance of breast milk" (Child and Maternal Health Division 1968, 124).

La Leche League International played a significant role in connecting breastfeeding and natural childbirth practices. In 1956, La Leche League was formed in Franklin Park, Illinois, by seven women. The name "La Leche" came from a shrine in St. Augustine, Florida, dedicated to a Spanish Madonna, Nuestra Senora de La Leche y Bueno Parto (loosely translated as Our Lady of Happy Delivery and Plentiful Milk). The league came to Canada in the early 1960s. The first groups started in Quebec and were followed by groups in Ontario and Alberta. By 1965, there were 5 groups in Canada (some of which are still in existence). By 1970, there were over 20 groups and 50 leaders; by 1976, 140 groups and 325 leaders (Audy 2004).

On 18 July 1968, the founder of the first group in the Toronto area wrote a letter to "Mrs. Thompson," the author of a women's advice column in *The Globe and Mail*. She described her own experiences, the mother-to-mother approach used by the league to support breastfeeding, and the early context of its formation:

> I am one of those women who always wanted to nurse her babies. I · got off to a terrible start in the hospital with our first baby, but one of my friends put me in touch with the then president of the Childbirth Education Association in Toronto. She had nursed four children and had taken upon herself the task of helping mothers who need another mother to give moral support and knowledge about the womanly art of breastfeeding. Within a week or so my sore nipples healed and our baby plainly preferred my milk to formula.

> I was so grateful to this mother that I asked her what I could do in
> return. She suggested that I form a La Leche League in Toronto. This
> I did a couple of years later (1965). In the meantime another woman
> formed a group in Weston, and since my group started, the mother who
> helped me has formed a league in Scarborough. There is one in Ajax,
> three in Hamilton, and also groups in Manitoba, Alberta, and Quebec.
> (Thompson 1968, W4)

The purpose of La Leche League was not to promote breastfeeding but to provide encouragement, information, and support to mothers who wanted to breastfeed. In part, the organization was a response to the dearth of information available on breastfeeding. According to one commentator, "There is no folklore in our society about breastfeeding so women who try it may feel isolated" (*Globe and Mail* 1964, W4). The league used a variety of formats to attempt to meet the needs of women. Mothers attended a series of home-based meetings led by a mother experienced in breastfeeding. At these meetings, women were able to share knowledge, gain a sense of connection to other mothers, and receive practical and emotional support for breastfeeding. The league also provided support by telephone and produced a manual entitled *The Womanly Art of Breastfeeding* (first published in 1958) (La Leche League International 1981).

When the league was formed, many of its ideas and perspectives were thought to be quite radical as they contrasted strongly with conventional medical wisdom. La Leche League challenged expert claims to breastfeeding with its mother-to-mother rather than physician-to-mother approach. Breastfeeding was not a medical issue but a "womanly art." The league valued the experience and wisdom of mothers rather than the expertise of physicians (Weiner 1994), and it challenged beliefs about the minimal difference between breastfeeding and bottle-feeding, arguing that there was an enormous difference. The league encouraged long periods of exclusive breastfeeding, delayed weaning, and later introduction of solids, and it argued against the use of feeding schedules and short feeding periods. It challenged "criticisms of breastfeeding ... from those who feel it's animal-like, and from puritan attitudes such as, 'if you nurse a baby getting close to a year it's not normal'" (*Globe and Mail* 1969). The league celebrated motherhood and the connection between mother and child and supported "good mothering through breastfeeding."

The "second wave" of feminist activity in Canada expressed dissatisfaction with scientific medicine and the devaluing of women's experiences (Clio Collective et al. 1987; Morrow 2007). Following the Second World War, it appeared that the early work of feminists on legal and political rights and opportunities for higher education and professional training had been partly achieved. Fertility rates for women in the late 1940s and throughout the

1950s accelerated, with the end of the war marking a return to domesticity (Pierson 1977; Prentice et al. 1988). However, feminist activity re-emerged with a vengeance in the late 1960s and early 1970s.

The immediate postwar period glorified women's roles as mothers and homemakers (Everitt 1998); however, by the 1960s, many women (primarily from the middle class) were questioning women's roles. The 1963 publication of Betty Friedan's *The Feminine Mystique* was considered by many to be a symbolic rebirth of feminism. This new wave of feminism brought attention to the lack of value placed on women's public and private nurturance (Black 1993). By 1967, women's rates of participation in the paid labour force had reached the same peak levels as they had during the Second World War. More and more women were experiencing the tension and strain of meeting high expectations both in the home and at work. Many lay organizations, such as Voice of Women and Toronto's New Feminists, worked to increase awareness of the impact of government policies on women's lives. Consciousness-raising and the mutual sharing of women's experiences led to discussions about solutions to women's common concerns. Throughout the 1960s and 1970s, women explored strategies for balancing work and motherhood and challenged the increasing trend towards everyday problems coming under medical jurisdiction.

Although the second wave feminist movement did not spend a lot of time discussing breastfeeding per se, it did highlight issues such as violence against women, abortion, and birth control. It drew attention to women's double roles and their work both inside and outside the home, and it raised issues about child care. It also worked to address the outright discrimination women faced while also recognizing issues relating to pregnancy and childbirth. The movement emphasized the importance of women's experiences and continued to challenge the institutional and political forces that shaped them (Clio Collective et al. 1987; Morrow 2007).

"Commerciogenic Malnutrition": International Interest in Breastfeeding and the Nestlé Boycott

For the most part, by the end of the Second World War, bottle-feeding with breast milk alternatives had been established as the norm in Canada, the United States, and, to a lesser extent, Europe. In the 1960s, partly as a response to declining birth rates in North America, infant formula companies turned their attention to less industrialized countries and intensified their promotion efforts (Ledogar 1975; The Bad News in Babyland 1972). Strategies used by infant formula companies included TV, billboards, radio, the distribution of free samples through doctors (who received gifts of equipment and research grants in exchange), and the use of "milk nurses" (i.e., women employed by the industry to visit new mothers in hospitals dressed in nurses' uniforms). Like earlier advertising messages in Canada, these promotional efforts suggested that formula use was supported by scientific medicine and that women's breast milk might be lacking in quality or quantity. Companies also played on the idea that, as breast milk alternatives were supposedly particularly good for sick and premature babies, they must also be good for healthy babies. In many colonized nations, infant formula became associated with the rich, the elite, and the modern, while breastfeeding was associated with the poor and the peasantry (Baumslag and Michels 1995).

Concerns about the decline of breastfeeding in developing countries occurred as early as the 1930s. In 1939 in Singapore, Dr. Cicely Williams made a Rotary Club presentation entitled "Milk and Murder." She argued that the increase in morbidity and mortality in infants in Singapore was directly related to the decline in breastfeeding and the use of inappropriate breast milk alternatives. Criticisms of the infant formula industry in developing countries continued to be published in the 1950s. These articles described a range of factors contributing to the decline of breastfeeding, including rapid social change, urbanization, the influence of Western ideas, and women's work that separated mother and child (Ermann and Clements 1984). Health workers, nutritionists, and missionaries warned about the detrimental effects of infant formula use. In the search for new markets, infant formula promotion efforts were encouraging mothers to abandon breastfeeding in places where there was insufficient cash for formula and bottles; a lack of sterilization equipment, fuel, and/or safe water; and high illiteracy rates, which precluded following the manufacturer's instructions. "'Bottle-baby disease,' the vicious–and often fatal–cycle of diarrhea, dehydration, and malnutrition ... was increasing in areas where previously the only real breastfeeding problem had been the death of a mother" (Baumslag and Michels 1995, 150).

In 1968, Dr. Derrick Jelliffe, at the time the director of the Caribbean Food and Nutrition Institute, coined the phrase "commerciogenic malnutrition" to describe the effects of the commercial promotion of infant feeding products. In 1970, Jelliffe and another international paediatrician, Bo Vahlquist, requested a meeting of the United Nations Protein Advisory Group (PAG) to discuss the problem.[2] This initial meeting was held behind closed doors and included twelve paediatricians, twelve industry representatives, and representatives from the UN, UNICEF, and the UN's Food and Agriculture Organization. The group continued to meet throughout the early 1970s to develop guidelines to address problems related to the increasing use of infant formula (Newton 1999).

Between 1973 and 1974, the issue moved beyond these quiet UN meetings and entered public discussion in a dramatic way. Public awareness of "commerciogenic malnutrition" had been increasing in the early 1970s through the educational efforts of development groups and churches. In 1973, the British magazine *New Internationalist* published an interview with two paediatricians, David Morley and Ralph Hendrikse, who had worked in Africa for many years. In March 1974, the British anti-poverty group War on Want published *The Baby Killer*, a pamphlet that was billed as an "Investigation into the Promotion and Sale of Powdered Milk in the Third World" and that highlighted the work of the Protein Advisory Group. *The Baby Killer* was translated into German by the Swiss Third World Action group (Arbeitsgruppe Dritte Welt), who renamed the report *Nestlé Kills Babies*. This report resulted in worldwide publicity and Nestlé filing a $5-million libel suit against the Third World Action Group.

In spite of publicity, law suits, and attempts at shareholder pressure, infant formula companies continued their marketing practices. Public awareness of the issue continued to grow, and a number of advocacy groups formed, including the Interfaith Centre for Corporate Responsibility. In Minneapolis, the Third World Institute at the Newman Centre, part of the University of Minnesota, organized study groups and talks about the issue. In many of the talks, a 1975 film entitled *Bottle Babies* was viewed. After seeing the film, many groups spontaneously called for a consumer boycott to challenge the apparent indifference of formula manufacturers. A student group at the University of Minnesota evolved into the Infant Feeding Action Coalition (INFACT). INFACT launched a boycott of Nestlé on 4 July 1977. Nestlé was chosen because it had the largest market share and, as a Swiss-based company, could not be influenced by shareholder resolutions. INFACT's (Chetley 1986) goal was to force Nestlé to halt all promotion of infant formula, including direct-to-consumer advertising, distribution of free samples to health care facilities and parents, promotion to health care workers, and the use of "milk nurses."

In early 1978, the boycott spread to Canada, New Zealand, and Australia. By 1980, it had spread to the United Kingdom; by 1981, to Sweden and West Germany; by 1982, to France. In Canada, organizations involved in the boycott included the Anglican Church of Canada, the United Church of Canada, the Canadian Religious Conference, the Canadian Nurses Association, the Toronto City Council, the Toronto Board of Health, and the Toronto Board of Education. Church groups in Canada were among the first advocacy groups to form around the issue. INFACT Canada grew out of the justice ministries of the Anglican Church and the United Church (Van Esterik 1989).

It is difficult to know the impact of the boycott on Nestlé. In 1979, Nestlé had 40 percent to 60 percent of the market in less industrialized countries, and world sales were $12 billion annually with 2 percent coming from infant formula sales (Hogan 1979a). At the time, Nestlé did not manufacture infant formula in Canada (Canadian Press 1980). However, in 1981, a Nestlé-commissioned market research survey in Toronto found that 30 percent of the population of two million people were aware of the boycott and that 10 percent were actively boycotting the company's products (Anonymous 1982a). Although the Canadian role in the boycott was relatively small, the Nestlé

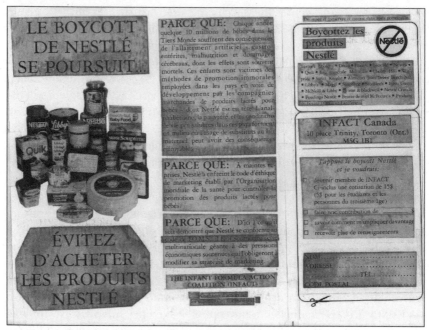

Figure 7.1   INFACT (Infant Feeding Action Coalition) Canada was formed at the end of the 1970s as a response to the international marketing practices of commercial infant formula manufacturers. Seen here is the French version of a Canadian Nestlé Boycott pamphlet. Image courtesy of INFACT Canada.

boycott is significant for a number of reasons. The issue of infant feeding resulted in the largest support for a boycott ever seen in North America. Furthermore, as a consumer movement, it drew attention to breastfeeding by focusing on how marketing of infant formula affects women's perceptions of their breasts, breast milk, and breastfeeding. And it raised questions about the acceptance and widespread use of infant formula (Van Esterik 1997).

"In Our Own Backyard": Bottle-Feeding in Aboriginal Communities

The Nestlé boycott raised awareness of the impact of infant formula in areas suffering poor socio-economic conditions, primarily in the developing world. But these conditions were not limited to countries abroad. Throughout the 1970s, reports on the detrimental effects of increasing use of infant formula in Aboriginal communities across Canada began to emerge. In a newspaper interview, Otto Schaefer commented on the parallels between the increasing uses of formula in developing countries and the increase in malnutrition, infection, and mortality occurring "right in our own backyard, the Canadian North" (*Globe and Mail* 1980, 5).

Throughout the 1960s and 1970s, research began to document the high infant mortality and infections rates in Aboriginal communities. One *Globe and Mail* article in 1981 drew attention to two studies demonstrating the impact of formula feeding on Aboriginal communities. A 1963 study cited showed that infant mortality rates in Aboriginal people could be reduced by one-third if babies were breastfed. Another study, which looked at Manitoba reserves between 1970 and 1974, reported that 60 percent of infant deaths on the reserves were due to respiratory infections and gastroenteritis (Kome 1981). A 1975 report by the Saskatchewan Council for International Co-operation estimated that the mortality rate of bottle-fed babies in Saskatchewan was 35 percent to 50 percent higher than that of breastfed babies (*Globe and Mail* 1980). In 1977, the Aboriginal infant mortality rate was twenty-six per one thousand live births, nearly double the rate in the general population (Kome 1981). A 1979 report released by the Anglican Church of Canada indicated that, as a result of bottle-feeding, Aboriginal infants were suffering higher rates of mortality, more hospital admissions, more gastroenteritis, and more middle-ear infections. It argued that, as Aboriginal women chose to bottle-feed, the risk of infant death increased by 40 percent (Hogan 1979b).

High rates of infant mortality were not the only concern resulting from increased bottle-feeding. Rates of otitis media, or middle-ear infections, were considered to have hit epidemic proportions in the 1970s. Estimates of the prevalence of ear infections in children in Arctic settlements were as high as 10 percent, with most children having had previous infections (Sallot 1979). Early explanations for these high rates had included examining the low level of humidity in northern climates, a lack of adequate health care, and genetic differences. Schaefer's studies in the 1970s demonstrated that bottle-fed Inuit infants were eight to ten times more likely to have otitis media than were breastfed infants. As breastfeeding duration increased, the risk of infection decreased. According to one article, "It's one of the major public health problems in the territories. And it's a problem caused by white people who convinced natives that it was better to bottlefeed their babies" (Sallot 1979, T8).

Rapid socio-cultural change was believed to be at the heart of the trend in the North towards bottle-feeding: "Dr. Spady points out that because of social upheaval, medical problems in the North are like those in developing countries. The infant death rates are the kind of thing one would expect. We're dealing to some extent with a developing country. It's called the Territories" (D. Jones 1980, 8). Contaminated water and an unstable supply of infant formula were two major concerns in the North. Sociologist Charles Hobart commented on the irony of having breastfeeding rates rise in southern Canada while they declined in northern Canada (D. Jones 1980). The increase in the use of infant formula mirrored the introduction of alcohol as well as processed and canned foods into Aboriginal people's diets. For some, the rise in the use of infant formula symbolized the changes occurring in Aboriginal communities (Neander and Morse 1989; Jasen 2002). Chief Ben Quill of Pikangikum in northwestern Ontario commented, "We no longer have our own midwives. Our mothers have to have operations to deliver their babies. Bottle-feeding makes many infants sick. Our elders say that is why the children do not respect their mothers. They are not brought up by their mothers, they are brought up by a cow" (Moore 1978, F4).

After studies in the 1960s and early 1970s consistently demonstrated a relationship between infant morbidity and mode of infant feeding, Schaefer and others in the North began to promote more and longer breastfeeding. They advocated a return to traditional infant feeding practices and attempted to counter new practices, such as giving infants sweets and drinks. During the 1970s, these efforts appeared to be quite successful. A study published in 1982 in the *Canadian Journal of Public Health* compared rates of breastfeeding in Inuit, First Nations, and non-Aboriginal mothers in the Northwest Territories between 1973–74 and 1978–79 (Schaefer and Spady 1982). During these years, the proportion of breastfed Inuit infants increased from 62 percent to 70 percent; breastfed First Nations infants increased from 33 percent to 43 percent; and breastfed non-Aboriginal infants increased from 49 percent to 68 percent. The mean duration of breastfeeding and the mean age at which bottle-feeding started also increased in all three groups over the five-year period. These findings paralleled the changes in breastfeeding rates in other parts of the country. On the other hand, the frequency of sweets consumption also increased in all three groups (Schaefer and Spady 1982). The study also found that the use of formula samples doubled in the Inuit and First Nations populations (5.1 percent to 9.9 percent and 15.5 percent to 32 percent, respectively) and remained high in the non-Aboriginal population (48.8 percent to 45.2 percent).

During the mid-1970s, Schaefer advocated for a solution to the apparent epidemic of intractable diarrhea in infants in babies on Baffin Island. Concern about high rates of anemia had resulted in a paediatric consultant at Montreal's McGill University issuing a policy that all babies on Baffin Island be given "supplemental iron." This resulted in an outbreak of diarrhea, which experts refused to acknowledge might be related to the iron supplements. When researchers at McGill University asked Health and Welfare Canada for $200,000 to help them find an answer to the epidemic, Schaeffer strongly advocated stopping the iron. This was done, and, two months later, there were no new cases; after a year, there were only a few sporadic cases. The iatrogenic epidemic was over (Hankins 2000). Schaefer continued to support introducing iron supplements after six months (Schaefer and Spady 1982).

The Revival of Breastfeeding

The data from the national survey provide a very accurate snapshot of breastfeeding practices in the late 1960s but little insight into whether or when the revival observed in the 1970s began. In contrast, data from a series of cross-sectional studies conducted between 1963 and 1973 (using

Table 7.1

Breastfeeding initiation rates by region, late 1960s and 1978

	Canada	BC	Prairies	Ontario	Quebec
1965–1971	26	41	33	33	11
1978	61	74	70	61	48
% increase between 1965–1971 period and 1978	135	80	112	85	336

Source: McNally, Hendricks, and Horowitz 1985; Myeres 1979.

mailed-out questionnaires and much less rigorously conducted than the national survey) indicate very little change in rates of initiation from 1963 to 1973 (McNally, Hendricks, and Horowitz 1985). However, the researchers reported that breastfeeding initiation rates across the country jumped from 36 percent in 1973 to 64 percent in 1979. In 1973, a marketing survey by Canada's Ross Laboratories reported that 35 percent of infants were breastfed during the first week of life. In 1976, surveys by Mead Johnson Company and Ross Laboratories found that 48 percent of infants in Canada were breastfed at the time of discharge from hospital (Canadian Paediatric Society Nutrition Committee and American Academy of Pediatrics Committee on Nutrition 1978; Canadian Paediatric Society 1978). A longitudinal survey conducted between 1977 and 1979 in Montreal and Toronto found that 71 percent of mothers initiated breastfeeding during the first week after birth (Yeung et al. 1981).[3]

However, breastfeeding initiation rates were not growing evenly across the country and in all population groups. In the 1960s, Quebec had the lowest rates, while British Columbia had the highest. By 1978, British Columbia's breastfeeding initiation rate had increased to 74 percent and was still the highest rate in the country. Quebec and the Atlantic provinces continued to trail behind the national average of 61 percent, with 48 percent of mothers initiating breastfeeding at birth. As is shown in Table 7.1, a revolution in infant feeding practices appears to have occurred during the 1970s in Quebec, where initiation rates increased by over 300 percent over the course of a decade or so. Changes in the Maritimes were also spectacular, with rates increasing by 220 percent during the same period (McNally, Hendricks, and Horowitz 1985).

The increase in breastfeeding rates also varied according to education. In 1977, McNally, Hendricks, and Horowitz (1985) found that more women with a higher level of education started and continued breastfeeding than did women with a lower level of education. Yeung et al. (1981) found that both father's and mother's education was statistically associated with breastfeeding–the higher the education, the more likely to engage in breastfeeding. In his survey of Toronto and Montreal mothers conducted between 1977 and 1979, of mothers who did not finish high school, 55.6 percent breastfed; of those who graduated from high school, 67.6 percent breastfed; of those who finished university, 80.1 percent breastfed; of those who finished graduate studies, 79.4 percent breastfed.

Breastfeeding duration rates were also increasing. A 1973 Ross Laboratories survey reported that 17 percent of infants were breastfed at three months and that 6 percent were breastfed at six months (Canadian Paediatric Society 1978). McNally, Hendricks, and Horowitz (1985) found that breastfeeding at six months increased from 17 percent in 1973 to 43 percent in 1979. And a survey conducted between 1977 and 1979 in Montreal and Toronto reported that 21 percent of mothers were breastfeeding at six months and 5 percent at twelve months (Yeung et al. 1981).

Parallel with the rise in breastfeeding rates was increasing support from public health and hospitals for breastfeeding initiation. Several local health departments and hospitals were favouring breastfeeding due to its convenience, cost, and immunological and nutritional benefits (Rozee 1976). Many physicians and nurses were advocating looser hospital rules, which encouraged rooming-in, sibling visits, and breastfeeding support (Bell 1979; Wallace 1980; Taggart 1976). Partly due to financial costs, the length of hospitalization following birth decreased in the 1970s to approximately five days (Prentice et al. 1988; Health Programs Branch 1975). Early discharge may have provided some mothers with the opportunity to be less dependent on feeding advice from their health care providers.

Official support for the revival in breastfeeding appeared to lag at the federal level. For example, the 1975 revised edition of *Recommended Standards for Maternity and Newborn Care* remained relatively neutral in its stance towards breastfeeding, although the authors did emphasize that a mother's request to breastfeed her child should be honoured. The authors supported the idea that infant feeding could improve bonding between mother and child: "The experience of being held for either breast or bottle-feeding is important for both mother and infant in providing emotional bonding ... In the case of breast feeding, the infant's sucking on the breast not only stimulates milk production by the infant's mother, but it also arouses her love for the infant and increases her confidence in herself as a mother. The mother finds relief of tension within the breast and the satisfaction of being loved, proving her dependability and gaining a feeling of competence" (Health and Welfare Canada 1975, 67). Interestingly, the authors commented on the phenomenon of bonding rather than on any other potential benefits of breastfeeding (e.g., nutrition, physical effects, and/or health outcomes).

For the most part, hospital feeding procedures following birth had changed relatively little since the late 1960s. According to the *Standards*, most infants should receive one to two feedings with sterile water following birth. After a few hours, breast- or bottle-feeding could be initiated.

La Leche League grew enormously during the 1970s. In 1970, there were 20 groups and 50 group leaders across the country. In 1976, there were 140 groups and 325 leaders (Audy 2004). Another report indicated that there were 300 branches of the league in Canada in 1977 (Cherry 1977). By 1981, there were 400 groups and 800 leaders. As well as continuing to provide mother-to-mother support through local groups, the Canadian La Leche League held its first national conference in 1972 at McMaster University in Hamilton, Ontario. The only La Leche League International Conference ever to be held outside the United States took place in Toronto from 14 to 16 July 1977: "Thousands of women from all over the world have put aside the prudishness, ignorance and medical indifference of the past and are now actively engaged in the promotion of the art of breast-feeding. La Leche League International drew 2,657 adult delegates to its annual conference in Toronto last year" (*Weekend Magazine* 1978). Approximately 900 infants under the age of three also attended the conference (Cherry 1977).

Nutrition in *The Canadian Mother and Child* (1979)

The third edition of *The Canadian Mother and Child* was edited in 1967 by Dr. Jean Webb and educational consultant Anne Burns (Lewis and Watson 1991/92). It was reprinted in 1968, 1969, 1970, 1971, and 1975. During these years, there were few changes in infant feeding advice. Breastfeeding was recommended for six months, solid foods were introduced at three months, and infants required supplements of vitamin C and D. The fourth edition of *The Canadian Mother and Child* was released in 1979 to coincide with the International Year of the Child. Although the newest edition reflected changes in attitudes towards contraception and parenthood, it remained relatively impartial on the subject of breastfeeding: "Because of the differences in infants, families and their circumstances, there is no one correct way of feeding all infants" (Canada, Department of National Health and Welfare 1979, 140).

As in previous editions, the authors of the 1979 edition recognized the value of breastfeeding and the fact that many mothers chose not to breastfeed: "Despite the great value of breast feeding, too few mothers breast feed their babies. They may not fully appreciate its importance and the advantages of breast milk over cow's milk; they may not be able to do so for medical reasons; often mothers are not sufficiently encouraged by the medical profession to breastfeed. It may not be possible to do so away from home, especially if mothers are working. In addition, it may be that mothers sense that breast feeding is not considered socially acceptable in their community"

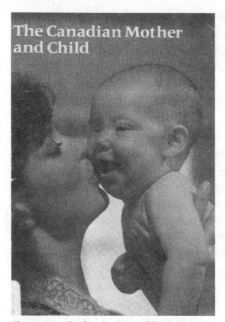

The Canadian Mother and Child

Figure 7.2   The fourth edition of *The Canadian Mother and Child* was released in 1979 to coincide with the International Year of the Child. The 1979 edition advised mothers to breastfeed exclusively for four to six months. *The Canadian Mother and Child*, 1979.

(Canada, Department of National Health and Welfare 1979, 150–51). The 1979 *The Canadian Mother and Child* advised mothers to breastfeed exclusively for four to six months (an increase of one to three months from the third edition) and to use vitamin D supplements.

The new edition also reflected the growing interest in nutrition in the 1970s, especially with respect to concerns about fats, sugar intake, and fortification. The first national survey on nutrition occurred in the early 1970s, and the links between nutrition and chronic disease were frequently discussed in policy arenas. The 1979 *The Canadian Mother and Child* commented on the importance of correct infant nutrition: "Towards these ends, greater attention is now being paid to encourage and help mothers breast feed their infants. Also, parents are encouraged to refrain from introducing solid foods too early, from over-feeding baby and giving him overly sweet formula and other foods" (Canada, Department of National Health and Welfare 1979, 140).

The manual described a variety of alternatives to breastfeeding, including commercial infant formulas (e.g., ready-to-feed formulas, concentrated formulas, and powdered formulas as well as traditional cow's-milk formulas). Different milk types required various forms of vitamin supplementation. Mothers using a canned evaporated-milk formula were supposed to supplement it with iron at four to six months. Mothers using a whole cow's-milk formula were to supplement with iron and vitamin C as well as vitamin D if the milk was not fortified. Mothers were warned, due to multiple nutrient deficiencies, not to use whole cow's milk, skim milk, or 2 percent milk to feed their infants (Canada, Department of National Health and Welfare 1979). Two percent milk and skim milk were becoming increasingly popular for adult consumption due to their reduced fat content. It was believed that many mothers assumed that if it was healthy for adults, then it would also be healthy for infants (Myres 1980).

Table 7.2

Changes in recommended length of breastfeeding, age of introduction of solids, and the suggested supplements in *The Canadian Mother and Child* (1923, 1940, 1967, 1979)

Year	Recommended length of breastfeeding	Age of introduction of solids	Suggested supplements
1923	9 months	10 months	Boiled water, from birth
			Fruit juice, from one month
1940	6 months	2 ½–3 months	Boiled water, from birth
			Cod liver oil, from second week
			Orange or tomato juice, from second month
			Iron, from 3 months (in food)
1967	6 months	2 ½–3 months	Vitamin C, from two weeks
			Vitamin D, from one week
1979	9–12 months	3 months	Vitamin C, from three weeks
			Vitamin D, from birth if breastfeeding (formula is fortified)
			Iron, from 4 months
			Fluoride, if not contained in water supply

"What Is Left besides the Poetry?": The Scientific Rediscovery of Breastfeeding

The field of nutrition was not the only science taking an interest in breastfeeding. In the 1970s, the pace of scientific research on breastfeeding increased. A paper in the middle of 1978 estimated that there had been over 150 papers on breastfeeding published in the preceding nine months (Myres 1979a). In the late 1970s, several professional health associations and scientific working groups began to issue official statements in renewed support of breastfeeding. In particular, two statements in 1978–the first an article entitled "Breastfeeding: What Is Left besides the Poetry?" by the CPS, the second a joint commentary by the CPS and the American Academy of Paediatrics (AAP)–were clear indications that the tide had turned. Scientific medicine clearly supported and recognized the superiority of breastfeeding.

Throughout the 1970s, discussions in the popular press and in medical journals examined the issue of breastfeeding. An abstract reprinted in the

Canadian Medical Association Journal entitled "Breastfeeding: Should It Be Recommended?" commented on how the value of breastfeeding had been proven forty to fifty years before. The author summarized the newly emerging research on the protection breastfeeding offered against gastrointestinal and respiratory infections and then asked, "Does our growing appreciation for the value of breast-feeding have any relevance today, particularly as formulas are now relatively safe bacteriologically?" (Gerrard 1975, 138). He argued that if we did not encourage breastfeeding, then physicians would continue to treat preventable and needless illnesses.

One Saskatchewan doctor encouraged physicians to stop being neutral about breastfeeding when speaking with mothers. Breastfeeding was clearly superior and physicians should advocate for the infant who was really an "innocent bystander" of his or her mother's decisions (Hollobon 1975, 12). A statement by the AAP received some media attention in Canada. The AAP committee on nutrition advised the public that formula was an adequate substitute for breast milk. It cautioned "against issuing dire warnings" to mothers who were not able to breastfeed their babies. However, doctors "should not unconsciously encourage a negative attitude toward breast-feeding" (Associated Press 1976, 11).

In January 1978, the nutrition committee of the CPS published a statement in the *Canadian Journal of Public Health* advocating exclusive breastfeeding for three to six months with a supplement of vitamin D. Later that year, in October, at the initiation of the CPS, the CPS and the AAP published a joint statement in the journal *Pediatrics*:

> For much of the population in developing countries, both economic and health considerations speak conclusively for breast-feeding. The physiologic role of breast-feeding has received less emphasis in the industrialized world because of low morbidity and mortality of bottle-fed infants, which has resulted from nutritional and technological advances in the formulation and manufacture of infant formulas as well as from the higher standards of housing, sanitation, and public health services in these countries. However, newer information suggests that significant advantages still exist for the breast-fed infant. (Canadian Paediatric Society Nutrition Committee and American Academy of Pediatrics Committee on Nutrition 1978, 591)

The evaluation of the scientific evidence for breastfeeding led to a discussion of ways of promoting the practice. Suggestions offered by the CPS nutrition committee for encouraging breastfeeding included education for children, nurses, physicians, and pregnant women. The fact that "breastfeeding is no longer routine in our hospitals" (Canadian Paediatric Society 1978, 17) was acknowledged: "Efforts should be made to change routine practices which are known to interfere with successful lactation. These include: the use of large amounts of sedation and/or anaesthesia during labour and delivery since they markedly impair sucking in the baby; separation of the nursing couple for the first 24 hours; a rigid 3–4 hourly schedule; and routine offering of supplementary bottles" (Canadian Paediatric Society 1978, 17–18). The committee also encouraged closer consultation between maternity services and members of La Leche League and the Human Lactation Centre (which was founded in 1975 to coordinate worldwide efforts to promote breastfeeding). It also made recommendations to work towards countering the influence of infant formula manufacturers. It acknowledged that many women work outside the home and advocated that all women receive a statutory maternity leave of twelve weeks and that government and industry should provide daycare close to work.

In 1979, as part of efforts to support the International Year of the Child, the Department of National Health and Welfare and the provincial departments of health made breastfeeding a priority issue. The CPS also adopted breastfeeding as its theme issue and established a task force to promote breastfeeding (Myres 1981). In 1979, the nutrition committee of the CPS, with the involvement of several consultants from the federal government and researchers as well as a liaison with the Canadian Dietetic Association, published another statement on infant feeding summarizing the scientific case for breastfeeding (Canadian Paediatric Society 1979). By the end of the decade, scientific medicine had clearly acknowledged the superiority of breastfeeding.

Conclusion

During the 1970s, nationally, breastfeeding initiation rates grew from approximately 25 percent to 65 percent. Interest in breastfeeding from lay organizations such as La Leche League and groups in the natural childbirth movement preceded the second wave of feminism in the late 1960s. The late 1960s and early 1970s marked a period in which women began to revive breastfeeding knowledge outside the sphere of scientific medicine. International interest and advocacy regarding the aggressive marketing strategies of infant formula companies in the developing world contributed to growing discussions among new mothers, health professionals, and government regarding the value of breastfeeding and ways to encourage it. However, by the time the scientific and medical community and state became re-engaged in issues of breastfeeding at the end of the 1970s, community interest in the practice had already taken off, and breastfeeding rates were increasing. The dramatic rise in breastfeeding in the 1970s appears to have been driven more by a variety of social, cultural, and political movements than it did from health professionals and the federal government, who did not get involved until the resurgence in breastfeeding was well under way in the next decade.

Chapter 8

Promoting Breastfeeding, 1980–90

A t the beginning of the 1980s, the federal government launched a national campaign to promote breastfeeding. This campaign brought together a range of activists, health professionals, and mothers, and it contributed to changing beliefs, values, and practices associated with breastfeeding. An article by Health and Welfare Canada official Tony Myres was published in the *Canadian Consumer* in 1979. In their introduction to the article, the editors of the magazine wrote, "In our guilt-ridden society, where breasts are exclusively identified with sex, breast-feeding has been relegated to the washroom in many locales. That this attitude is wrong is easy enough to say; changing it will not be easy, as A.W. Myres points out. Time, perhaps, to bring babies suckling at their mothers' nippies off the pages of National Geographic and into Canadian society" (Myres 1979b, 12). In the 1980s, breastfeeding promotion became part of ongoing efforts by health professionals to gain support for breastfeeding, international initiatives to regulate the infant formula industry, and the growing family-centred childbirth movement. Unlike in the 1920s, in the 1980s the promotion campaign was directed at all women and occurred at a time when a strong movement towards breastfeeding had already been initiated. It also garnered support from health organizations, health professionals, and La Leche League.

A National Promotion Campaign

Following the release of the 1978 CPS position paper in the *Canadian Journal of Public Health*, the federal government launched a national campaign to promote breastfeeding. With the endorsement of eight professional societies that were members of the Canadian Science Committee on Food and Nutrition, this paper was considered "a catalyst for the generation of a national commitment to the promotion of breastfeeding" (Myres 1988, 101). The task force assigned to the campaign included members from the Society of Obstetricians and Gynaecologists of Canada, the Department of National

Health and Welfare, and La Leche League Canada. National strategies for the promotion of breastfeeding included (1) improving the quality, timing, and targeting of breastfeeding information to both health care professionals and the public; (2) stimulating professional support for breastfeeding within the health care system; (3) forming national alliances from government, professional, and voluntary sectors to create a national emphasis on breastfeeding; (4) supporting mothers' groups and citizen coalitions; (5) developing a national advocacy position to culminate in a national policy position on breastfeeding; and (6) monitoring and influencing patterns of breastfeeding in Canada through policies and practice (Myres 1988).

The national campaign to promote breastfeeding was launched in 1979. Although this represented the federal government's first visible support for breastfeeding since the 1920s, some individuals in Health and Welfare Canada and the CPS had shown interest in breastfeeding promotion in the early 1970s. However, it was thought that, without a strong, authoritative position paper from the medical profession, national programming to support breastfeeding would fail: "It was believed that if first the medical profession could be influenced to be more supportive in motivating women to breastfeed and secondly, that if this was followed up with practical and helpful advice, a significant step forward would be made which would have a cascading effect throughout the health care system" (Myres 1988, 101).

Subsequently, the first phase of the national campaign focused on increasing professional awareness of breastfeeding. Without professional and institutional support, it was admitted that mothers' knowledge about the value of breastfeeding would do little to increase actual breastfeeding rates (Myres 1979b). The professional awareness campaign took the form of an information kit directed at health professionals, including physicians, public health nurses, and hospital staff. The kit included the 1979 CPS/AAP position paper, a paper on the practical management of breastfeeding, a fact sheet on breastfeeding, a fact folder on La Leche League, and a contact sheet containing provincial sources of information and teaching aids. The kit also contained a poster that could be used in offices, clinics, and waiting rooms and letters of endorsement from the minister of National Health and Welfare and the president of the CPS (Myres, Watson, and Harrison 1981).

In November 1979, 40,000 kits were distributed to health professionals across the country. By March 1980, another 23,000 were distributed in response to requests (Myres, Watson, and Harrison 1981). One of the primary goals of the professional awareness campaign was to increase the knowledge and skills of health professionals. Although there were few studies of physician knowledge of breastfeeding, one study in British Columbia showed physicians scoring highly with regard to the encouragement of breastfeeding (it is possible that this correlated with the high rates of breastfeeding initiation in British Columbia) (Myres 1981). Other goals included increasing contact between professionals and La Leche League and encouraging health professionals to "advertise" breastfeeding by utilizing the kit's poster. An evaluation of the program found that 90 percent of public health nurses but only 50 percent of physicians and hospitals received the kit. The professionals who did receive the kit found it to be helpful and used it for self-education and for counselling mothers. There was a high degree of interest in receiving further information on other aspects of infant feeding as well as a desire for a practical booklet that could be shared with mothers (Myres, Watson, and Harrison 1981; Myres 1983).

Such a booklet was already in development. Following the professional awareness program, a public information campaign began. The campaign used a variety of mechanisms to promote breastfeeding to mothers and the general public. A booklet containing information on breastfeeding for new mothers was developed in partnership with the CPS and La Leche League and was published under the joint authorship of these two organizations. The cover of the booklet had the same image as did the cover of the professional awareness kits–a woman breastfeeding. Entitled "Breastfeeding" and adapted from La Leche League International materials ("Why Breastfeed Your Baby" and "When You Breastfeed Your Baby"), the booklet described some of the benefits of breastfeeding but focused on providing practical advice, addressing emotional challenges, and suggesting where to get support (see Figure 8.1).

The original purpose of the booklet was not to influence the decision to breastfeed but, rather, to ensure that mothers who chose to breastfeed had the necessary information for successful breastfeeding. Thus, mothers who were immediately postpartum were the target audience. When considering which distribution method would have the greatest impact, the Department of Health and Welfare Canada examined the successes of the infant formula industry in reaching mothers (Myres 1983). The department chose to use a hospital distribution system and collaborated with the commercial marketing company Gift-Pax Canada to distribute the booklet to new mothers in hospital. Beginning in March 1981 and continuing until 1983, over 300,000 copies were distributed to individual mothers each year. An evaluation of the booklet found that one of its most noteworthy messages for mothers was "The more you nurse, the more milk you will have." This message was key in addressing concerns about the adequacy of a mother's milk supply and the relationship between anxiety and the inhibition of the letdown reflex. The direct distribution of the booklet to new mothers in hospital was discontinued in 1983 but was re-established in a different form in 1985: the booklet was redesigned into a magazine entitled *Chatelaine's New Mother* and was distributed to the majority of Canada's maternity hospitals (Myres 1988).

In addition to written materials, the Department of National Health and Welfare also chose to develop audiovisual resources in order to promote

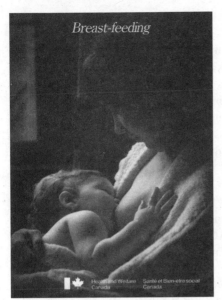

Figure 8.1 Breastfeeding ... the best start in life. This image was used as a logo for the breastfeeding promotion campaign in the early 1980s. Cover image of the *Breastfeeding ... the best start in life* pamphlet in the Breastfeeding Information Kit, Public Health Agency of Canada, 1985. Reproduced with the permission of the Minister of Public Works and Government Services Canada, 2008.

breastfeeding in group situations. Taking advantage of the partnership between the federal government and the National Film Board (NFB), the department purchased numerous copies of the film *The Breastfeeding Experience*, which was then distributed to libraries across Canada. In 1982, the first Canadian film on breastfeeding, *A Moveable Feast*, was produced and was again purchased by the Department of National Health and Welfare and made available through the NFB. The department and the NFB also collaborated on developing a French-language film on breastfeeding: *Le doux partage* was released by the NFB in 1983. It was estimated that by 1988, 150,000 health professionals and new or expectant mothers had viewed these films (Myres 1988), which were part of public discussions and changing views on breastfeeding. As one article commented on responses to *A Moveable Feast*, "Because breastfeeding has traditionally had negative connotations, the subject has been cloaked in silence. As a result, even the most informed and enthusiastic women reveal that they came in for a few surprises, and it's hard to avoid feeling that most men seem vaguely uneasy about the whole process" (Finlayson 1982, F8).

After the initial distribution of the booklet, the Department of National Health and Welfare utilized two other distribution methods. As it was well known that decisions about breastfeeding were generally made prior to birth, the department distributed the booklet to health professionals. In March 1981, a sample copy of the booklet and a "Dear Doctor/Colleague" letter was mailed to physicians, hospitals, and public health units across the country. In 1981, the subsequent demand for sample copies of the booklet required that a further 300,000 copies be printed. The booklet also accompanied video rentals from the NFB. It was available on request, and many of the provinces also requested permission to reprint it. By 1984, over 550,000 copies were distributed (Myres 1983).

Implementing the WHO Code—or Not

During the 1970s, public awareness and concern about the marketing of infant formulas continued to grow. One of the outcomes of this awareness and advocacy was the Nestlé Boycott, which had started in 1977 and continued into the 1980s. Another outcome was the development of an international code to regulate the promotion of baby foods. The federal government and various Canadian advocacy groups participated in the events leading up to the development of the WHO/UNICEF Code of Marketing of Breastmilk Substitutes (the WHO Code) in May 1981. The federal government endorsed the· code and various initiatives, and throughout the 1980s it attempted to implement the code's provisions.

The publicity surrounding the Nestlé Boycott in the United States eventually came to the attention of Senator Edward Kennedy. Kennedy, the chairman of the Senate Subcommittee on Health and Scientific Research, decided to hold a hearing in May 1978 on the promotion of infant formula in developing countries. The congressional hearings intensified public awareness of the issues (some parts were televised) and led to heated discussion and debate. At one point, Oswaldo Ballerin, president of Nestlé Brazil, stated, "The U.S. Nestlé Company has advised me that their research indicates that this [boycott] is actually an indirect attack on the free world's economic system. A world-wide church organization, with the stated purpose of undermining the free enterprise system, is in the forefront of this activity" (Baumslag and Michels 1995, 160). This statement was greeted with laughter and Kennedy's response that a boycott was a "recognized tool in a free democratic society."

After the hearings, Kennedy concluded that unilateral action by the U.S. government against American-based infant formula companies might not be the best course of action. He suggested that an international problem required an international solution (Chetley 1986). He referred the issue to the World Health Organization (WHO), with a recommendation to the director-general, Dr. Halfdan Mahler, that a special meeting be convened under the WHO. The WHO/UNICEF Meeting on Infant and Young Child Feeding was held in October 1979 and included representatives from government, industry, non-governmental organizations (NGOs), and various professionals. This unique meeting resulted in a "blue book" containing a series of recommendations to promote and protect breastfeeding. These recommendations were endorsed by the World Health Assembly in May 1980. One of the recommendations was for the development of an international code of marketing conduct for the formula industry. Another outcome of the meeting, which occurred outside the official proceedings, was the formation of the International Baby Food Action Network (IBFAN). IBFAN was founded on 12 October 1979 and included representatives from six NGOs, including INFACT, Oxfam, War on Want, Arbeitsgruppe Dritte Welt (Third World Action Working Group), and the Interfaith Center on Corporate Responsibility.

Table 8.1

Summary of international code of marketing of breast milk substitutes

- No advertising of these products to the public.

- No free samples to mothers.

- No promotion of products in health care facilities.

- No company mothercraft nurses to advise mothers.

- No gift or personal samples to health workers.

- No words or pictures idealizing artificial feeding, including pictures of infants, on the labels or Products.

- Information to health care workers should be scientific and factual.

- All information on artificial infant feeding, including labels, should explain the benefits of breastfeeding, and the costs and hazards associated with artificial feeding.

- Unsuitable products, such as sweetened condensed milk, should not be promoted for babies.

- All products should be of a high quality and take account of the climatic and storage conditions of the Country where they are used.

Source: Health Canada 2000.

On 21 May 1981, the thirty-fourth World Health Assembly adopted the International Code of Marketing of Breast-milk Substitutes, which aimed to "provide safe and adequate nutrition for infants, by the protection and promotion of breastfeeding, and by ensuring the proper use of breast milk substitutes when these are necessary, on the basis of adequate information and through appropriate marketing and distribution." The code imposed strict guidelines that prohibited the promotion of infant formula to the public, the promotion of infant formula through health care systems, and direct contact between formula companies and mothers. It also ensured the proper labelling of all products, describing the benefits of breastfeeding and the dangers of infant formula (see Table 8.1). The WHO urged all member states to translate the code into national legislation, regulations, or other suitable measures; to involve all concerned groups in its implementation; and to monitor compliance. The code was intended as a *minimum* requirement, and individual governments were encouraged to strengthen its provisions.

The Canadian government endorsed the code. Although some parts of it were directed at developing countries, the aspects most relevant to Canada related to professional support for breastfeeding, hospital policies and practices, and the direct marketing of infant formula through sample donations. In terms of implementation, Canada did not translate the WHO Code into legislation (e.g., through the Food and Drugs Act), preferring to support voluntary agreements. Myres (1981), a senior program officer in the Department of National Health and Welfare, commented on the role of the federal government in applying the WHO Code, arguing that, at the federal level, the government's role in health was confined to sharing fiscal arrangements for health care and health promotion activities as defined by the British North America Act, according to which the delivery of health care and services is determined by the provincial government. It appeared that the federal government would not implement most aspects of the code.

The devolution of hospital policy to the provincial and local levels was a critical point with regard to the WHO Code provision that received the most attention in Canada: the distribution of free samples of infant formula in hospitals. In 1981, the *Globe and Mail* conducted a cross-Canada survey. Quebec was the only provincial government willing to enforce the aspects of the code that applied to Canada: "Some provinces will rely on moral suasion. Others are not willing to interfere with hospital autonomy and a couple of provinces don't want to step on the toes of free enterprise" (Makin 1981, 5). Quebec used legislation to end formula distribution, but the rest of the provinces intended to leave decisions up to individual hospital boards (*Globe and Mail* 1981). By 1981, in the relatively few hospitals under federal jurisdiction (primarily in the Yukon and Northwest Territories), the distribution of free samples was discontinued (Myres 1981).

Discussions regarding the implementation of the WHO Code paralleled growing research on how infant formula marketing affected the duration of breastfeeding. Researchers at Montreal General Hospital conducted a randomized, controlled clinical trial that provided new mothers with free sample packs of infant formula prior to discharge. Packets included a bottle, a can of ready-to-feed formula, a can of formula powder, a reusable plastic nipple, and three small information booklets. The researchers found that "sample" mothers were less likely to be breastfeeding at one month (78 percent versus 84 percent) and more likely to have introduced solid foods by two months (18 percent versus 10 percent). This finding was particularly significant when three groups of women were considered–first-time mothers, mothers with little education, and mothers who reported postpartum illness (Bergevin 1983).

More conclusive evidence came from the first national survey of Canadian infant feeding patterns (Health and Welfare Canada 1985). The 1982 survey was implemented due to a lack of nationally available data and a desire to respond to requests from the WHO and other international organizations as well as citizen and action groups for information on Canadian action to support the WHO Code. The survey revealed that 71 percent of all mothers received a free sample of commercial infant formula in hospital. There appeared to be regional differences, with rates being higher in Alberta and lower in Manitoba and Saskatchewan. The survey examined the age at which breastfeeding stopped in relation to whether or not mothers received a formula sample. Within the first month, almost three times as many mothers

Graph 8.1

Breastfeeding and age when first used supplement of infant formula in relation to receipt of free formula sample, Canada, 1982

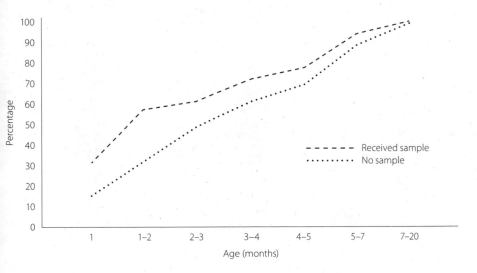

Source: Breastfeeding and Age When First Used Supplement of Infant Formula in Relation to Receipt of Free Formula Sample, Canada, 1982. *Canadian Infant Feeding Patterns: Results of a National Survey, 1982,* included in the Breastfeeding Information Kit, Public Health Agency of Canada, 1985. Reproduced with the permission of the Minister of Public Works and Government Services Canada, 2008.

gave up breastfeeding in the "sample" group as in the "no sample" group. Mothers who received a sample were much more likely to introduce formula sooner than were mothers who did not receive a sample. Further, the sample that mothers received in hospital had a clear influence on the brand choice of the first formula used. The donation of a particular brand of infant formula by a hospital resulted in the choice of that brand by 80 percent to 90 percent of mothers.

Although the federal government had taken the stance that it could not directly influence the provinces to adhere to the WHO Code, Health and Welfare Canada developed a hospital awareness kit to encourage changes in hospital policies and practices. With input from La Leche League, UNICEF Canada, the Health League of Canada (a citizens' coalition of the WHO), and various professional organizations, the hospital awareness kit was designed to target key health professionals within the hospital system. The advocacy kit contained an interpretive guide to the WHO Code, a research study from the *Lancet* on the influence of formula samples on the duration of breastfeeding, and other tools designed to facilitate change (Myres 1988). It was distributed in March 1985. A 1989 survey found that 75 percent of health

Graph 8.2

Type of formula first introduced by breast-feeding mothers in relation to the brand of sample received from the hospital, 1982

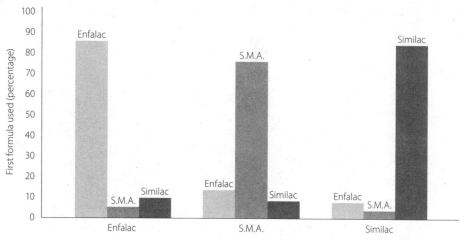

Brand of free sample received from hospital

Source: Type of Formula First Introduced by Breastfeeding Mothers in Relation to the Brand of Sample Received from the Hospital. *Canadian Infant Feeding Patterns: Results of a National Survey, 1982,* included in the Breastfeeding Information Kit, Public Health Agency of Canada, 1985. Reproduced with the permission of the Minister of Public Works and Government Services Canada, 2008.

professionals were aware of the WHO Code and had received information through federal educational initiatives. However, a 1992 survey found that this national campaign had only a small impact on professional practices: 11.7 percent of health professionals had discontinued giving out formula company literature to new or expectant mothers, and 25 percent had stopped giving mothers formula samples (INFACT Canada 2001).

New Trends: Culture, Place, and Formula

By 1982, breastfeeding initiation and duration rates had increased dramatically across the country. A national survey undertaken by Health and Welfare Canada in 1982 reported a national breastfeeding initiation rate of 69.4 percent (Health and Welfare Canada 1985) compared to 60 percent in 1978 (McNally, Hendricks, and Horowitz 1985) and 26 percent in 1965–71 (Myeres 1979). Most of the growth in breastfeeding initiation occurred between the early and the late 1970s (Graph 8.3). The second spurt in initiation rates, from 1978 to 1982, unlike the dramatic resurgence of the 1970s, was small and even across the regions.

Between 1977 and 1982, McNally, Hendricks, and Horowitz (1985) found that, as in prior surveys, while more women with higher levels of education

Graph 8.3

Breastfeeding initiation rates by region, 1965–71, 1978, 1982

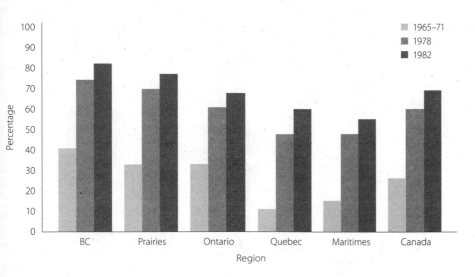

Source: Breastfeeding initiation rates by region, 1965–71, 1978, 1982. *Sources:* Health and Welfare Canada 1985; McNally, Hendricks, and Horowitz 1985; Myeres 1979.

started and continued breastfeeding than did women with lower levels of education, the gap in breastfeeding initiation rates between these groups also narrowed. Breastfeeding among women who were least educated grew more rapidly than it did among better-educated women, increasing by 58 percent from 1977 to 1982. In contrast, among the two categories of women who were most educated (women who had attended or completed college and women who had attended or completed university), breastfeeding increased more slowly, at 22 percent and 18 percent, respectively, over this five-year period (McNally, Hendricks, and Horowitz 1985). As in earlier national surveys, in 1982 there remained a clear east-west gradient, with the lowest rates in the Maritimes (57.6 percent) and the highest rates in British Columbia (82.9 percent) (Health and Welfare Canada 1985).

Duration rates also appeared to be increasing. In 1973, McNally, Hendricks, and Horowitz (1985) reported that 31 percent of mothers breastfed for at least four months; in 1982, 59 percent of mothers breastfed for at least four months. They found that, in 1982, the duration of breastfeeding tended to be shorter in Quebec and the longest in British Columbia and the Prairies. The national 1982 survey also suggested that overall duration was increasing across the country: 28 percent of all mothers stopped breastfeeding within the first two months, while 75 percent stopped within six months. It also found regional

Graph 8.4

National breastfeeding initiation and duration

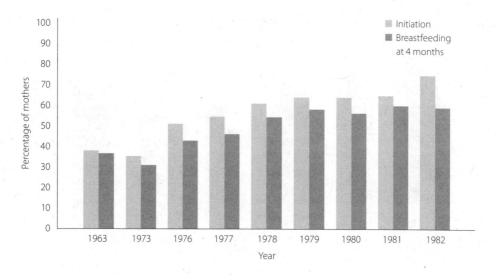

Source: National Breastfeeding Initiation and Duration Rates, 1963–1982. Based on data from McNally, Hendricks, and Horowitz 1985.

differences in breastfeeding duration, albeit slightly different from the findings of McNally, Hendricks, and Horowitz. Duration tended to be longer in the Prairie provinces and shorter in the Atlantic region and British Columbia (Health and Welfare Canada 1985). Overall, "nationally, nearly twice as many mothers were breastfeeding in hospital in 1982 as in 1963 and for each mother breastfeeding at 6 months in 1963, 4.4 mothers were doing so in 1982" (McNally, Hendricks, and Horowitz 1985) (see Graph 8.4).

Data on infant mortality at the end of the nineteenth century had suggested differences in breastfeeding practices between francophone and various anglophone groups. The 1982 national survey found that 55 percent of French-speaking women in Canada initiated breastfeeding, compared to 73 percent of English-speaking mothers (Myres 1988). Other evidence suggested that breastfeeding among francophones was generally less prevalent than it was among other groups (Health and Welfare Canada 1990). For example, a study in New Brunswick in 1982–83 found that approximately 20 percent more English than French infants were breastfed at birth, and this difference was maintained for up to six months. The authors of the study believed that this was a reflection of socio-economic status, as most mothers of French background were of a lower socio-economic status than were mothers with an English background (Beaudry and Aucoin-Larade 1989). However, other studies conducted at the time (and as clearly shown in the infant mortality studies that focused on nineteenth-century Montreal) suggest that these differences were also likely strongly related to cultural factors.

A longitudinal study between 1977 and 1979 in Montreal found that 77 percent of the anglophone mothers in Montreal attempted to breastfeed, compared to 61 percent of the francophone mothers. In Ottawa-Carleton in 1984, the average rate of breastfeeding initiation was 76 percent. This study, like others, showed that social class was related to feeding choice: mothers of higher social class were more likely to breastfeed. As well, a higher proportion of anglophone mothers breastfed their infants (81 percent) than francophones (59 percent) or mothers who were neither anglophone nor francophone (75 percent). Echoing the studies conducted in Montreal in the nineteenth century (see Chapter 1), although more than one-third of the mothers in this last group were in the lowest socio-economic status (SES) category, their breastfeeding initiation and duration rates were much higher than those of the francophone mothers who were socio-economically better off (Greene-Finestone et al. 1989). A 1992 study in the Sudbury area also found that anglophone mothers tended to breastfeed longer than did francophone mothers (Bourgoin et al. 1997).

Promotional messages in the 1980s attempted to convey three key concepts: "to promote breastfeeding, to favour prepared infant formula as the best alternative to human milk, and to stress the potentially deleterious effects of early weaning to unmodified cow's milk and solid foods" (Myres 1980, 11). The 1982 national survey provided information on trends in solids introduction and type of breast milk alternatives used by non-breastfeeding mothers. The survey found that almost 30 percent of breastfed infants had been introduced to cow's milk or formula supplement by one month and that 45 percent had been introduced to it by 2 months (Health and Welfare Canada 1985). Twenty-five percent of these mothers used cow's milk, while 75 percent used commercial infant formula. For bottle-fed infants, 98.4 percent of infants began with commercial infant formula. Approximately 60 percent of these infants had stopped formula feeding by six months. When infants were switched from their first formula, 82 percent were introduced to cow's milk, while 18 percent were switched to another type of commercial infant formula. Whole cow's milk and 2 percent milk were the most common types of milk introduced (Health and Welfare Canada 1985). The survey also showed differences in the age of introduction of solids between infants who were breastfed and infants who were bottle-fed. Twenty percent of breastfed infants were introduced to solids by two months, while 40 percent of bottle-fed infants were introduced to solids by two months. However, by six months, there was little difference between the two groups, and most infants (86 percent to 90 percent) had been introduced to solids (Health and Welfare Canada 1985). Overall, more infants were being introduced to commercial infant formulas than was the case in the late 1960s, and the median age of introduction of solids was increasing.

Tradition and Change: Breastfeeding Trends in the Aboriginal Population

National studies describing infant feeding practices in the 1960s found that the Aboriginal population had the highest rates of breastfeeding in Canada. However, by the early 1980s, government officials were concerned that many First Nations women were not breastfeeding and that those who were breastfeeding were doing so for a short period of time. This interest stemmed from concern about high rates of infection, which had been highlighted in the 1970s, and a desire to promote a return to traditional practices. Consequently, in 1982, the Medical Services Branch at Health and Welfare Canada developed the National Database on Breastfeeding among Indian and Inuit women.

In 1962, 69.4 percent of First Nations women breastfed their infants—only slightly higher than the 63 percent observed in 1983. In the general population, breastfeeding initiation rates increased from 200 percent to 300 percent in this twenty-year period, depending on region and SES. By 1982, in all regions of Canada breastfeeding initiation rates were higher among non-Aboriginal than among Aboriginal women (Graph 8.5).

The survey examined the infant feeding practices of all First Nations and Inuit infants receiving services from the Medical Services Branch in Canada in 1983 (Stewart and Steckle 1987). It found that 63 percent of First Nations infants and 70.7 percent of Inuit infants were breastfed at birth and that 0.4 percent of First Nations infants and 48.6 percent of Inuit infants were breastfed at six months. The report described the high adoption rate among Inuit infants (approximately 20 percent were adopted). Of the Inuit infants who remained with their mothers, approximately 88.9 percent were breastfed. Interestingly, as with national rates, there was considerable variation in rates of breastfeeding initiation and duration across the country among First Nations women. Rates were highest in the Yukon, followed by the Northwest Territories, and then there was a gradient through the provinces, increasing from east to west.

Research shows that, in the 1970s and 1980s, the situation for Aboriginal women (both First Nations and Inuit) in the Northwest Territories was much different than it was for Aboriginal women in the rest of Canada. For example, surveys in the Northwest Territories in the 1970s showed that breastfeeding initiation and duration rates were increasing in the Inuit population (Schaefer and Spady 1982). In 1973–74, 21.4 percent of infants were breastfed until six months, and this increased to 44 percent by 1978–79. This trend continued into the 1980s, especially with respect to duration as, by 1983, 48.6 percent of Inuit women breastfed until six months (Stewart and Steckle 1987).

In the Northwest Territories, unlike in the rest of Canada, duration and initiation rates increased in the First Nations population. In 1973, 33 percent of First Nations mothers in the Northwest Territories initiated and 5 percent breastfed to six months. By 1983, 74 percent initiated and 34 percent were still breastfeeding at six months (Stewart and Steckle 1987). Changes in the Territories during this period included an intense breastfeeding promotion

Graph 8.5

Breastfeeding Initiation in the non-Aboriginal and First Nations populations by region, 1982

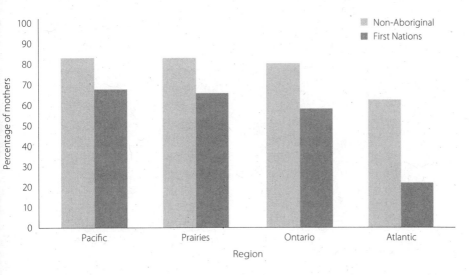

Source: Breastfeeding initiation in the non-Aboriginal and First Nations populations by region, 1982. Based on data from the National Database on Breastfeeding among Indian and Inuit Women, cited in McKim et al. 1998.

campaign, the encouragement (in the few hospitals in the Territories) of early contact between mother and infant in maternity wards, and the prohibition of formula samples in the two large federal hospitals that served the Territories. As well, the government advised the private hospital to stop accepting formula from various companies (*Globe and Mail* 1980).

In other parts of the country, there is some evidence that the downward trend in breastfeeding observed among Aboriginal women at this time was stopped and even reversed, possibly paralleling changes in broader Canadian society. For example, one study of breastfeeding in the Mohawk Nation on the Territory of Kahnawake, Quebec, showed an increase in breastfeeding initiation from 45 percent in 1978 to 64 percent in 1985–86. Breastfeeding duration also increased, from 20 percent to 29 percent at three months and from 7 percent to 24 percent at six months, during this time. These rates corresponded to rates in the First Nations population and general rates in Montreal and Quebec. Interestingly, the study suggested that "breastfeeding is an expression of lifestyle, that breastfeeding rates in both 1978 and 1985/1986 paralleled the lifestyle changes of the surrounding dominant society and that professional advice to the pregnant mother seems unimportant" (McCaulay, Hanusaik, and Beauvais 1989, 180). In both 1978 and 1985–86, mothers who

Graph 8.6

Breastfeeding rates among Indian and Inuit women compared with overall Canada rate, 1988

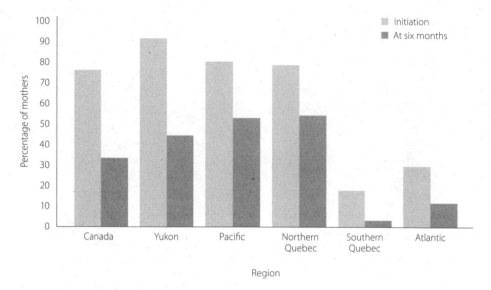

Source: Breastfeeding Rates among Aboriginal Women and General Population, 1988. Rates cited in McKim et al. 1998.

identified as adhering to the traditional Mohawk Longhouse way of life almost always breastfed. Extended family also seemed to have an important influence on infant feeding decisions. However, many aunts, grandmothers, and great-grandmothers supported bottle-feeding as it was the practice they had adopted in previous generations.

The dramatically high rates of breastfeeding initiation and duration among Aboriginal people in the Northwest Territories in the 1970s and early 1980s was likely due to the influence of hospital policy changes (given the few hospitals in the Territories, it is likely that effective changes in their promoting breastfeeding would have a wide regional effect) in conjunction with concerted efforts to promote breastfeeding. While, as is shown in the Mohawk example, other parts of Canada may have shown similar positive changes, in general, by the early 1980s, rates of initiation were declining among Aboriginals and, for the first time in several decades, were less than they were for non-Aboriginal women. By the late 1980s, rates of breastfeeding in the Aboriginal population varied considerably across the country (see Graph 8.6).

Family-Centred Maternity and Newborn Care

Strong interest in natural childbirth and family-centred maternity care continued into the 1980s. Since the 1960s, family-centred practices, such as rooming-in, breastfeeding, birthing rooms, and support for prenatal classes, were increasingly promoted in the professional literature. Research was beginning to show that many conventional maternity practices were ineffective, expensive, or harmful. In the 1980s, public support for home birth, midwifery, and patient's rights began to grow. Due to public pressure and a professional desire to improve quality of care, many routine maternity and newborn care practices (such as shaving of pubic hair and making women deliver infants lying on their backs with their feet in stirrups) were being questioned.

At the federal level, the Canadian Institute of Child Health took a leadership role in promoting family-centred maternity care in Canadian hospitals. Breastfeeding, and maternity practices that supported it, became a part of the dialogue on family-centred maternity care. Many hospital practices were recognized as influencing breastfeeding success. These included minimal drug use during labour, rooming-in, frequent and flexible feeding schedules, skin-to-skin contact between mother and infant in the delivery room, and the elimination of formula supplements (Health and Welfare Canada 1987; Post 1981).

The Canadian Institute of Child Health conducted two surveys, one in 1980 and the other in 1985, in order to examine changing maternity care practices. Across Canada, the researchers surveyed nursing directors who worked in hospitals that had more than twenty births a year. Five hundred and sixty-seven hospitals were selected, and approximately 392 (69 percent) responded to the detailed questionnaire. The 1980 survey reported that 68 percent of the hospitals surveyed had no active program to promote breastfeeding (Post 1981). It also provided information on other maternity practices that affected breastfeeding, including the use of pain medications, rooming-in, permitting the infant to take the breast in the delivery area, and allowing the infant to stay with the mother after birth. Overall, the survey found that many medical interventions that were lacking in clear clinical benefit were widespread across the country. The survey also found that many practices varied by province and hospital size. For example, 75 percent of larger hospitals gave analgesia/anesthesia to most patients, while only 41 percent of smaller hospitals did so. As well, 65 percent of larger hospitals were more family-centred, especially with regard to having the father in the delivery room and having the infant stay with the mother after birth (Post 1981). In terms of practices that influence breastfeeding success, 82 percent of hospitals allowed for infants to be put to the breast in the delivery area, while 70 percent permitted the infant to stay with the mother for one hour after birth (Post 1981). Rooming-in was increasingly requested by mothers, and most hospitals in the survey allowed it for at least a few hours a day. The survey findings demonstrated that the number of hours that mothers spent

Table 8.2

Number of hours infant spent with mother in hospital with rooming-in programs vs. hospitals with non-rooming-in programs in 1980

Number of hours infant spent with mother	Percentage of infant/mother pairs in each time category	
	Non-rooming-in program	Rooming-in program
0–4	24.0	3.0
5–12	44.2	21.3
13–18	6.6	30.7
19–24	4.3	39.8

Source: Post 1981.

with their infants varied greatly, depending on whether the hospital had a rooming-in program (Post 1981) (see Table 8.2).

The survey also revealed provincial variation in maternity practices. For instance, the use of analgesia and anesthesia was higher in central and eastern Canada than it was on the Prairies and in the West. Also, "some provinces (Saskatchewan, Manitoba, New Brunswick, and Newfoundland) reported considerably less, i.e., 56–70 percent of hospitals allowing breastfeeding in the delivery room as compared with British Columbia (98%) and Alberta (92%). These percentages were consistent across hospital sizes within the provinces" (Post 1981) (see Table 8.3). This is an interesting finding, given that breastfeeding rates in the 1980s showed a similar east-west trend. Although many practices did not show such great variation across provinces, support for midwifery displayed a clear trend: "There are more nurse midwives working in Alberta (63%) and British Columbia (83%) than the rest of the country. This is especially true when compared with Ontario (45%) and Quebec (12%)" (Post 1981). While numerous factors were influencing maternity practices, the findings did suggest that some practices tended to "cluster" in certain hospitals and parts of the country. It is difficult to know whether or not these "clusters" contributed to actual breastfeeding rates.

Overall, the researchers commented, "Our 1980 survey indicated wide variation in maternity practices between hospitals across the country. Policies were for the most part rigid, with many procedures applied routinely and without much question. Many services appeared downright traditional" (Hanvey and Post 1986, 28). In response, the Canadian Institute of Child Health initiated several activities to contribute to change and dialogue regarding maternity practices. Some of these initiatives included a review by provincial health associations, the production of a twenty-eight-minute

Table 8.3

Provincial variations in hospital practices that influenced breastfeeding initiation in 1980

Hospital practice	BC	AB	SK	MB	ON	QC	NB	NS	NL	Avrg.
Infants put to breast in delivery room	98%	92%	70%	68%	98%	84%	69%	84%	56%	82%
Infants with mother for one hour after birth	88%	67%	68%	57%	74%	66%	44%	78%	22%	70%

Source: Adapted from Post 1981. PEI, NWT, and Yukon excluded due to small sample size.

Health and Welfare Canada video entitled *Childbirth ... The Changing Sounds,* and the publication of *Family-Centred Maternity and Newborn Care: A Resource and Self-Evaluation Guide* for hospital obstetrical units.

In 1985, the institute conducted another survey of 636 nursing directors in order to assess progress in moving towards a family-centred model (Hanvey and Post 1986). Once again, 69 percent of the hospitals responded, perhaps indicating that this was still an important issue for nurses. Many hospitals were using more permissive language in their policies, moving from words such as "allow," "permit," and "require" to "offer," "choose," and "support." While hospital practices were continuing to change, controversial practices such as perineal shaves, enemas and suppositories, electronic foetal heart monitoring, and episiotomies remained widespread. Seventy-three percent of hospitals reported using Demerol, while 53 percent offered epidural anesthesia (and, in 17 percent of these units, more than half of the women received an epidural). The majority of hospitals offered some rooming-in, with 54 percent of the units having twenty-four-hour rooming-in (Hanvey and Post 1986). Eighty-six percent of units facilitated putting the baby to the breast as soon as possible after birth, and 92 percent of units allowed breastfeeding on demand. There was a trend towards providing combined care, where a nurse was assigned to a mother-infant pair rather than one nurse being assigned to the mother and another to the infant. This form of care aided in facilitating breastfeeding. Forty-one percent of units provided combined-care nursing. Supplementation with formula or glucose water was known to confuse infants, as breast nipples and bottle nipples require different sucking mechanisms. Even though supplements were not required for nutritive purposes, 71 percent of units normally gave babies supplementary drinks, and 49 percent gave glucose and water (Hanvey and Post 1986).

In 1987, *Family-Centred Maternity and Newborn Care: National Guidelines* was published, replacing 1975's *Recommended Standards for Maternity and Newborn Care*. The new guidelines firmly supported breastfeeding and recognized that, in the past, it had lacked institutional support: "Human breast milk is the optimal form of nutrition for newborn infants. In a society which has gone through at least one generation of formula feeding, the reinstitution of breastfeeding requires active support from health professionals" (Health and Welfare Canada 1987, 67). They commented specifically on the practice of quickly switching mothers to formula feeding when difficulties arose with breastfeeding, and they condemned supplemental feeding: "There is no need for routine supplemental feedings of either water or cow's milk formula for breastfeeding infants. If a new mother is too tired or ill to breastfeed, she may request that a supplemental feed be given. However, this should be the exception, not the rule" (Health and Welfare Canada 1987, 72).

The guidelines embraced family-centred care and demonstrated a firm commitment to questioning routine obstetric practices. They also encouraged flexibility in hospital practices and discussed the appropriate use of medical interventions. Their intent was to provide direction rather than rigid standards: they were in no way meant to violate the autonomy of each institution. Like the WHO Code, the guidelines could only be implemented at the provincial and/or local level. They recognized that the principles of family-centred maternity care were generally agreed upon but that implementation was challenging.

As the 1980s continued, more and more research demonstrated how maternity practices influenced breastfeeding, which provided more weight to advocacy efforts and contributed to changing attitudes and practices. As an example, a study in New Brunswick showed that babies who were put to the breast within twelve hours of birth were breastfed five to six weeks longer than were those who were put to the breast later (Beaudry and Aucoin-Larade 1989). A study of the outcomes of 1,001 midwife-attended home births in Toronto between 1983 and 1988 found that exclusive breastfeeding at twenty-eight days postpartum was 98.6 percent (Tyson 1991). Although these rates may reflect the beliefs and values of women who elected to have a home birth, they also suggest that low rates of medical intervention were better for breastfeeding outcomes.

The Campaign Closes

Through the 1980s, Canada was heavily involved in the international campaign to regulate the infant formula industry. Following the passage of the WHO Code in 1981, Nestlé signed an agreement with the International Nestlé Boycott Committee stating that it would develop marketing policies that were consistent with the code. The boycott was suspended in 1984, and, after a six-month trial period, it was officially halted. By the time the boycott ended, national boycott groups had formed in ten countries, and over one hundred organizations, including INFACT Canada, were part of the International Baby Formula Action Network (IBFAN).

While international rhetoric was strong, by 1988 only seven countries had implemented the WHO Code as law. In Canada, there was an attempt at industry self-regulation. Health and Welfare Canada accepted a new industry code on the marketing of breast milk substitutes produced by the Canadian Infant Formula Association (CIFA). This voluntary agreement with the formula industry was much weaker than was the WHO Code (Van Esterik 1989), and complaints about advertising were neither registered nor responded to (INFACT Canada 2001; Canadian Home Economics Association 1997; Newton 1999). Following widespread violations of the WHO Code, the Nestlé Boycott was reinstated in 1988. Groups in Canada, the United States, the Philippines, and Australia expanded the boycott to include American Home Products (Wyeth), the second largest manufacturer of infant formula in the world. WHO and UNICEF have never monitored the WHO Code. In Canada, INFACT Canada took on the role of monitoring code compliance.

By the end of the 1980s, the federal campaign to promote breastfeeding came to a close. Beginning with the professional awareness campaign at the end of 1979, the federal government developed and distributed breastfeeding information for mothers, collected data on infant feeding practices, worked to change professional and hospital practices that undermined women's abilities to breastfeed, and supported lay organizations and advocacy groups. The campaign had succeeded in bringing national attention to breastfeeding, forging new alliances, and ensuring consistent information for both health professionals and mothers across the country. Rather than solely encouraging mothers to breastfeed, the campaign focused on addressing factors that influenced breastfeeding success. However, at the end of the decade, as the rates of breastfeeding appeared to be plateauing, the marketing practices of the infant formula industry remained unregulated in Canada and abroad, and hospital practices to support breastfeeding varied considerably across the country. As well, some public health professionals and researchers were drawing attention to how promotion efforts, both nationally and regionally, had overemphasized the nutritional and medical benefits of breastfeeding and had neglected women's experiences and the context of their infant feeding decisions. While acknowledgement of the scientific medical value of breastfeeding had increased dramatically, the socio-cultural conditions that supported successful breastfeeding continued to lag behind.

One of the accomplishments of the national promotion campaign was the forging of new alliances between the federal and provincial governments and between professional and lay groups. The federal campaign acknowledged the importance of health professionals and hospital practices in influencing breastfeeding success. In doing so, it recognized that providing mothers with education was not enough to change infant feeding practices: "Any woman who is interested in breastfeeding should be strongly encouraged to do so. But pressing an unwilling mother into breastfeeding will not do mother or child any good and a decision to bottle-feed must be respected and supported ... If health professionals motivate mothers to breastfeed and then do not follow up with the kind of support and practical advice that contributes so greatly to the success of breastfeeding, then they have, inadvertently, failed in their responsibilities" (Myres 1980, 12).

One of the most interesting partnerships occurred between the federal government, the CPS, and La Leche League Canada. With the revival of breastfeeding at the end of the 1970s, these three groups, with their varying perspectives, came together to work to support breastfeeding. Under the leadership of the state, the maternalist, experiential perspective of La Leche League and the scientific and medical perspective of the CPS blended to form a unified voice in many of the educational materials distributed to mothers. La Leche League had moved from its radical roots in the 1960s and was now accepted by the scientific medical community. Throughout the campaign, the federal government had worked to support and strengthen lay groups and to increase health professional awareness and appreciation for the wealth of skill and knowledge that these groups possessed.

Interestingly, while many medical practices associated with pregnancy and childbirth were being reappraised and less medical intervention in childbirth was being advocated, infant feeding moved firmly back into the domain of scientific medicine. After having abandoned breastfeeding in the first half of the twentieth century, paediatrics now took on a new role in guiding health professionals and new mothers in proper infant feeding. Some would argue that scientific medicine was now validating and acknowledging what women's groups like La Leche League had known for decades. In 1986, Health and Welfare Canada, in conjunction with the CPS, published a guide entitled *Feeding Babies: A Counselling Guide on Practical Solutions to Common Infant Feeding Questions* for health professionals and new mothers. This guide was meant to complement the position paper issued by the CPS in 1979 on aspects of infant feeding and was intended to contribute to the development of consistent and practical advice by health professionals.

At the end of the decade, breastfeeding rates appeared to be reaching a plateau. Unpublished data reported in Maclean (1990) and Nolan and Goel (1995) reveal that national breastfeeding initiation rates were approximately 80 percent. From 1982 to 1987, Ross Laboratories reported that breastfeeding rates shifted up and down by only three to four percentage points. In 1987, 80 percent of women sampled initiated breastfeeding. At two months, 66 percent of infants were breastfed; at four months, 47 percent; at six months, 32 percent (personal communication, cited in Maclean 1990, 10).

Although breastfeeding initiation rates were quite high at 80 percent, this figure disguised underlying differences in breastfeeding across the country and in various socio-demographic groups. National data had revealed clear differences in breastfeeding practices between French- and English-speaking mothers and between Aboriginal groups and the general population. They had also revealed a distinct east-west gradient across the country. Other studies showed how breastfeeding was consistently associated with a range of socio-demographic factors. Among other things, breastfeeding rates were known to be higher if mothers were well educated, were from a higher socio-economic background, were married, were older, did not smoke, attended prenatal classes, had previously breastfed, were motivated to breastfeed, had supportive family members, had a healthy newborn, and had the opportunity to nurse after birth (Morse and Harrison 1987). Yet, these variables explained very little about women's decisions, and many health professionals who promoted breastfeeding made assumptions based on these indicators.

Consequently, several public health professionals and researchers were calling for more appreciation for the complexity of women's lives and the context in which infant feeding decisions were made. Heather Maclean conducted a four-year study of 122 Toronto women's experiences of breastfeeding at the end of the 1980s. She commented that an understanding of the context in which breastfeeding occurred could help make sense of why not all women breastfeed or why they breastfeed for short periods of time–in spite of breastfeeding's apparently endless benefits:

> Much of the professional literature on breast feeding has stressed edu-
> cation as a strategy to help women breast feed for longer periods of time.
> Without denying the importance of education, this emphasis may be
> displaced. Breastfeeding takes place in a social milieu that promotes
> and idealizes breast feeding. This same milieu encourages women to
> believe that everything in life is in their control. It idolizes the super-
> woman; it glamorizes paid work and undervalues domestic work; it
> glorifies women's breasts as sex objects but abhors public displays of
> breastfeeding; it reveres thin bodies over maternal shapes; and it rel-
> egates the responsibilities of child bearing and rearing to the private
> realm of the family. (Maclean 1990, 5)

Others pointed out that most of the past two decades of research on the benefits of breastfeeding had come from nutrition and epidemiology per-spectives. While the federal campaign had recognized the numerous envi-ronments that can influence breastfeeding, including hospital, home, and society, most provincial and local promotion programs had narrowed their focus to an exclusive emphasis on education. Many professionals assumed that, when presented with information on the benefits of breastfeeding, mothers would logically choose to start and to continue breastfeeding: "Cultural values and assumptions guide behavior. The failure of the 'health culture' to influence breast-feeding behavior worldwide can be accounted for if one examines the biomedical bias of past research and the cavalier attitude of practitioners who attempt to impose their biases on their clients" (Morse 1989, 223).

This "cavalier attitude" was leading to some inappropriate promotion efforts. The author of a study of historical and present-day infant feeding practices among the Woodlands Cree of northern Alberta commented, "In an attempt to foster breastfeeding, an article in the *Canadian Journal of Public Health* in 1987 recommended that Native mothers be encouraged to nurse their infants immediately after delivery. Such recommendations are contrary to traditional practices in this region and also to a worldwide practice of withholding colostrum from the infant. Furthermore, medical personnel interpret the immediate postpartal refusal to nurse as a desire not to breastfeed at all, rather than realizing that the mother may wish to delay the first breastfeeding for 24 to 36 hours" (Neander and Morse 1989, 194). Breastfeeding was not an isolated phenomenon: it was a personal and emotionally charged activity influenced by a complex array of psychological, structural, and cultural factors. Although the 1970s and 1980s had been a period of enormous change in values and beliefs associated with infant feeding, many promotion efforts were not attentive to the contexts that were essential to successful breastfeeding. While the value that scientific medicine placed on breastfeeding was growing, promotion efforts very often continued to oversimplify the complexity of women's lives, their decision making, and the diversity of their breastfeeding experiences.

Conclusion

By the end of the 1980s, nearly 75 percent of Canadian mothers were initiating breastfeeding. Under the leadership of the federal government, efforts to promote breastfeeding were occurring across the country. In addition to developing educational materials for mothers, the federal government also recognized the importance of gaining strong support for breastfeeding from the medical profession. As a signatory to the WHO Code, the federal government recognized the impact of hospital and infant formula marketing practices on women's abilities to breastfeed. Through awareness and education campaigns targeted at health professionals and key professionals within hospitals, the government attempted to develop voluntary guidelines to meet the provisions of the WHO Code. In 1982, the magazine *New Internationalist*, in their review of government action on implementing the WHO Code, commented, "Canada's official attitude is 'education not legislation.'" They also noted the support of the Toronto City Council for the Nestlé Boycott: "You couldn't buy a cup of Nescafe in a city government facility in Toronto even if you wanted to" (Anonymous 1982b, 110). By the end of the decade, the WHO Code was implemented, albeit incompletely.

Breastfeeding was part of the shift towards family-centred maternity care. In response to strong consumer interest and shifts towards natural childbirth, the federal government developed new standards, which addressed a range of issues, including breastfeeding. The campaign to promote breastfeeding had numerous successes, although it is difficult to know the extent to which the increase in breastfeeding rates can be attributed to it. As Myres (1988, 111) comments,

> The results to date should not be interpreted as a direct result of efforts at the national level. However, the leadership role played by the Federal Government in forging national alliances and in establishing a policy position supported by the implementation of projects, has resulted in an increased prominence being given to breastfeeding by provincial governments, local communities, and professional and lay groups. What the national programme did, in effect, was to focus a national emphasis on breastfeeding in a very tangible and visible way, and in so doing, stimulated, complemented, and reinforced programme efforts at other levels.

While the most rapid period of increase in breastfeeding occurred in the late 1970s, prior to the national promotion campaign, it is likely that federal efforts in the 1980s aided in strengthening and maintaining these gains. The national campaign also officially recognized the social and cultural shifts in infant feeding practices and attitudes in the 1970s. With the authority and approval of the state and scientific medicine, the national campaign contributed to the commitment of resources towards increasing breastfeeding practices and the development of policies which supported these new trends.

Chapter 9

Protecting, Promoting, and Supporting? 1990–2000

In 1990, a journalist in the *Vancouver Sun* commented, "'Breast is best.' That's the well-worn adage spouted by nearly everyone who knows about feeding Baby. What could be better than Mother Nature's own elixir, custom made to nourish infants and packaged in portable and attractive containers? No one has anything bad to say about breastfeeding. But actions speak louder than words" (Priest 1990, 1). During the 1990s, the federal government continued to recognize the value of breastfeeding through WHO/UNICEF agreements on breastfeeding and other international agreements to support the well-being of the child. These commitments resulted in pockets of money and resources being available to support breastfeeding initiatives throughout the 1990s. However, while the official commitment to promoting breastfeeding remained strong, the actual commitment of resources, attention, and advocacy paled in comparison to the campaign of the 1980s.

Breastfeeding promotion strategies continued to focus on education regarding the benefits of breastfeeding, the effects of hospital practices, and the marketing practices of the formula industry. While on one hand, promotion efforts expanded to consider broader influences on breastfeeding practices by addressing attitudes towards breastfeeding in public, they also narrowed their focus by shifting to promoting breastfeeding in select target groups or mothers who were perceived as "high risk" for not breastfeeding. Without the implementation of the WHO Code, the marketing practices of the formula industry remained unregulated in the 1990s, while at the same time these became more aggressive as formula companies shifted to direct marketing to mothers as a strategy to increase their market share. As well, controversies over the acceptability of breastfeeding at work, the threatened closure of Canada's last milk bank, and the use of vitamin D supplements suggested that a "culture of bottle-feeding" still predominated. And, the apparent universal agreement that breastfeeding was "the one best way" contrasted with the results of national surveys in 1994 which revealed that breastfeeding initiation rates had changed minimally since the last national survey in 1982.

Protecting, Promoting, and Supporting

In the early 1990s, the WHO and the United Nations Children's Fund (UNICEF) coordinated a series of international meetings to support breastfeeding. In 1989, the WHO and UNICEF had issued a joint statement entitled "Ten Steps to Successful Breastfeeding" (the Ten Steps; see Table 9.1). This document listed ten practices and policies that hospitals should adopt to successfully encourage and support breastfeeding. In August 1990, UNICEF and the WHO, with the support of the United States Agency for International Development and the Swedish International Development Agency, sponsored a meeting of policy-makers entitled "Breastfeeding in the 1990s: A Global Initiative." The meeting was held in a converted orphanage in Lo Spedale degli Innocenti in Florence, Italy, and included representatives from over forty countries (but not Canada). The statement emerging from the two-day meeting was entitled the Innocenti Declaration on the Protection, Promotion and Support of Breastfeeding. The declaration reflected the content of the original background document prepared for the meeting and the views of the participants.

The Ten Steps were one of the recommendations of the Innocenti Declaration, which also emphasized the global importance of breastfeeding and the responsibility of all governments to protect, promote, and support it:

> As a global goal for optimal maternal and child health and nutrition, all women should be enabled to practise exclusive breastfeeding and all infants should be fed exclusively on breast milk from birth to 4–6 months of age.... Attainment of this goal requires, in many countries, the reinforcement of a "breastfeeding culture" and its vigorous defence against incursions of a "bottle-feeding culture." This requires commitment and advocacy for social mobilization, utilizing to the full the prestige and authority of acknowledged leaders of society in all walks of life. Efforts should be made to increase women's confidence in their ability to breastfeed. Such empowerment involves the removal of constraints and influences that manipulate perceptions and behaviour towards breastfeeding, often by subtle and indirect means. (WHO and UNICEF 1990)

The declaration also listed several goals that all member states were to accomplish by 1995, including appointing a national breastfeeding coordinator, establishing a multi-sectoral breastfeeding committee, and ensuring that all maternity facilities practise the Ten Steps to Successful Breastfeeding, uphold the WHO Code, and enact legislation to protect the

Table 9.1

Ten steps to successful breastfeeding

Every facility providing maternity services and care for newborn infants should:

Step 1: Have a written breastfeeding policy that is routinely communicated to all health care staff.

Step 2: Train all health care staff in skills necessary to implement this policy.

Step 3: Inform all pregnant women about the benefits and management of breastfeeding.

Step 4: Help mothers initiate breastfeeding within a half-hour of birth.

Step 5: Show mothers how to breastfeed, and how to maintain lactation even if they should be separate from their infants.

Step 6: Give newborn infants no food or drink other than breast milk, unless medically indicated.

Step 7: Practice 24-hour rooming in.

Step 8: Encourage breastfeeding on cue.

Step 9: Give no artificial teats or pacifiers (also called dummies or soothers) to breastfeeding infants.

Step 10: Foster the establishment of breastfeeding support groups and refer mothers to them on discharge from the hospital or clinic.

Source: WHO and UNICEF 1989.

breastfeeding rights of working women. The declaration was endorsed by all governments present.

A few months later, at another meeting convened by UNICEF, the idea of giving recognition to hospitals (which followed the Ten Steps) emerged. In June 1991, the WHO and UNICEF launched the Baby-Friendly Hospital Initiative (BFHI) in Ankara, Turkey. This initiative was a structured approach to implementing the Ten Steps and the WHO Code at a hospital level (Naylor 2001; Phillipp and Merewoord 2004). Maternity facilities that successfully followed the Ten Steps were designated as "Baby-Friendly." Parallel to the launch of the BFHI was the formation of a new international breastfeeding advocacy organization, the World Alliance for Breastfeeding Action (WABA), which was formed in February 1991. As an umbrella for a global network of organizations and individuals, WABA was committed to the Innocenti Declaration and to protecting, promoting, and supporting the right of all children and mothers to breastfeed. Core members included La Leche League International and IBFAN.

At the same time as the Innocenti Declaration was being developed, another international agreement was being developed by the United Nations. This one also had implications for breastfeeding promotion. On 20 November 1989, the United Nations General Assembly adopted the Convention on the Rights of the Child. Based on the belief that children under the age of eighteen require special consideration and protection of their human rights, the convention, in fifty-four articles and two optional protocols, described basic standards and obligations towards children. As a convention, this agreement was biding on governments and ensured that they had a legal, not just a moral, obligation to fulfill the commitments described in it. Article 24 described the obligations of government to diminish infant and young child mortality and to combat disease and malnutrition: "States Parties ... ensure that all segments of society, in particular parents and children, are informed, have access to education and are supported in the use of basic knowledge of child health and nutrition, the advantages of breastfeeding, hygiene and environmental sanitation and the prevention of accidents" (Office of the United Nations High Commissioner for Human Rights 1990).

Throughout the 1990s, the Canadian government continued to participate in a series of international governmental conferences that had implications for breastfeeding. These included the Plan of Action of the International Conference on Nutrition in Rome (1992), the Programme of Action of the International Conference on Population and Development in Cairo (1994), and the Platform of Action of the World Conference on Women and Development in Beijing (1995). But the international conference that had the most impact on breastfeeding policies in Canada was the World Summit for Children held in September 1990. The World Summit helped shape federal government policies with respect to children throughout the 1990s, and it contributed to renewed support and interest in breastfeeding.

Brighter Futures

With the encouragement of UNICEF, Canada was one of six initiating nations to assist in the preparation for the first world summit to focus on children. The 1990 World Summit was the largest gathering of world leaders to consider the situation of the world's children, and it brought together seventy-one heads of state along with eighty-eight other national representatives. At the end of the summit, each of the participating countries signed the World Declaration on the Survival, Protection and Development of Children, with an accompanying plan of action. The Innocenti Declaration was endorsed at the summit, and its operational targets became part of the summit's goals for the year 2000.

The World Summit helped shape Canada's federal policies with respect to children for the next decade. Following its endorsement of the Declaration on the Survival, Protection, and Development of Children and a Plan of Action, the federal government initiated a National Plan of Action entitled "Brighter Futures." This five-year, multi-departmental initiative represented an investment of $500 million over five years (Government of Canada 2002). It included over thirty different steps and programs to address the well-being of children, particularly young children at risk and their families. As a follow-up to the Brighter Futures Initiative, the government introduced the Child Development Initiative in May 1992 (Canadian Heritage 2007)). The Child Development Initiative committed $500 million from 1992 to 1997 to address

Table 9.2

Members of the Expert Working Group on Breastfeeding

- Aboriginal Nurses Association of Canada
- Breastfeeding Support Service, Lethbridge Regional Hospital
- Canadian Confederation of Midwives
- Canadian Dietetic Association
- Canadian Hospital Association
- Canadian Institute of Child Health
- Canadian Medical Association
- Canadian Nurses Association
- Canadian Paediatric Society
- Canadian Perinatal Regionalized Coalition
- Canadian Pharmaceutical Association
- Canadian Public Health Association College of Family Physicians Task Force of Children's Health
- Federal/Provincial/Territorial Group on Nutrition
- Health Canada
- INFACT Canada
- La Leche League Canada
- Ligue La Leche
- Legal Representative
- Province Perinatal Program, Newfoundland
- Society of Obstetrics and Gynaecologists of Canada
- UNICEF Canada
- Vancouver Breastfeeding Centre

Source: Expert Working Group on Breastfeeding 1993.

the well-being of children, especially those five and under. Breastfeeding became a key area in child health promotion (Moxley et al. 1997).

Throughout the 1990s, the federal government enacted a variety of initiatives and activities to support its international commitments to the well-being and rights of children. These included the ratification of the Convention on the Rights of the Child (1991), the announcement of a proposed child benefit in the federal budget (1992), the National Children's Agenda (1997), the National Child Benefit (1998), and the Early Childhood Development Agreement (2000). The focus on early child development and healthy families provided much of the impetus for breastfeeding initiatives during the 1990s. Funds for breastfeeding promotion came primarily through the 1992 Child Development Initiative, but breastfeeding issues were discussed and included in a range of federal initiatives.

One of the immediate results of the 1990 World Summit was the organization of a breastfeeding task force by Health Canada in 1991. The first meeting occurred in October 1991 and included thirty representatives from the infant formula industry, government, advocacy groups, and health associations. The major outcome of this first meeting of the task force was the recommendation to continue to meet and discuss breastfeeding promotion in Canada. At the second meeting of the task force, the participants did not include representatives from the formula industry. As the objective of the meeting was "moving forward by consensus rather than confrontation," the group chose to provide industry representatives with a copy of the meeting summary. At the meeting, the name of the task force was changed to the Expert Working Group on Breastfeeding. Health Canada agreed to provide $25,000 for annual meetings.

Between 1991 and 1996, the mission, goals, and objectives of the group became formalized. As a national committee supported by Health Canada, the Expert Working Group took on the role of being the national authority on breastfeeding, as described in the Innocenti Declaration. The group's mission was to protect, promote, and support breastfeeding within Canada as the optimal method of infant feeding. Throughout the 1990s, the Expert Working Group provided input into various Health Canada initiatives to support breastfeeding. It also continued to support breastfeeding at the provincial level and through various professional associations. In terms of resources, Health Canada continued to support the annual meetings. However, the majority of the work accomplished by the individuals of the Working Group appeared to have occurred in addition to their existing professional commitments, through their ability to gain support and resources from other local sources or through their own additional voluntary commitments of time and energy.

Breastfeeding Anytime, Anywhere

In Health Canada's *National Plan of Action for Nutrition*, breastfeeding was recommended as the preferred method of infant feeding for the protection and promotion of health of infants, children, and women. Throughout the 1990s, Health Canada produced a variety of publications, including *A Breastfeeding Advocacy Kit*; *A Breastfeeding Poster Series*; *A Breastfeeding Media Kit*; two pamphlets entitled *10 Great Reasons to Breastfeed* (1998a) and *10 Valuable Tips for Successful Breastfeeding* (1998b); *Breastfeeding: A Selected Bibliography and Resource Guide* (1997); *Breastfeeding in Canada: A Review and Update* (1998c); and *Multicultural Perspective of Breastfeeding in Canada*. As well, a revised edition of *The Canadian Mother and Child* was published in 1991 with a new title: *You and Your Baby*.

One of the earliest breastfeeding activities in the 1990s involved a survey on attitudes towards breastfeeding. The survey included twelve focus group discussions across the country, with participants ranging from ex-

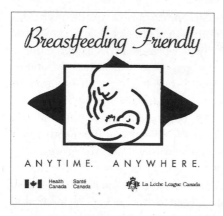

Figure 9.1   Logo from Health Canada's 1994 social marketing campaign. The Breastfeeding Friendly logo indicated that breastfeeding was welcome and encouraged on the premises. Breastfeeding Friendly logo, Public Health Agency of Canada (n.d.). Reproduced with the permission of the Minister of Public Works and Government Services Canada, 2008.

pectant teenagers to immigrants to male partners of pregnant women. It revealed that most women were aware of the benefits of breastfeeding; however, many thought that breastfeeding was far from natural. Discussions included the view that breastfeeding was restrictive as it did not provide women with a break from their child. And many women found it embarrassing to breastfeed in public. Some women were uncomfortable about breastfeeding in front of their male partners in their own home. According to the report, "Many of the mothers remained housebound or restricted in their movements while breastfeeding. The reticence to breastfeed in public comes from a number of sources. For some, it is primarily a matter of self-image (i.e., their discomfort with their own body); for others it seems to be primarily in reaction to the behavior of others–people they know or strangers" (Samuel 1997).

An appreciation for the need to change the culture or environment in which women were breastfeeding led to Health Canada's developing a five-year social marketing campaign. In 1994, the federal government launched a five-year campaign to promote breastfeeding, with annual spending ranging from $70,000 to $90,000. In 1994, Health Canada ran a $90,000 advertising campaign to make breastfeeding in public places socially acceptable (Canadian Press 1994b). The campaign included a series of "Breastfeeding Anytime, Anywhere" posters, which focused on the lifestyles of the general public, including teens. The posters included variations of slogans such as "Who Said (a Day at the Mall, a Day at the Park, Time with Friends) Was Impossible?" Health Canada also aired commercials during the 1994 Commonwealth Games and the program *Spilled Milk*. A logo was developed that was used to designate certain shopping malls, stores, and restaurants as "Breastfeeding Friendly." In 1995, Health Canada developed a media kit for distribution through La Leche League and Ligue La Leche to communities interested in conducting a breastfeeding promotion campaign.

Responses to the promotion campaign were mixed. Most health professionals were supportive of it. The general public often had strong opinions, as is demonstrated in a series of letters in the *Ottawa Citizen* in October 1994. Gordon Ford's "letter of the day" commented:

Health Canada proclaims in a TV commercial that breast feeding in public is a normal and perfectly acceptable form of behavior. I do not agree
with this and would be very surprised if the majority of Canadians did
so. I would like to know on what basis the department arrived at this
moral judgment and what moral authority it has to spend $90,000 in tax
dollars trying to force such a judgment on Canadians. Breast feeding is
something that should be encouraged and is a highly desirable method
of properly nourishing babies ... Breast feeding is a natural body function, the same as urinating and defecating, but please not in public.

The author suggested that if breastfeeding is to occur in a restaurant, then
there should be non-breastfeeding areas, just as there are non-smoking areas.

The following day, two citizens responded to Ford's letter. Alessandra
Fylyshtan (1994) responded as follows:

Breastfeeding is not like urinating or defecating and that is a perception
that desperately needs to change. Monday's Letter of the Day is an
excellent example of why Health Canada's breastfeeding promotion is
worth every penny of the $90,000 it spends ... If a baby is given a bottle
in a restaurant nobody in the restaurant thinks twice but why is the
better form of nourishment given this shameful treatment? It appears
to me that this is because people are either comparing it to bathroom
functions and or assuming there is something sexual about it. How
pathetic. My advice for people who can't handle the sight of an innocent
baby having its lunch: go eat in the bathroom.

Clearly, gaining support for breastfeeding in public still had a long way to go.

The Responsibility of the Health Care System

The 1981 WHO Code and the 1989 WHO/UNICEF joint statement *Protecting,
Promoting and Supporting Breastfeeding* emphasized the critical role of
health care workers in promoting successful breastfeeding. In the 1990s,
breastfeeding advocates from a range of professional backgrounds worked
to produce national guidelines on breastfeeding for health care providers
and continued to work towards changing hospital practices that discouraged
breastfeeding initiation and duration. These efforts were also paralleled
by the emergence of lactation consultants–a new coterie of breastfeeding
specialists.

In 1993 and 1996, the Canadian Institute of Child Health produced *National
Guidelines for Health Care Providers*. The intent of the guidelines was to bring
together representatives from nursing, medicine, and nutrition as well as lactation consultants and consumers to standardize breastfeeding knowledge.
The guidelines emphasized that breastfeeding was the normal and superior

method of infant feeding: "As part of a family-centred approach, breastfeed-ing is viewed as a healthy phenomenon of childbearing" (Canadian Institute of Child Health 1996, 6). The documents acknowledged that the decision to breastfeed was influenced by a variety of factors and recognized that health care providers can affect that decision. The underlying philosophy of the guidelines is as follows: "Parents have the right to make informed decisions about the method of feeding their infants and require accurate information about the benefits of breastfeeding and the hazards of not breastfeeding, in order to do so. Health care providers have a responsibility to encourage breastfeeding by providing accurate, consistent information, dispelling myths and misinformation and guiding women towards this method of nutrition for their babies" (Canadian Institute of Child Health 1996, 10). This philosophy encouraged "informed choice." It also suggested that health care providers should not take a neutral stance with respect to infant feeding deci-sions: "Negative or neutral attitudes towards breastfeeding from health care providers help to undermine women's chances of reaching their breastfeed-ing goals. Because bottlefeeding is often considered the norm in our culture, any neutrality by health care professionals about infant feeding may in fact be perceived as support for bottlefeeding" (Jones and Green 1996, 7).

Hospital practices and the aggressive marketing of the infant formula industry interfered with a woman's ability to make an informed decision. A 1993 survey examined whether hospital practices across the country were consistent with the WHO Code, the Ten Steps, and the Baby-Friendly Hospital Initiative (Levitt et al. 1996). The researchers found the following patterns:

- 58.4 percent of hospitals reported having a written policy on breastfeeding
- 75.7 percent of hospitals did not provide artificial teats or pacifiers
- 23.8 percent of hospitals reported routinely giving sample packs containing formula to breastfeeding mothers; 17.8 percent stated that they were only given on request, and 58.4 percent said they were never given
- 61.1 percent of hospitals reported routinely giving sample packs containing formula to formula-feeding mothers; 8.5 percent stated that they were only given on request, and 30.4 percent said they were never given
- 82 percent of hospitals had an exclusive contract with a formula company
- 45.9 percent of hospitals responded that breast-fed babies were usually given other liquids
- 89 percent of hospitals responded that all beds could be used for rooming-in; 65.2 percent reported that infants were with their mothers nineteen to twenty-four hours per day

- 97.1 percent reported that newborns were allowed to breastfeed on demand
- 57.9 percent stated that they had a policy of offering mothers information on breastfeeding support groups or advice on breastfeeding

They also found variations across the country:

- 50 percent of the hospitals in Quebec and New Brunswick gave formula samples to breastfeeding mothers, compared with 8 percent in Ontario and 10 percent in British Columbia
- rooming-in was more common in the western provinces than in Quebec and eastern Canada; breastfeeding rates were 10 percent lower at hospitals that allowed fewer than sixteen rooming-in hours or no rooming-in
- hospitals in the Prairie provinces and the Atlantic provinces were significantly less likely than were those in Ontario to have a policy for giving newborns no food or drink other than breast milk
- hospitals in Quebec were significantly less likely to have policies supporting nineteen to twenty-four hours of rooming-in per day
- hospitals in British Columbia and the Prairies were slightly less likely than were those in Ontario to have a policy of offering mothers information on breastfeeding support groups or advice on breastfeeding at discharge
- hospitals in the Prairies and in Quebec were more likely to give sample formula packs to breastfeeding and formula-feeding mothers

Overall, only five hospitals met the criteria for the "Baby-Friendly" designation (Dunlop 1995), and all five were in Ontario.

In the early 1990s, lay support for breastfeeding was quite strong in Canada. Throughout the 1980s and 1990s, La Leche League continued to grow. In 1978, La Leche League Canada had its own logo; in 1985, it incorporated and elected its first board of directors; and in 1987, it became an affiliate of La Leche League International by signing the Agreement of International Principles of Cooperation. At the same time, the Canadian French-speaking groups became their own affiliate—Ligue La Leche. In 1976, the league had 140 groups and 325 leaders in Canada. By the early 1990s, there were nearly 300 groups and about 640 leaders.

At the same time as the growth of La Leche League, a lactation consultant designation emerged. Lactation consultants were breastfeeding specialists who could provide professional support to mothers. In the mid-1980s, Canadians began to write the International Board Certified Lactation exam. Many of the first lactation consultants came from a health background, especially nursing, or were La Leche League leaders. Many greeted the emergence of this new specialty with mixed feelings. Lactation consultants could play an important support role for women who were experiencing breastfeeding difficulties and who could not get the knowledge they required from other health professionals. However, this new profession also supported the idea that breastfeeding required expert advice and education. The number of lactation consultants grew throughout the 1990s, and by 2002, there were 1,191 lactation consultants in Canada (Canadian Institute for Health Information 2004b).

"Competing with Women's Breasts": New Industry Marketing Strategies

The 1993 survey revealed that over 80 percent of Canadian hospitals had exclusive contracts with formula manufacturers. For the most part, formula manufacturers followed the voluntary industry code produced by the Canadian Infant Formula Association (CIFA). In the late 1980s, three companies—Mead Johnson, Ross Abbott, and Wyeth—dominated the infant formula market in Canada. Marketing consisted mostly of the distribution of sample packs of formula through exclusive contracts with hospitals and endorsements from health professionals. In the 1990s, this approach to marketing began to change as another formula company, Nestlé, entered the Canadian market. By the end of the 1990s, direct marketing to mothers was the new industry strategy for increasing market share.

In 1990, Nestlé entered the infant formula market in Canada after working to establish a product known as Carnation Good Start in the United States. There, Nestlé had been charged in nine states for misleading and deceptive advertising that presented Carnation Good Start as a new formula that offered a remedy for colic and allergies (Sterken 2002). Throughout the early 1990s, the other three formula companies continued their bidding wars in their attempts to negotiate contracts with hospitals and to provide them with free formula. In order to maintain market share and brand loyalty (93 percent of mothers were known to continue to use the formula brand they were provided with in hospital), companies induced hospitals with large amounts of money and/or gifts. There were several contracts that received media attention. In 1989, Abbott Laboratories offered $500,000 to Grace Hospital in Vancouver in a bidding war with Bristol-Myers for the privilege of donating formula supplies for three years. Baumslag and Michels (1995) reported that, at Grace Hospital, the largest birthing facility in Canada, 85 percent of mothers expressed a desire to breastfeed; however, by the second day, 75 percent of infants were given glucose water or formula. In 1993, Women's Health College, a Toronto teaching hospital, and Mead Johnson Canada signed an agreement that gave the hospital $1 million towards a $7.5 million renovation of its perinatal unit plus an annual $35,000 grant for a hotline for breastfeeding mothers. Mead Johnson would also provide the hospital with free formula. Elisabeth Sterken from INFACT commented that the company was essentially "buying the right to compete with women's breasts" (*Gazette* 1993). At Isaac Killam Hospital in Halifax, Ross Laboratories offered to pay $1 million to the Doctor's Hospital (Baumslag and Michels 1995). Meanwhile, Mead Johnson signed a five-year deal with the Royal Columbian Hospital in British Columbia. Following the announcement of this deal, the B.C. Health Minister slammed the agreement and called for hospitals to refuse free supplies (Baby Milk Action 1993).

However, Nestlé, as a newcomer to the Canadian market, could not take this approach to marketing. It began advertising in Canadian parenting magazines, on "shelf talkers" in store aisles, by asking mothers to register for "clubs," through advertising at physicians' offices, and through tear-outs in magazines (INFACT Canada 2002a; Sterken 2002). Nestlé also began contacting mothers directly through Canada Post. Mothers received free mailings and free formula throughout pregnancy and a year after birth. Soon, the other companies began to follow Nestlé's example. Finally, in the early 1990s, Nestlé launched an anti-trust complaint with Industry Canada against its competitors. CIFA was disbanded and all bets were off (Sterken 2002).

Throughout the 1990s, there was an increasing shift by infant formula companies toward direct marketing to mothers rather than relying on regular advertising (Canadian Press 1994a). Cheryl Levitt, co-chair of the Expert Working Group, commented, "Recently, a new infant-formula marketing strategy has evolved in which formula advertising and business reply cards for free cases of infant formula are distributed to expectant mothers through physicians' obstetric offices. In Canada, there are reports of direct advertising and sample distribution to women themselves as well as prenatal classes sponsored by formula manufacturers" (Levitt 1995). A survey of York region (within the Greater Toronto Area) found that 45 percent of mothers had received formula gift packs even though the hospitals denied allowing such gifts. In one hospital, professional staff did not give out samples, but the formula company gave them to Women's Auxiliary volunteers to take when they visited new mothers (Dunlop 1995). When hospitals refused to distribute samples, formula companies targeted doctors or drugstores. In 1997, 54 percent of women in a sample of mothers in Hamilton-Wentworth received coupons for formula in the mail. Many mothers were frustrated by these marketing tactics. They would fill out a form for parenting information or coupons and receive unsolicited formula samples (Canadian Press 1994a). In other cases, marketers would buy the names of new mothers from hospitals and send women samples and coupons or target mothers in doctors' offices, prenatal classes, maternity wards, and maternity clothing stores (Kryhul 2000).

For the most part, infant formulas, regardless of price, are very similar to each other as their contents are regulated by the Food and Drugs Act (regulations to control the nutritional composition of formulas were first promulgated in 1976). As the birth rate in Canada is relatively stable and the market share among the few competing companies that manufacture infant formula changes minimally, there are few ways for formula manufacturers to increase profit. One strategy used by manufacturers is to add nutrients and supplements to formula and argue that this product more closely resembles mother's milk.[1] One example of this was reported in the media in 1996, when Ross Products introduced Similac Advance formula in Canada. Similac Advance was purportedly fortified with iron, which did not lead to constipation, and contained nutrients found in breast milk that helped the baby's immune system to develop. The new formula was described as "clinically proven to offer benefits previously associated only with breast milk" and was part of a direct marketing blitz, which included the provision of free samples, invitations to join a "relationship club" called Similac Welcome Addition Club, and nutrition seminars for members (Canadian Press 1996). Similac Advance was sold at 5 percent to 10 percent above the price of regular Similac (Heinrich 1996). Following the introduction of Similac Advance, Mead Johnson filed a lawsuit against Ross Products (Canadian Press NewsWire 1996). In November 1996, an Ontario judge ruled that Ross Products was required to change its promotional campaign. Mead Johnson, the producer of Enfalac, was apparently pleased about the decision.[2] The previous year, Mead Johnson was required to remove a claim that said "modeled after mother's milk" (Canadian Press NewsWire 1996).

In the late 1990s, it became more challenging for formula manufacturers to ensure their market share from contracts with hospitals. In 1995, B.C. Women's Hospital, Canada's largest obstetrical facility, became the first hospital to refuse free supplies of infant formula (INFACT Canada 1995). All infant formula would have to be paid for—at an estimated cost of $60,000. In a 1999 ruling in Quebec, Mead Johnson lost its legal challenge of a system that allowed hospitals to offer turns to the three major manufacturers to provide free supplies, which the company claimed was causing it a yearly loss of $10 million (International Baby Food Action Network 2001).

The Purpose of Breasts: Sex or Food?

The Breastfeeding Anytime, Anywhere campaign was designed to encourage mothers and the general population that breastfeeding in public was acceptable. One of the core beliefs underlying the view that breastfeeding was "disgusting" or "inappropriate" in public was a perception that breasts were innately sexual. Throughout the twentieth century, breasts had become increasingly viewed as sexual organs. While it was acceptable to see breasts in a sexual light (whether in the media or in public settings), it was often not acceptable to see them as being for the purpose of nourishing infants. Negative views of breastfeeding had long been acknowledged as a barrier to successful breastfeeding. In the 1990s, reports of the difficulties that women encountered breastfeeding in public continued. However, in 1997, a decision by the B.C. Human Rights Tribunal in the case of *Poirier v. British Columbia* led to the first legal decision on breastfeeding issues in Canada. This case provided legal protection for women who chose to breastfeed in public. It also signified a legal shift from viewing breasts solely as sexual objects to viewing them as also for feeding infants. The case was very important, as it raised interesting questions about how breastfeeding could be combined with paid work (Arneil 2000).

Although rates of breastfeeding had grown dramatically, particularly during the 1970s and early 1980s, and the benefits of breastfeeding were widely acknowledged, women in the 1990s continued to report challenges to breastfeeding in public (Cox 1997; Braungart 1990; Woodard 1997). Women described being asked to leave shopping malls, department stores, and restaurants by owners or security guards. Many women felt harassed, receiving leers and sexual remarks as well as angry stares (Woodard 1997). In some situations, women were forced to retreat to the washroom to feed their babies. Other women commented on how they were not permitted to feed their babies at public pools because food was not allowed there (Haley 2001). Mary Anne Domarchuk in Nanaimo, British Columbia, was asked to stop breastfeeding her eight-month-old son at her daughter's Valentine's Day school lunch. She was informed that the school was private property and that it was her duty to protect the public interest ((INFACT Canada 1996).

Interestingly, objections to breastfeeding in public came from *both* men and women. Many believed that breasts were primarily sexual organs that should remain covered in public, as exposing them could be perceived as offensive or sexually provocative. This stands in contrast to the pressures many women felt to present their breasts as attractive yet respectable (Arneil 2000; Yalom 1997). Figure 9.2 provides an example from INFACT Canada's breastfeeding promotion campaign, the goal of which was to address the multiple purposes of breasts and to raise awareness of societal beliefs that created barriers to breastfeeding. However, objections to breastfeeding in public were not limited to the general population: they also extended to health professionals, the very individuals who were supposed to support and promote breastfeeding. In the mid-1990s, members of the BC Baby Friendly Network visited fifteen communities and conducted focus groups with parents, nurses, and physicians. They found attitudinal barriers to breastfeeding in every community: "These attitudinal barriers, which exist among health professionals as well as the general public, were identified by every community as the most significant factor limiting informed choice and effective support for breastfeeding" (Jones and Green 1996, 7).

All of these tensions and pressures came to the attention of the B.C. Human Rights Commission in 1997 with the case of *Poirier v. British Columbia*. In December 1990, Michelle Poirier returned from a four-month maternity leave to her job as a speech writer with the B.C. Ministry of Municipal

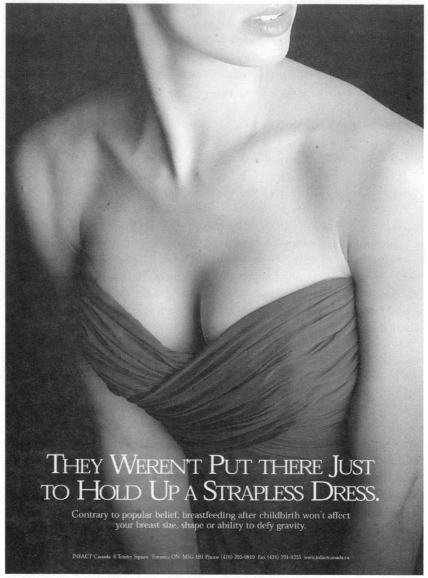

They Weren't Put there Just to Hold Up a Strapless Dress.

Contrary to popular belief, breastfeeding after childbirth won't affect your breast size, shape or ability to defy gravity.

INFACT Canada 6 Trinity Square Toronto, ON M5G 1B1 Phone (416) 595-9819 Fax (416) 591-9355 www.infactcanada.ca

Figure 9.2   INFACT Canada poster suggesting multiple purposes for breasts. Image courtesy of INFACT Canada.

Affairs, Recreation and Housing. With the agreement of her supervisor and co-workers, Poirier made arrangements to have her baby brought to her at lunch to be breastfed in her cubicle over her lunch break (*Poirier v. British Columbia* 1997). In March 1991, the ministry sponsored a series of noon-hour seminars in honour of International Women's Week. Michelle attended two sessions. The first session offered a film on women's working conditions in the 1940s and 1950s, while the second focused on a new social movement, the "men's movement." Following the second session, the ministry received complaints from several individuals, mostly women, that Michelle had breastfed in a "mixed" audience of men and women (INFACT Canada 1997). Michelle was advised that the ministry was developing a policy about children in the workplace and was asked to breastfeed her child off-site for two weeks until the controversy had died down. In April, another noon-hour presentation was scheduled. Michelle was told that she could neither bring her daughter to the presentation nor receive compensatory time off work to attend to her breastfeeding needs.

In February 1992, Michelle filed a complaint with the B.C. Council for Human Rights (BCCHR), insisting that she had been denied a service available to the public (contrary to Section 3 of the B.C. Human Rights Act) and that she had been discriminated against with regard to the terms and conditions of her employment (contrary to Section 8) (INFACT Canada 1997). In 1997, the B.C. Human Rights Tribunal found that the B.C. Ministry of Municipal Affairs, Recreation and Housing had discriminated against Michelle Poirier because of her sex when it refused to allow her to breastfeed her child in the workplace: "The Tribunal finds that discrimination because of breastfeeding is discrimination because of sex. Only women breastfeed and restrictions on when and where women can breastfeed affect only women ... Ms. Poirier was faced with the choice of refusing a direct request from her supervisor or breastfeeding away from work. She was also required to choose between attending work-related seminars and breastfeeding her child" (*Poirier v. British Columbia* 1997, D/87).

In many ways, the decision was a victory, as it supported Poirier's right to breastfeed at work and could serve as a precedent for protecting other women who chose to breastfeed in public. It marked a shift away from the view that the exposure of women's breasts in public was inherently sexual (Law, 2000). However, the case also raised some other questions. The decision in favour of Michelle Poirier was based on the principle of accommodation (Arneil 2000): "The Ministry did not reasonably accommodate Ms. Poirier" (*Poirier v. British Columbia* 1997, D/87). The principle of accommodation suggests that equality between the sexes merely requires accommodating difference. According to Arneil (2000, 367), "Accommodation, while providing the basis for victory in the *Poirier* ruling and others, creates two central difficulties for women: the unthinking acceptance of existing norms, and the tendency to minimize the differences between men and women." It is possible that the ministry could have accommodated Poirier by simply providing her with the opportunity to express, or pump, her breast milk. In the United States, the prevalence of corporate lactation programs suggest that breast-pumping is the primary means of accommodating breastfeeding mothers. While the *Poirier* case highlighted the importance of breastfeeding, it put the responsibility

Table 9.3
Women's breastfeeding rights chart

Province/ territory	Is a woman's right to breastfeeding in public protected?	Is a women's right to breastfeed at her work place protected?	Have there been complaints and what was the outcome?	Has public education been carried out or is it planned?
British Columbia	YES	YES	YES – Michelle Poirier	NO
Alberta	YES (qualified)	YES (qualified)	YES – Resolved through the women acknowledging that lack of discretion is a problem, and the facility acknowledging that they could have offered solutions such as discreet are or covering.	NO – Information provided on request
Saskatchewan	YES	YES – As per Poirier decision of the Supreme Court of BC.	NO	YES – Although there is not specific campaign on breastfeeding, it is mentioned in their general overview presentation.
Manitoba	NOT ABSOLUTELY "The code states that employers should make reasonable accommodations for any individual whose needs are based on...section 9 (2). The important word is 'reasonable'. The right to	NOT ABSOLUTELY	YES – Two women have received settlements. One was denied the right to breastfeed in a shopping mall, the other on public transportation. A third will be heard later this year.	YES – Although there is no campaign that deals specifically with breastfeeding, information is included in a number of educational programs and initiatives for their website.

breastfeed is not absolute and an employer or service provider has the right to attempt to show that it may be unreasonable or an undue hardship to accommodate a woman who wishes to breastfeed."

Ontario	YES	YES	Protected by Freedom of Information and Privacy Legislation	YES – Their new policy relating to pregnancy and breastfeeding was released October 99, and more is planned.
Quebec	YES	No complaint and therefore no precedent. But if one was received they would look at it "very closely."	YES – In 1996 a woman was asked by a security guard to leave a mall. Discrimination was proven under articles 10, 15, 4 and 39 of Quebec's Charter of Human Rights and Freedoms. Plaintiff settled for $2500.	Not at this time, but there is good awareness because of media coverage of the 1996 complaint.
New Brunswick	VERY LIKELY	VERY LIKELY	NO – No formal complaints. A few informal complaints which have been resolved.	NO – "It is my impression that New Brunswick is very positive and welcoming of breastfeeding due to the good work of out public health department and La Leche League."
Nova Scotia	YES – A new policy has just been approved.	YES	YES – Their new policy was developed as part of the settlement.	YES – In partnership with public health, a campaign is in place to educate breastfeeding advocates, government officials, employers, retail operators and the general public about the new policy.

Table continues

Table 9.3 Continued
Women's breastfeeding rights chart

Prince Edward Island	YES	POSSIBLE – AS discrimination in employment on the bass of sex is prohibited.	NO
Newfoundland	YES	POSSIBLE – Family status is not protected, but a woman may have grounds to file a complaint alleging sex discrimination.	NO
Northwest Territories	Did not answer this question	Did not answer this question	NO
Yukon	YES	YES – As per Poirier decision of the Supreme Court of BC	YES – A woman was denied permission to take breaks at certain time in order to breastfeed her child. It was resolved informally with the employer agreeing to accommodate her needs.
			Did not answer this question
			NO – Due to human and financial resource constraints.

Source: INFACT Canada 2000.

for determining "reasonable accommodation" on the employer. In other words, the Ministry of Municipal Affairs, Recreation and Housing could have accommodated Michelle Poirier in any way it chose as long as her daughter was fed. Yet breastfeeding is not equivalent to expressing breast milk: "The response of the BC government to the ruling is evidence of the failure to recognize the importance of the physical bond between infant and mother for many women" (Arneil 2000, 369). The principle of accommodation does not distinguish between the practice of breastfeeding and the provision of breast milk to infants.

Although a variety of human rights conventions, including the Convention on the Elimination of All Forms of Discrimination against Women (1979), the Convention on the Rights of the Child (1991), and the International Labour Organization's Convention on Maternity Protection (1919, 1952) all protected women's right to breastfeed to some extent, the *Poirier* case represented the first Canadian legal challenge on the basis of human rights. Each province has a human rights code that protects women from discrimination on the basis of sex. In 2002, INFACT published a national chart describing the status of women's rights with regard to breastfeeding in public.

National Surveys Reveal ... Breastfeeding Practices at the End of the 1990s

In the mid-1990s, the first national survey data on breastfeeding since the 1980s became available. The 1994 National Population Health Survey (NPHS) asked mothers of children under the age of five whether they breastfed their youngest child. The 1994/95 National Longitudinal Survey on Children and Youth (NLSCY) asked about breastfeeding for children ages zero to twenty-three months at the time of the survey. In 1994, both surveys showed that national breastfeeding initiation stood at 73 percent. Surprisingly, this resembled the national rates of breastfeeding reported in the early 1980s. In terms of duration, 40 percent of mothers breastfed for fewer than three months. In 1982, 17 percent of mothers stopped breastfeeding at two months, and 41 percent stopped breastfeeding at four months (Health Canada 1998c). Breastfeeding rates appeared to have increased minimally in the past decade.

These two surveys also found that there were still regional trends in breastfeeding and that women with higher education still breastfed more than did women with lower education. Interestingly, differences in breastfeeding according to income level were not so dramatic. The NPHS found that initiation rates in low/low-middle-income women were 61 percent, while the rates for middle- and upper-middle/high-income women were 76 percent and 78 percent, respectively. The NLSCY found that 68 percent of low/low-middle-income women breastfed, while 69 percent of middle-income and 78 percent of upper-middle/high-income women breastfed. However, while lower-income women initiated breastfeeding at lower rates, they also tended to breastfeed for longer durations (Health Canada 1998d).

Table 9.4
Select maternal characteristics and breastfeeding initiation and duration rates in Canada 1994–95 from the National Population Health Survey and National Longitudinal Survey on Children and Youth

Demographic Characteristics	Percentage of Mothers			
	Initiation		Breastfed for fewer than 3 months	
	NPHS	NLSCY	NPHS	NLSCY
Ages				
All ages	73	73	38	41
<25	67	66	63	56
25–29	72	73	45	42
>29	75	77	31	33
Marital status/family type				
Married/two parents	74	75	34	60
Single/lone parent	66	65	66	38
Other	76	N/A	49	N/A
Region				
Atlantic	53	60	51	43
Quebec	54	56	43	46
Ontario	78	80	38	41
Prairies	86	83	30	34
British Columbia	87	85	39	39
Income level				
Lowest/lower-middle	61	68	51	53
Middle	76	69	39	40
Upper middle-high	78	78	33	36
Education				
High school or less	63	63	49	52
Some post-secondary	76	76	38	42
University	93	81	—	32
Immigrant status				
Immigrant	82	84	50	39
Non-immigrant	71	71	35	40

Source: Health Canada 1998d.

The NLSCY, first launched in the 1990s, continued to collect data on children and their families in Canada throughout the decade. Rates of breastfeeding initiation increased throughout the 1990s, from 73 percent in 1994–95 to 78.5 percent in 1996–97 to 81.9 percent in 1998–99 (Dzakpasu 2003). Interestingly, the greatest percentage change in these years occurred in the two provinces with the lowest and highest rates of breastfeeding. In Quebec, breastfeeding initiation increased from 56.7 percent in 1994–95 to 71.0 percent in 1998–99. In British Columbia, rates increased from 87.9 percent in 1994–95 to 95.2 percent in 1998–99. Initiation rates in Quebec surpassed rates in the Atlantic provinces in the 1990s. Although initiation rates for the Atlantic provinces increased minimally from 60.8 percent in 1994–95 to 64.5 percent in 1998–99 (Dzakpasu 2003), dramatic changes did occur. Prince Edward Island had a large increase between 1994–95 and 1996–97, from 61 percent to 73 percent (Statistics Canada 2001a).

Duration rates increased slightly across the country, with 58.7 percent of women breastfeeding for more than three months in 1994–95 and 63.0 percent doing so in 1998–99. Duration rates increased in all provinces except Quebec, where they remained stable, and had the biggest increase in British Columbia, where they went from 60.3 percent in 1994–95 to 69.2 percent in 1998–99 (Dzakpasu 2003). While initiation rates plateaued between the mid-1980s and mid-1990s, they were beginning to increase at the end of the decade. Duration rates, however, seem to have increased only slightly.

The Breastfeeding Committee for Canada and the Baby-Friendly Initiative

In 1996, Health Canada funding for the annual meetings of the Expert Working Group on Breastfeeding, which had started in 1991 following the World Summit for Children, ended (Coutts 1997). Members of the Working Group decided to continue to work together to promote breastfeeding across the country. In 1996, the Expert Working Group on Breastfeeding parted ways with Health Canada and became the Breastfeeding Committee for Canada (BCC). By 2000, the BCC had developed bylaws and was recognized as a national not-for-profit corporation. Like the Working Group, the BCC remained a multi-sectoral national breastfeeding committee. Its vision, mission statement, and objectives remained similar to those of the Working Group. The BCC's vision was "to establish breastfeeding as the cultural norm for infant feeding within Canada" and its mission statement indicated that it intended "to protect, promote, and support breastfeeding in Canada as the normal method of infant feeding." However, unlike the Working Group, the BCC relied on "soft," unstable funding from a series of grant proposals to Health Canada.

In 1996, the BCC identified the WHO/UNICEF Baby-Friendly Hospital Initiative as a primary strategy for the protection, promotion, and support of breastfeeding in Canada. The BCC became the national authority for the Baby-Friendly Hospital Initiative and, in November 1997, developed the Baby-Friendly Initiative Action Plan. In 1998, the BCC launched the Baby-Friendly Initiative (BFI) at a conference in Vancouver entitled "Breastfeeding: Stepping into Baby-Friendly." Hosted by the BC Reproductive Care Program, the conference had the goal of providing health care professionals, policy-makers, and government representatives with the theory and practical skills needed to

Table 9.5

Seven-point plan for the protection, promotion, and support of breastfeeding in community health care settings

1. Have a written policy that is routinely communicated to all staff and volunteers.

2. Train all health care staff in skills necessary to implement policy.

3. Inform pregnant women and their families about the benefits and management of breastfeeding

4. Support mothers to establish and maintain exclusive breastfeeding to six months.

5. Encourage sustained breastfeeding beyond six months with appropriate introduction of complementary foods.

6. Provide a welcoming atmosphere for breastfeeding families.

7. Promote collaboration between health care providers, breastfeeding support groups and the local community.

Source: Breastfeeding Committee for Canada 2002.

implement the BFI in Canada. The conference, coined as the "Breastfeeding Conference of the Decade" by the Canadian Lactation Consultant Association, attracted widespread interest. Over 500 delegates attended, including a federal government representative, a B.C. Ministry of Health representative, UNICEF, and various academics. Other attendees were breastfeeding advocates, health care practitioners, educators, consumers, administrators, and policy-makers as well as researchers representing a variety of health disciplines and all levels of government from all provinces and territories.

The name "Baby-Friendly Hospital Initiative" was changed to "Baby-Friendly Initiative" (BFI) to "reflect the continuum of care for breastfeeding mothers and babies outside the hospital environment." The BCC recognized that non-hospital health care facilities and broader communities needed to be involved in the implementation of the BFI. Other than the United Kingdom, Canada was the only country to expand the focus of the Baby-Friendly Hospital Initiative. The BCC adapted the United Kingdom's "A Seven Point Plan for the Protection, Promotion, and Support of Breastfeeding in Community Health Care Settings," turning it into "The Seven Point Plan for the Protection, Promotion, and Support of Breastfeeding in Community Health Services" (see Table 9.5). This plan was to be used to designate both hospitals and community health services as "Baby Friendly" (see Table 9.6).

Due to the structure of the Canadian health care system, the BCC was forced to work in committees at the provincial and territorial levels. This being the case, progress in implementing the BFI has been uneven and, without stable funding, it has also been slow. In the late 1990s, BCC worked to develop the structures and mechanisms for promoting, assessing, and designating hospitals as "Baby Friendly." Research throughout the decade supporting the benefits of the BFI remained strong, however. One study at the Boston Medical

Table 9.6

Ten steps to baby-friendly communities

Step 1: UNICEF designates all community hospitals delivering maternity services as "Baby Friendly."

Step 2: All health care facilities promote, protect, and support breastfeeding.

Step 3: Health care institutions work together to increase the availability of breastfeeding support.

Step 4: The community is informed as a whole about the benefits of breastfeeding and the risks of not breastfeeding

Step 5: Attitudes are addressed within the community that perceive bottle-feeding as the norm and provide education directed at changing these attitudes.

Step 6: Communities recognize the importance of supporting the mother-baby relationship.

Step 7: Education is provided about breastfeeding as the natural and normal method of infant feeding.

Step 8: All public and private facilities, including parks and recreation centres, restaurants, and stores, support the need to be mother- and baby-friendly.

Step 9: Work settings promote breastfeeding through the provision of extended maternity leave and/or provide facilities for mother to express milk and maintain their breastfeeding relationship.

Step 10: Support is given to women who do not meet their breastfeeding goals so as to resolve their feelings and to find the most suitable alternative.

Source: Ten Steps to Baby-Friendly Communities, Public Health Agency of Canada, 2002. Reproduced with the permission of the Minister of Public Works and Government Services Canada, 2008. Adapted from F. Jones and M. Green, *British Columbia Baby-Friendly Initiative: Resources Developed Through the BC Breastfeeding Resources Project* (Vancouver: BC Baby-Friendly Initiative, 1996).

Centre reported breastfeeding initiation rates before, during, and after Baby-Friendly policies. In 1995, before the initiative, initiation rates were 58 percent; in 1998, after the initiative, they were 78 percent; and in 1999 they were 87 percent. Exclusive breastfeeding rates increased from 6 percent to 29 percent to 34 percent (Philipp et al. 2001).

By 1999, there was only one hospital in Canada that qualified for Baby-Friendly status: Hôpital Brome-Missisquoi-Perkins Hospital in Quebec. Another forty-nine hospitals had indicated that they had an interest in being designated Baby-Friendly or were at some stage of changing maternity practices (Breastfeeding Committee for Canada 2002b). Worldwide, by 2000, 132 countries and nearly 15,000 hospitals had joined the Baby-Friendly Hospital Initiative. Only 300 of these hospitals were in the industrialized world, with the United States having twenty and Canada having one (Wah 2000).

Actions Speak Louder Than Words

While it appeared that all sectors of the health care system supported breastfeeding, several events in the late 1990s suggested that there was perhaps still a need for a "vigorous defence against incursions of a 'bottle-feeding culture'" (WHO and UNICEF 1990). At the end of the decade, controversies erupted between breastfeeding advocates and several professional health associations, including the Dieticians of Canada, the CPS, and the Society of Obstetricians and Gynaecologists.

In the late 1990s, there were several reports of advertisements in Canadian medical journals that violated the WHO Code. In the mid-1990s, letters to the editor in the journal *Canadian Family Physician* debated whether accepting advertisements from the formula industry, which violated the WHO Code, was a sign that the College of Family Physicians was giving in to strong industry pressures or whether physicians were entitled to scientific information from the formula industry. After a new series of advertisements, the college formally endorsed the WHO Code and stopped accepting advertisements that did not comply with it (Reid 1996). In 1997, an article in the *Globe and Mail* commented on a letter that Bev Chalmers, a researcher at the Centre for Research in Women's Health at the University of Toronto, sent to the *Journal of Obstetricians and Gynaecologists of Canada*. The journal had recently included an advertisement that showed a formula-fed infant that, quite literally, had stars in its eyes (Coutts 1997).

Other controversies erupted from the suggestion that exclusive breast-feeding in the first months of life was not enough to maintain the health and well-being of infants. In 1998, the CPS, the Dieticians of Canada, and Health Canada released a document entitled *Nutrition for Healthy Term Infants*. This publication provided infant feeding guidelines for health professionals and recommended that exclusive breastfeeding be encouraged for at least four months, followed by the continuation of breastfeeding along with complementary foods for up to two years and beyond. The guidelines also recommended that all infants, regardless of feeding method, receive a vitamin D supplement. Advocates argued that vitamin D supplementation was definitely recommended in select cases, but they disagreed with the overall recommendations. Universal supplementation of breastfeeding with vitamin supplements suggested that breast milk was not adequate, and this undermined mothers' belief in the value of breastfeeding. Another example of the lack of conviction in the adequacy of breast milk emerged in other medical discussions. One 1998 article entitled "Feeding Premature Infants after Hospital Discharge" and published in the *Journal of the Canadian Paediatric Society* suggested that premature infants required either commercial premature infant formulas or breast milk and supplements. Formula and breast milk were viewed as equivalent, and the risks of formula to premature infants were not adequately recognized. The idea that breast milk was not adequate was also encouraged by the formula industry. For example, Mead Johnson published an advertisement in the *Canadian Family Physician* that depicted a breastfed infant along with the statement: "Right now this baby could be looking at a vitamin D deficiency" (Habib 1999).

Human milk banks were another area of controversy. In the mid-1980s, there had been nineteen milk banks in Canada (Sauve et al. 1984). Throughout the

1980s, across North America, a number of milk banks closed due to concerns about viral transmission, especially HIV/AIDS (Sterken 2004; F. Jones 2003). By the end of the 1980s, there were only eight or nine milk banks in North America and only one in Canada (F. Jones 2003). Throughout the 1990s, Canada's only milk bank, located at B.C. Children's Hospital in Vancouver, was threatened with closure due to the CPS's negative comments about milk banking and a lack of funding. In this same decade, after safety concerns were adequately addressed, the number of milk banks began to grow in countries such as the United States, Britain, Norway, France, and Brazil (Habib 1997). In Canada, however, the influential CPS published a 1995 position paper advising against the routine use of human milk and wet-nursing. As Frances Jones (2003, 315) commented, this position paper essentially condemned "donor milk banking, [blending it] with the quite distinctly different activities of blood banking and wet nursing." Although the CPS's statement was later withdrawn, support for milk banks did not increase in Canada as it did in other countries. Five years later, rather than questioning the lack of material resources and support that the last remaining milk bank received, an editorial in the *Canadian Medical Association Journal* commented on how the milk bank cost $100,000 to run and provided milk to only twenty infants (Sibbald 2000; Cosh 2000).

Making Informed Decisions

In the 1990s, breastfeeding promotion and advocacy shifted towards ensuring that all women were able to make informed decisions about infant feeding. Hospital practices, aggressive marketing by the infant formula industry, and societal attitudes towards breastfeeding in public were three factors that were seen to be impairing women's abilities to make informed choices and to successfully breastfeed in the long-term. Breastfeeding promotion programs shifted from universal programs targeted at all mothers towards programs targeted at "high-risk" groups. Many promotion programs continued to be based on the principle that mothers merely needed information about the scientific merits of breastfeeding in order to make an appropriate decision. Often, in the process of convincing mothers of the benefits of breastfeeding, health promotion professionals created a romantic view of breastfeeding– one that did not necessarily reflect women's actual experiences.

Survey after survey demonstrated that particular groups of mothers were less likely to breastfeed than others. Breastfeeding promotion programs in the 1990s began to target these "high-risk" groups, including low-income mothers, young mothers, and immigrant mothers (Doran and Evers 1997; Barber et al. 1997). One of the most novel approaches to increasing breastfeeding in low-income women occurred in the province of Quebec. In 1994, the government of Quebec found that only 9 percent of women on welfare were breastfeeding while 60 percent of women in the general population were doing so. Consequently, the provincial government decided to increase income assistance premiums to women who breastfed and to cease paying for infant formula (International Women's Rights Watch 1994). For the past twenty-five years, Quebec had paid supplements to breastfeeding mothers and subsidized the cost of infant formula. In March 1994, the province raised the breastfeeding allowance from $15 per month to $37.50 per month and reduced the subsidy for formula. It was estimated that there were 7,000 women in Quebec who had infants under the age of six months. The program would cost the province $3.8 million a year, and it was to be financed with money saved by the reduction in formula subsidies. To prevent abuses, the government required that women provide an affidavit from their doctor's office or their local income security office (Farnsworth 1994).

Immigrant mothers were another "high-risk" group upon which the federal government increasingly focused. In 1997, Health Canada published *Multicultural Perspective of Breastfeeding in Canada.* This publication was developed in order to provide cross-cultural awareness and, hence, culturally sensitive breastfeeding support services. It examined breastfeeding norms and practices in various cultural groups in Canada. There was a strong belief in the breastfeeding promotion community that breastfeeding was a dominant practice in the country of origin for many immigrants. Yet, when women immigrated to Canada, they were believed to switch to bottle-feeding due to their perception that formula was the dominant and preferred form of feeding in Canada. The switch to formula feeding was considered to be a component of the acculturation process. Interestingly, the results from the 1994 NPHS and NLSCY surveys suggested that significantly more immigrants than non-immigrants initiated breastfeeding. Both surveys found that approximately 83 percent of immigrant mothers initiated breastfeeding, while only 71 percent of non-immigrant mothers did so (see Table 9.4). However, duration rates were higher in the non-immigrant population, with 50 percent of immigrants breastfeeding for fewer than three months and only 35 percent of non-immigrants doing so. One 1993 study in Vancouver found variations in breastfeeding initiation and duration between various ethnic groups. The researchers found that infant feeding practices did not vary according to the length of time that the mother had lived in Canada. It was unclear to what extent other socio-demographic variables (e.g., age, education, marital status) might have explained these differences. Such socio-demographic variables could reveal other factors that influence breastfeeding practices, such as greater social support or a more flexible schedule (Williams, Innis, and Vogel 1996).

In 1991, a revised edition of *The Canadian Mother and Child* entitled *You and Your Baby* was co-published by Douglas and McIntyre and Health and Welfare Canada. When discussing infant feeding decision making, the authors wrote, "Whether to breast-feed or bottle-feed your baby is a personal decision that should not be made lightly. Before making up your mind, learn about each method. What are the advantages and disadvantages? After gathering the facts, you and your partner can make the right decision for you" (Nonesuch and Health and Welfare Canada 1991, 127). The book discussed the advantages and disadvantages of both breastfeeding and formula feeding and provided a range of options: "How long should I nurse my baby? You may choose to nurse for a number of weeks, or up to twelve months, or even longer" (Nonesuch and Health and Welfare Canada 1991, 135). Underlying *You and Your Baby* and many of the breastfeeding promotion materials produced by Health Canada during the 1990s was the principle that mothers needed appropriate information regarding the infant feeding choices that were available to them.

Most research had indicated that women make their infant feeding decisions prior to conception or in their first trimester of pregnancy. Numerous studies had examined the relative impact of various social influences (e.g., family, health professionals, media) on women's decisions, with inconclusive results. The National Population Health Survey found that health professionals (24 percent), a woman's partner (15 percent), and a woman's family (13 percent) were the most frequently cited influences on women's decisions. Health professionals had the most influence on young women, immigrant women, women with upper-middle- and high-class incomes, and rural women (Maclean 1998). Yet most mothers reported that they made an autonomous decision to breastfeed, with nearly 50 percent of the women surveyed indicating that "no one" influenced them. Clearly, it is difficult, if not impossible, to make truly autonomous decisions when one is born into and lives within a particular socio-cultural milieu. Yet, this finding challenges the assumption that mothers make deliberate and active decisions about infant feeding. Further, Maclean (1990) found that nearly half of her sample of mothers claimed that the decision to breastfeed was not really a decision at all as there was simply no question as to what they would do; the other half described a more deliberative process, which involved reading and talking with women and health professionals (Maclean 1998, 1990).

Throughout the 1990s, promotion materials generally presented breastfeeding in a positive light. The *National Guidelines for Health Care Providers* (1996) listed nearly three pages of benefits and no disadvantages. In practice, many mothers and health professionals painted a rosy and simple picture of breastfeeding. For example, it was described as convenient, as there was no need to sterilize bottles or heat things up: one could simply leave the house without prior thought. Little attention was given to the fact that mothers would find it challenging to be apart from their child for long periods without expressing and pre-planning and that they would be the only ones who could provide nourishment for the first few months after birth. One of the benefits commonly emphasized was that breastfeeding would help mothers lose weight following birth (Wall 2001). While many professionals acknowledged that breastfeeding can be uncomfortable or difficult, promotional materials suggested that all of these problems could be overcome with a little support: "It is important to understand that the first few weeks are the learning period for both of you, and that time, patience, and humour will solve many problems" (Health Canada 1998b).

In her analysis of breastfeeding education materials throughout the 1990s, Wall (2001, 604) commented, "an emphasis on the unique, intimate, and embodied connection between mother and child is combined with efforts to convince women of the benefits of breast milk for their babies and technical advice that will help them to better manage their bodies in this regard." An emphasis on the benefits of breastfeeding avoided contributing to messages that supported formula feeding (e.g., bottle-feeding is not only convenient but also less messy). The difficulty with trying to "sell" breastfeeding to mothers was that it focused on the benefits of breastfeeding rather than on the risks of infant formula. Rather than truly assuming that breastfeeding was the normal method of infant feeding, health promotion materials took a defensive stance, focusing on the merits of breastfeeding and avoiding the subject of infant formula altogether. Ironically, the formula industry often used scientific evidence on the merits of breastfeeding to promote its own products (e.g., "just like mother's milk!"). Perhaps more troubling was the refusal to acknowledge the incongruity between health promotion materials, mother's ideals, and women's actual experiences. The "Breastfeeding Anytime, Anywhere" campaign attempted to convince mothers and the public that breasts should not be considered sexual in the context of breastfeeding, with posters proclaiming messages such as, "Who Said a Day at the Mall Was Impossible?" As Wall (2001, 598) points out, "to the extent that such representations lend authority to women's right to breastfeed in public, they are indeed helpful. They can also, however, act to deny women's experiences."

In the 1990s, breastfeeding promotion efforts targeted mothers who were less likely to breastfeed. The decision not to breastfeed was often perceived as a deliberate choice resulting from a lack of education or from women not trying hard enough to overcome barriers. Ironically, considering all the structural barriers to breastfeeding, these high-risk groups were, in all likelihood, comprised of the same mothers who had the least resources with which to successfully breastfeed. While breastfeeding was indeed a personal choice, the philosophy of informed choice promoted by health care providers did not sufficiently acknowledge the structural constraints on breastfeeding. Mothers who were not comfortable breastfeeding in public were often given advice on the type of clothing that might render breastfeeding a discreet activity (Canadian Institute of Child Health 1996). However, overcoming this kind of social pressure often requires women to have personal resources other than merely the right wardrobe. Similarly, while the stance of the Quebec government towards allowances for breastfeeding mothers suggested a shift towards a "breastfeeding culture," where breastfeeding was assumed to be the norm, this initiative more closely resembled social coercion than informed choice. Often, it was not personal preference that governed women's infant feeding choices but, rather, whether they had access to material resources. Practically, the Quebec breastfeeding allowance may have covered food expenses for women's additional caloric needs while breastfeeding. While many initiatives in the 1990s addressed "the removal of constraints and influences that manipulate perceptions and behaviour towards breastfeeding, often by subtle and indirect means" (WHO and UNICEF 1990), promotion efforts also continued to focus on providing education to mothers, in the hope of providing women with the knowledge and confidence to make the decision to breastfeed and to overcome the structural barriers that inhibited breastfeeding success.

Conclusion

In the 1990s, the Canadian government committed to "protecting, promoting, and supporting" breastfeeding through a variety of international agreements. In particular, initiatives to support breastfeeding evolved out of widespread interest, and they focus on the health and well-being of children. The federal government's most visible efforts to support breastfeeding included developing health promotion materials, funding the Expert Working Group on Breastfeeding (which later evolved into the Breastfeeding Committee for Canada), developing a social marketing campaign to encourage breastfeeding in public, and including breastfeeding in national discussions of child well-being and in the development of national surveys.

The federal government did not take further action to implement the 1981 WHO Code or to regulate the marketing practices of the formula industry. In 2000, infant formula sales across Canada were approximately $140.3 million (Kryhul 2000). Throughout the 1990s, marketing practices shifted from targeting hospitals and health professionals to targeting mothers directly through advertising, direct mailings, and free samples. Although UNICEF and the WHO had developed the Baby-Friendly Hospital Initiative in 1991, Canada did not become involved with this campaign until 1998. The campaign was launched by the Breastfeeding Committee for Canada, a national, multi-sectoral organization that received minimal financial support from the federal government and that worked via committee at the provincial and territorial levels. By 2000, 132 countries and nearly 15,000 hospitals worldwide had joined the Baby-Friendly Hospital Initiative. At the end of the decade, Canada had only one baby-friendly hospital (Wah 2000; Canadian Institute of Child Health 1996).

Increasingly, women were being challenged to see their breasts as more than just sexual organs. The social marketing campaign Breastfeeding

Anytime, Anywhere encouraged mothers and the general population to see breastfeeding as an acceptable public activity. As well, the 1997 decision by the B.C. Human Rights Tribunal in the case of *Poirier v. British Columbia* led to the first legal decision on breastfeeding issues in Canada. This decision not only supported women's right to breastfeed in public but also raised questions about how breastfeeding could be combined with paid work.

Breastfeeding promotion efforts shifted towards targeting high-risk groups of mothers (i.e., those who were less likely to breastfeed). Many of these efforts focused on educating women about the benefits of breastfeeding and strategies for overcoming difficulties. While the value of breastfeeding seemed to have universal support, controversies over vitamin supplements, the need for breast milk banks, and the relationship between various health professional groups and the formula industry contradicted the value that, publicly, many health professionals placed on breastfeeding. At the end of the decade, national breastfeeding initiation rates hovered just above 80 percent.

Part 4

At Equilibrium: Into the Twenty-First Century

Chapter 10

Continuities and Change: Breastfeeding in Canada at the Turn of the Twenty-First Century

O ver the past 150 years, rates of breastfeeding have declined and increased dramatically. Breastfeeding initiation rates in Canada fell from near universal levels at the beginning of the twentieth century to less than 25 percent at mid-century and returned to just over 80 percent at the turn of the twenty-first century. Changes in breastfeeding practices have been accompanied by changes in the availability and promotion of breast milk alternatives, the transmission of breastfeeding knowledge and skills, and the individual and societal value placed on breastfeeding and breast milk. In Canada, the practice of breastfeeding shifted from a private issue to a public concern at the end of the nineteenth century. Throughout the twentieth century many important influences on existing breastfeeding practices and policies emerged. At the beginning of the twenty-first century, as new social trends and values emerge, discussions of the importance and meaning of breastfeeding have grown and breastfeeding continues to receive interest, attention, and support from individuals, professionals, activists, mothers, and various social movements.

Breastfeeding Rates in Canada in 2003

In 2003, the Canadian Community Health Survey (CCHS) became the first national survey since the 1960s to collect data on exclusive breastfeeding rates. The CCHS measured the prevalence and duration of breastfeeding in women aged fifteen to fifty-five who had had a baby in the past five years. According to the survey, 85 percent of women attempted to breastfeed their child. Of the women who initiated breastfeeding, 22 percent had stopped by the end of the first month. Fewer than half the women (47 percent) breastfed for six months or more, and fewer than half of these women (17 percent) breastfed exclusively for six months or more (Millar and Maclean 2005). In 2003, a strong east-west gradient in breastfeeding initiation and duration persisted. Initiation rates ranged from 63 percent in Newfoundland and

Graph 10.1

National breastfeeding initiation trends, 1965–2003

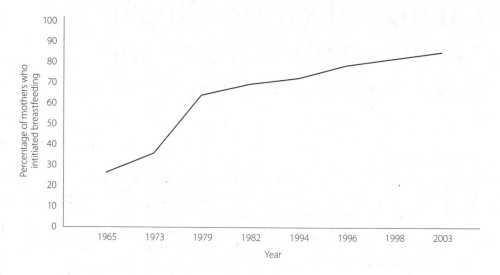

Source: Compiled from data found in Myres 1979; McNally, Hendricks, and Horowitz 1985; Health Canada 1985; Dzakpasu 2003; Millar and Maclean 2005.

Labrador to 76 percent in Quebec to 86 percent in Saskatchewan to 93 percent in British Columbia. Exclusive breastfeeding at six months ranged from 9 percent in Newfoundland and Labrador to 18 percent in Ontario, Manitoba, and Saskatchewan to 28 percent in British Columbia. The 2001 Aboriginal Peoples Survey revealed that breastfeeding rates in the Aboriginal population had also been increasing throughout the 1990s. Breastfeeding initiation was approximately 73 percent in 2001. Although initiation rates varied little between First Nations, Inuit, and Metis mothers, duration rates did. The average duration of breastfeeding for Inuit children was fifteen months, compared with eight months for First Nations and seven months for Metis children (Statistics Canada 2001b).

At the beginning of the twenty-first century, the majority of mothers in Canada were initiating breastfeeding at rates that resembled those at the beginning of the twentieth century. Since the 1960s, when breastfeeding rates were at their lowest, initiation and duration rates have been increasing. Between the late 1960s and early 1980s, breastfeeding initiation rates accelerated rapidly; rates plateaued nationally at about 75 percent for just over a decade. Initiation rates began to increase again in the mid-1990s from about 75 percent to about 85 percent in 2003. Duration rates have also increased over the past forty years, although at a much slower pace. The growth of exclusive breastfeeding practices has lagged behind the increase in duration rates. Only one in six mothers breastfed exclusively for six months in 2003. National breastfeeding rates hide a wide range of variation in breastfeeding practices across the country, including across social classes and across provinces. In many parts of Canada, particularly in British Columbia and in several social groups, initiation rates are very high. Consequently, growth in breastfeeding is mainly possible in terms of duration and exclusivity. While the rise and fall of breastfeeding in Canada has followed a pattern similar to that found in other Western countries, at the beginning of the twenty-first century, Canadian rates remain lower than those in Europe and Australia, although considerably higher than those in the United States (Callen and Pinelli 2004).

Alternatives to Mother's Milk:
From Cow's Milk to Breast Milk Banking and Commercial Infant Formula

The decline and rise of breastfeeding rates over the twentieth century have been accompanied by changes in the availability of alternatives to mother's milk in Canada. The majority of alternatives to breast milk were based on cow's milk. However, these alternatives were derived from various cow's-milk products, ranging from fresh whole cow's milk to canned evaporated and condensed milk to "ready-to-feed" commercial infant formulas. The popularity of many breast milk alternatives has changed over time, partly as a result of differences in cost, safety, and accessibility. Marketing, technological advances, and the societal value of breastfeeding have also driven the development and popularity of various alternatives. While many products used to feed infants are often called "breast milk substitutes," breast milk alternatives are still considered only to resemble–not replicate–mother's milk. Since the 1930s, milk banks have provided women who were not able or willing to breastfeed the opportunity to obtain breast milk for their infants.

Mead Johnson, Abbott Ross, Wyeth, and Nestlé continue to dominate the worldwide market for infant formula in the 2000s. In the late 1980s, with their ties to hospitals and physicians, Mead Johnson and Abbott Ross dominated the Canadian market. In the early 1990s, Nestlé entered the Canadian market. In 2005, approximately $191 million of milk formula was sold. The three dominant companies were Abbott Laboratories (makers of Similac and Isomil), Mead Johnson Nutritionals (makers of Enfamil and Enfalac), and Nestlé Canada (owners of Carnation and makers of Good Start and Alsoy). As of 2008, Wyeth's infant formula business in Canada belongs to Nestlé (Wyeth's brands include SMA and S-26). At present, most formula sold in Canada is manufactured in the United States or Europe: only Abbott Laboratories manufactures formula in Canada.

Data on the safety of infant formula in Canada is difficult to obtain. In the United States, between 1983 and 1993, there were twenty-two recalls of formula (Baumslag and Michels 1995). Since 2000, there have been several media reports on infant formula safety in Canada. In March 2000, Nestlé Canada voluntarily recalled its Good Start liquid concentrate when temperature fluctuations in its manufacturing process could not guarantee sterility of the products (Bertin 2000; Canada NewsWire 2000). In 2004, Mead Johnson recalled Enfalac Pregestimil Hypoallergenic Infant Formula as it contained an incorrect size of scoop that could cause over-concentration of the formula and thus result in medical problems (Canadian Press NewsWire 2004). In 2006, the Canadian Food Inspection Agency issued a warning about a can of Mead Johnson powdered infant formula containing what appeared to be detergent (Canadian Food Inspection Agency 2006). As well, because powdered infant formula is not commercially sterile, it can be contaminated. After outbreaks in neonatal intensive care units in the United States, Canada, and some European countries, there are ongoing concerns about *Enterobacter sakazakii* infection and powdered infant formula.

In 2005, there were three kinds of formula available on the market: powdered, liquid, and ready-to-feed. Powdered formula represented 91 percent of the market while liquid formula represented 9 percent. The price of formula varies, with powdered formula being the cheapest and ready-to-feed formula being the most expensive (Netscribes 2005). In addition to the major brand names, there are several "value-priced" products available in Canada. Unilac, a Canadian company, sells formula through retail outlets, including Zellers. Parent's Choice is sold in Wal-Mart and President's Choice is sold in The Real Canadian Superstore (Loblaws). As all these products are governed by the Food and Drugs Act, there are no major nutritional differences between store brands and name brands. However, name brands can cost two to three times more than store brands, especially when brand names including essential fatty acids are compared (Lowry 2004).

The inclusion of essential fatty acids such as ARA (arachidonic acid) and DHA (docosahexaenoic acid) are a recent development in infant formula marketing. Both ARA and DHA are found in breast milk, and some studies have suggested that ARA and DHA have positive benefits with regard to a variety of child development outcomes. Although birth rates are declining in Canada, a 2006 report on baby foods commented that formula sales were expected to increase by 2 percent in 2005. This predicted increase was attributed to the launch and popularity of fatty-acid-fortified formulas (Euromonitor International 2006). The "trendiness" of functional foods also appears to be extending to baby foods. Products such as Nestlé Baby Cereal Add Milk (dried baby cereal that can be mixed with breast milk or infant formula) are becoming popular. In terms of regulation, additives like ARA and DHA are permitted in infant formula as the current regulations allow any compound found in breast milk to be added to formula (Committee on the Evaluation of the Addition of Ingredients New to Infant Formula 2004).

In the 2000s, commercial infant formula is the dominant alternative to mother's milk, although evaporated milk continues to be used in some low-income groups. The popularity and accessibility of milk banks have also declined since the 1930s. During the 1950s and 1960s, when breastfeeding rates were at their lowest in Canada, there was a decline in interest in milk banks. The 1980s saw Canada's milk banks close due to fears about HIV/AIDS, until only one of the twenty-three remained. The milk bank at B.C. Children's and Women's Hospital in Vancouver is part of the Human Milk Banking Association of North America and follows the association's guidelines for the collection, processing, and distribution of donor milk. In 2002, the milk bank distributed 33,399 ounces of donor milk (F. Jones 2003); in 2004, 255 babies received milk from the bank (Nicholson 2005).

However, Canada's only milk bank is not accessible to most mothers. It is hospital-based and primarily provides milk for hospital patients, including premature infants, formula intolerant infants, and infants of HIV-positive mothers. Infants within British Columbia and other infants at risk across Canada can also use the milk bank. While the milk is technically donated and distributed for free, milk bank recipients have to pay a processing fee of approximately three dollars for 2.5 ounces. In 2006, an article in the *Toronto Star* reported on a family that found the Vancouver milk bank on the Internet (Kopun 2006). The family spent $160 per week on breast milk plus $100 to have it delivered (packed in ice) by courier. Some families attempt to obtain donor milk from an American milk bank, and this can cost over $20,000.

While breast milk banks may provide the preferred alternative to mother's milk, they are currently underfunded and inaccessible to most mothers in Canada. Commercial infant formulas regulated by the Food and Drugs Act are what is predominately used in Canada. Evaporated milk, once the most widely used form of cow's milk in infant formulas, is rarely used now except by some low-income groups (Friel 1997). Although the Canadian birth rate is declining, the commercial formula industry remains a growth industry dominated by a handful of competitors. Technological advances have improved the nutrient quality of infant formulas, yet they still bear little resemblance to mother's milk. As well, while not nearly as extreme as in the early twentieth century, concerns about the safety and suitability of existing infant formulas remain.

Breastfeeding Knowledge and Skills: Shifting Domains

The manner in which women have acquired knowledge and skills about breastfeeding has changed over the past 150 years. For most of the twentieth century, breastfeeding has fallen under the jurisdiction of scientific medicine. In some circumstances, the state has encouraged lay support groups, like La Leche League, that valued women's knowledge and experiences. One of the consequences of socio-demographic change (e.g., immigration, declining fertility, hospitalization of childbirth, migration) in conjunction with long-term scientific and medical involvement in infant feeding has been the "deskilling" of mothers, with the result that many women do not have the practical knowledge or social support to breastfeed successfully. Unfortunately, over much of the twentieth century, professional support has often been absent or problematic for women attempting to breastfeed.

In the 2000s, breastfeeding has remained under the jurisdiction of scientific medicine. Indeed, in the 1990s, two new groups of professionals became more prominent in their involvement with breastfeeding: the Dieticians of Canada and lactation consultants. In the mid-1980s, Canadians began to write the International Board Certified Lactation exam, and the number of lactation consultants grew throughout the 1990s. By 2002, there were 1,191 lactation consultants in Canada (Canadian Institute for Health Information 2004b).

The popularity of La Leche League has also diminished since the 1990s. In 1976, the League had 140 groups and 325 leaders in Canada. In the early 1990s, the size of the organization peaked, with nearly 300 groups and about 640 leaders. As of October 2003, there were 1,169 members in La Leche League Canada. It is estimated that during 2002–3 over 460 volunteer leaders conducted approximately 450 monthly education sessions and fielded 35,000 phone calls and e-mails from mothers, health professionals, and others (Ayre-Jaschke 2004). In 2004, the league had 188 groups and 466 leaders (Audy 2004).

The relationship between the state and scientific and medical professionals has changed over the past century. Often, the state has utilized physicians and health professionals as "gatekeepers" to enact various infant feeding policies. For example, during the Second World War, parents could only obtain evaporated milk rations with a medical prescription or certificate from a physician, public health nurse, or a recognized healthy agency (Canadian Press 1943). Similarly, in 1994, mothers in Quebec on income assistance could receive a breastfeeding allowance provided that they had an affidavit from their doctor's office (Farnsworth 1994). In 2006, mothers could access the milk bank at B.C. Children's Hospital with a doctor's prescription. At other times, the state has been less autonomous and has been unable to enact infant feeding policies without considering scientific and medical professionals and other interest groups. The national campaign to promote breastfeeding, initiated in 1979, was delayed until the government could ensure widespread support and consensus on the value of breastfeeding from medical authorities. The government also recognized the influence of health professionals in creating environments supportive of breastfeeding.

For most of the twentieth century, scientific medicine has been dominant in shaping and influencing the transmission of knowledge and skills about breastfeeding. Although some of the strongest advocates of breastfeeding have emerged from the health professions, for the most part, the involvement of scientific medicine in issues of infant feeding has negatively influenced breastfeeding outcomes. The lack of support for breastfeeding has sometimes been passive, with professionals espousing an attitude of indifference towards breastfeeding. It has also been quite active, with professionals encouraging the abandonment of breastfeeding when difficulties occur and/ or disseminating misleading information. While all health professionals can potentially influence breastfeeding outcomes, the knowledge, attitudes, and skills of physicians have received the most attention in the past two decades as medical doctors enjoy elevated status among health professionals. They are also assumed to be knowledgeable about infant feeding. The need for breastfeeding education for physicians has been recognized for decades. Research has also shown that many physicians remain unconvinced about the merits of breastfeeding and that poor advice and lack of knowledge or interest in breastfeeding is widespread (Burglehaus and Sheps 1997). The greater number of women entering the profession do not seem to have influenced practices considerably. Indeed, most female residents and self-employed physicians receive only a few weeks or months of maternity leave, which is often an enormous barrier to continued exclusive breastfeeding (Lent et al. 2000; Bowman 2005). As well, there remains a long-standing suspicion of the relationship between physicians and the infant formula industry and of industry involvement in providing education materials and seminars for physicians.

In recent years, there have been a number of controversies regarding breastfeeding advice disseminated by authoritative medical bodies, and this has raised questions about their commitment to breastfeeding promotion. In 1996, the Canadian Paediatric Society released a statement on infant feeding claiming that breast milk alone was not adequate for preterm infants. It also compared human donor milk to wet-nursing and argued that the sterilization process that makes human donor milk safe also destroys the properties that make breast milk superior to infant formula. The statement clearly advised against the use of human donor milk and advocated for reallocating resources currently dedicated to human milk banks. Overall, it suggested that infant formula was an appropriate choice for many women who experienced difficulties breastfeeding (Canadian Paediatric Society 1996). In 2004, the CPS issued an advisory against bed-sharing, the practice of infants sharing a bed with their parents, due to concerns about entrapment and suffocation. While questions were raised about the appropriateness of health authorities dictating sleeping arrangements that may be rooted in long-standing cultural practices, the lack of attention to evidence suggesting that bed-sharing facilitates breastfeeding raised the ire of breastfeeding advocates (Bueckert 2006; Ball 2003; McKenna, Mosko, and Richard 1997).

In the 1920s, the federal government publication *The Canadian Mother's Book* recommended providing all infants with two to three drops of cod-liver oil from the age of two weeks to ensure adequate vitamin D intake. Over eighty years later, questions about the need for vitamin supplements for breastfed infants still remain. In 1998 and 2005, Health Canada, the Dieticians of Canada, and the CPS released statements recommending that all breastfed, full-term infants in Canada receive a daily vitamin D supplement of 10 µg (400 IU). Statements about the need for vitamin supplementation continue to suggest that breast milk alone is not adequate to nourish an infant and encourage mothers to question the quality of their breast milk. In the case of vitamin D, breastfeeding advocates argue that sunshine and mother's vitamin D levels are sufficient to ensure an adequate supply for infants and that universal recommendations of vitamin D supplements are not an appropriate strategy for addressing the rare case of rickets in Canada.

Over the twentieth century, demographic change and changes in the social organization of daily life resulted in fewer opportunities for women to gain from other women the skills to successfully breastfeed (Ryan and Grace 2001). Institutional structures based on scientific medical authority have, for the most part, replaced mother-to-mother learning. Although, since the 1960s, La Leche League has supported breastfeeding in Canada, at the beginning of the twenty-first century most new mothers remain dependent on expert sources of breastfeeding knowledge and support.

The Value of Breastfeeding

The federal government has valued breastfeeding over the past century for various reasons. Initial interest in promoting breastfeeding emerged in the 1920s due to concerns about infant mortality. The end of the 1970s marked a renewed period of government interest in and support of breastfeeding. In the 1970s, breastfeeding was especially valued for its nutritional, immuno-logical, and psychological benefits for both mother and infant. Breastfeeding emerged in policy discussions in the 1990s as part of a greater emphasis on early childhood development and population health. In the 2000s, there appears to be growing interest in breastfeeding as a result of new and grow-ing research showing a relationship between breastfeeding and childhood obesity (Kirkey 2005; Cohen 2006) and the relationship between nutrition and chronic disease. The 2004 report *Improving the Health of Canadians* (Canadian Institute for Health Information 2004a) includes five strategies to prevent obesity: breastfeeding is listed first. Ongoing breastfeeding promo-tion efforts increasingly list decreased risk of developing obesity as another benefit of breastfeeding.

The popularity of breastfeeding has been closely linked to changes in social values. In the 1920s, as women were exploring new roles in society, the bottle began to symbolize women's autonomy, offering convenience and flexibility. In contrast, with the emergence of the natural childbirth movement and the women's health movement, breastfeeding symbolized freedom from scientific and medical authority. The perception that bottle-feeding offers a more flexible, comfortable, and predictable lifestyle persists in the twenty-first century, particularly in the marketing messages of the formula industry (Van Esterik 1994). Values relating to parenthood have also shifted. Beginning in the 1940s, fathers were increasingly involved in infant care. And many women see bottle-feeding as one way to receive support from their partners in caring for children.

In the past decade, new forms of activism and social movements concerned with sustainability, anti-corporatism, and food security have included breastfeeding in their discussions. Breastfeeding is viewed as an ecologically sound, complete, and safe food source. Infant formula, in contrast, contributes to environmental contamination with the consumption of materials and production of waste (INFACT Canada). Controversies over the merits of genetically engineered ingredients in food have extended to infant formula and baby foods and have raised questions about the potential impact of genetically engineered products on infants (Habib 2002). Disasters such as Hurricane Katrina have highlighted how formula fosters dependence on external food sources, while breastfeeding does not (Payne 2005). In an editorial in *Public Health Nutrition*, editor Marilyn Tseng suggests that breastfeeding could be considered part of the "slow food movement," which resists the growth of fast food and high-paced lives, with their detrimental impact on local food traditions and food choices. She comments on the global shift away from the practice of individuals growing and preparing their own food in favour of purchasing food: "Infant formula is the earliest possible introduction to buying food for consumption ... Breast milk is locally grown, authentic, unprocessed and certainly time-intensive" (Tseng 2006, 667). A renewed emphasis on anti-consumerism stands in contrast to the consumerism of the 1930s, when good motherhood was associated with the purchase of "modern" products, including bottles and related infant feeding products. These types of concerns are also present in government policy. The subject of breastfeeding was included in "Canada's Action Plan for Food Security: A Response to the World Summit." The summit was held in 1996, and the plan was formed in 1999. It stated, "For the majority of infants, breastfeeding is the most important guarantee of food security. It ensures a safe, secure and nutritionally complete food source" (Agriculture and Agri-Food Canada 1998, 2003, 1999).

In the past decade, several researchers and breastfeeding advocates have attempted to quantify the value of breastfeeding by calculating its health benefits and economic savings. For example, Beaudry, Dufour, and Marcoux (1995), in a retrospective study in New Brunswick, examined the relationship between infant feeding method and gastrointestinal and respiratory infections. The researchers found that, after controlling for socio-economic status, infant's age, mother's age, and maternal smoking, gastrointestinal illnesses were 47 percent lower in breastfed infants and respiratory illnesses were 34 percent lower. Another study using data from Scotland and the United States examined the cost of health care services for lower respiratory tract illnesses, otitis media, and gastrointestinal illness in formula-fed infants in the first year of life (Ball and Wright 1999). The researchers found that there were 2,033 excess office visits, 212 excess days of hospitalization, and 609 excess prescriptions for these three illnesses per 1,000 never-breastfed infants compared with 1,000 infants exclusively breastfed for at least three months. These additional health care services cost the managed care health system between $331 and $475 per never-breastfed infant during the first year of life. In 2002, INFACT Canada calculated the hospitalization costs for infants admitted with acute respiratory disease and asthma. The total hospitalization cost of infants under the age of one admitted for acute respiratory disease across Canada was $38,587,535; for asthma, the costs were $36,416,587 (INFACT Canada 2002b).

While some researchers have used economic analyses to explore the costs and benefits of breastfeeding, others have used them to highlight women's reproductive and unpaid work. Since 1993, the Norwegian National Council has included human milk output in its annual reports on national food production (Smith 1999). While this approach may be considered offensive to some individuals and may be seen as contributing to "putting a price on something that is priceless," it does make visible women's reproductive contributions (Smith and Ingham 2005). Smith (1999) calculated that, in 1992 in Australia, women produced 33 million kilograms of breast milk and that this was worth US$1.5 to $1.6 billion. This accounted for 0.5 percent of the GDP, or 6 percent of private spending on food (Smith and Ingham 2005; Smith 1999). Smith pointed out that, at present, national GDP increases if more infant formula is sold but not if breastfeeding is increased (Smith and Ingham 2005).

Since the 1930s, with the emergence of milk banks (which superseded the historical use of wet nurses), there has been increasing attention paid to the benefits of breast milk rather than breastfeeding. In 2002, Van Esterik (2002, 257) commented, "Paradoxically, the more breastfeeding is valued the more it may be embedded in rules and pattern of interactions unconnected to infant feeding. The more we know about all the desirable properties of the product, the greater its potential to be commodified, and the more breastfeeding may become regulated or embedded in coercive practices." In the 2000s, the value that many individuals and groups place on breast milk appears to be contributing to an increasing trend towards the commodification of breast milk.

In the 2000s, the demand for donated human breast milk has been increasing in response to the increasing value placed on breast milk (Pearce 2007; Tully, Lockhart-Borman, and Updegrove 2004). Donor milk is being used for purposes ranging from supplementing mother's own milk to therapy for infants after surgery to providing milk for adopted infants whose parents want to ensure optimal growth. Because of breast milk's IgA content, it is useful for immunologically deficient adults, and there is growing interest in using donor milk for cancer therapy (Tully, Lockhart-Borman, and Updegrove 2004). In Canada, where there is currently only one milk bank, efforts are being made to set up milk banks in Quebec, Alberta, Saskatchewan, Nunavut, and Ontario (Kopun 2006).

Historically, breast milk was viewed as a commodity. When milk banks first emerged in the 1930s, women could sell their breast milk in order to earn money. Eventually, this view of breast milk shifted as formula feeding became more popular and breast milk was donated mainly by middle-class women (Golden 1996). With increasing public awareness of the value of breast milk, it appears that the view of breast milk as a commodity is re-emerging–this time within a highly complex corporate food and drug environment.

Prolacta Bioscience, a new organization in California, is challenging the view of breast milk banks as being a philanthropic endeavour. In 2005, Prolacta started selling its own brand of breast milk, called Prolact-22, for low birth weight babies–at ten times the price of milk available from milk banks. Prolacta has also begun to develop a highly sophisticated donation and collection system in hospitals across the United States, causing some to worry that the new collection system may pressure women into donating. Some are asking whether it is ethical for mothers to donate and then to have the hospital and Prolacta profit from this donation (Picard 2005; Bernhard 2005; Ensor 2006).

At the same time, reports from across Canada and the United States describe the development of a "breast milk black market." Using American figures, enough breast milk from a milk bank for one infant for six months could cost as much as $18,000 (even though the price of breast milk from milk banks is intended only to cover processing fees). As a response to this, women on the Internet and in classified ads are developing "milk sharing" networks, where they share, swap, and sell breast milk. Women also appear to be forming their own networks with family members and close friends. An article in the *Globe and Mail* on the return of the wet nurse described the experience of one mother:

> When Toronto mother Janet Belray was diagnosed with breast cancer in her right breast, a mastectomy and chemotherapy ended her six-month-old son's breastfeeding at least a year earlier than she'd intended. A close friend organized six "milk mamas," including one woman Ms. Belray had never met, to pump for baby Julian until he was 11 months old. "It was the single most amazing thing these women could have done for me," says Ms. Belray, who celebrated her milk donors at a "weaning" brunch at a Toronto restaurant. (quoted in Pearce 2007, L1)

While many women are happy to donate their milk to needy infants, others believe that they should be compensated, like sperm or egg donors. While Prolacta is selling breast milk concentrate for forty-eight dollars an ounce, mothers on the Internet are selling their breast milk for one dollar to $2.50 an ounce (Austin 2006). Another report suggests that mothers who cannot afford the price of milk banks can purchase unpasteurized breast milk for ten to twenty dollars a litre (Anonymous 2005).

However, unlike with historical wet-nursing, where an infant would receive milk from one woman, the sale of breast milk results in one infant receiving milk from multiple women. In 2006, Health Canada released a warning about the sale and distribution of human milk obtained from the Internet or sold directly by individuals (Health Canada 2006; F. Jones 2006a). The advisory highlighted concerns about the transmission of disease (e.g., HIV, staphylococcus aureus) through breast milk, especially where medical information is lacking, as well as risks from improper handling and storage. Thus far, there has been minimal discussion of the need for regulation or whether informal mothers' networks should be allowed to thrive as they have done historically.

The valuable properties of mother's milk have certainly been recognized by the infant formula industry, particularly in the development and marketing of infant formulas. At the end of the nineteenth century, scientists were experimenting with strategies for "humanizing" cow's milk through the addition of substances such as lactic acid, lemon juice, barley water, and sodium bicarbonate. At the beginning of the twenty-first century, scientists and industry are increasingly using biotechnology to create formulas that, purportedly, more closely resemble breast milk. Attempts to replicate mother's milk through the addition of substances also found in human milk have contributed to debate about the actual benefits and safety of these products. Most recently, research is emerging on the use of probiotics (bacteria that colonize the intestine and aid in digestion) and prebiotics (substances such as fructo-oligosaccharides and galacto-oligosaccharides, which make the environment in the gut more conducive to the survival of probiotic bacteria) in infant formulas (Sommer 2005). Currently, Martek Biosciences is the only company licensed by the U.S. Food and Drug Administration to sell the "proprietary blend" of nutritional oil that contains DHA and ARA (Anonymous 2004). In addition to the questionable process of marketing these infant formulas as mimicking breast milk, the addition of DHA and ARA raises questions about who can own these products. Is it possible for a corporation to own or patent chemicals that are naturally found in breast milk? Further, researchers have shown that federal regulatory processes for evaluating the safety of food ingredients in conventional foods are not adequate for ensuring the safety of these new types of ingredients in infant formulas (Committee on the Evaluation of the Addition of Ingredients New to Infant Formula 2004).

One of the most startling applications of new biotechnologies to infant feeding has unnerving similarities to the premise of a science fiction novel. In the late 1990s, researchers developed the ability to genetically modify mammary-specific genes in cows. This technology has been fuelled by commercial interests, and it has been suggested that modifying bovine mammary glands could result in altering the composition of cow's milk. Further, it might just be possible to produce a milk that resembles human breast milk, which could then supplement or replace infant formula (Wall, Kerr, and Bondioli 1997).

Herman was the first transgenic dairy bull (Anonymous 2000). A human gene was spliced into Herman to produce milk with human proteins, lysozyme, and lactoferrin. Rather than having to add lactoferrin to infant formula, Herman's female progeny were intended to produce these proteins at a lower cost. This product was initially intended to be launched in 1996. Following widespread protests, the product was redefined as containing modified lactoferrin and sold for different purposes (Van Esterik 2000). Another report from the late 1990s described Wyeth as working with PPL Therapeutics in Virginia to develop a "completely humanized milk product where you would milk a cow and almost any human milk would come out ... We now have a mini-herd of transgenic cattle that are making human alphalactalbumin ... in their milk" (quoted in Martyn 2003, p. 213).

Conclusion

At the beginning of the twenty-first century, the majority of mothers in Canada do not breastfeed exclusively for long periods of time. Even in the province of British Columbia, which has had the highest rates of breastfeeding since the 1960s, in 2003 only 50 percent of women breastfed exclusively for at least four months. The rise and fall of breastfeeding in Canada is related to enormous transformations in the economic, political, and social organization of life. One significant change has been the decline of informal methods for the sharing of breastfeeding knowledge and skills. Public institutions, in particular the health care system, currently provide practical and emotional support to new mothers learning to breastfeed. For most of the twentieth century, breastfeeding has fallen under the jurisdiction and expertise of scientific medicine, which has often not encouraged successful breastfeeding. Over the past century, there have been a variety of alternatives available to women who were unable or chose not to breastfeed. By the end of the twentieth century, commercial infant formula had become the most widely used alternative. Science and industry continue to apply new technological developments to replicate the properties of mother's milk. In the 2000s, individuals and groups have increasingly recognized the benefits of breast milk. The demand for milk banks and the development of informal selling and sharing of breast milk are raising new concerns about the regulation of breastfeeding and breast milk.

Chapter 11

Using the Past to Look Forward: Breastfeeding Policy for the Twenty-First Century

W hile the twenty-first century offers a new context for the development of breastfeeding policy, existing policy continues to be based on precedents and perspectives from earlier times. In this chapter we consider the lessons learned from our century-long description of breastfeeding and breastfeeding policy and offer guidance, based on an understanding of this history, for breastfeeding policy in the twenty-first century.

Looking Back: Eighty Years of Federal Breastfeeding Policy

A review of federal breastfeeding policy over the past eighty years reveals a variety of strategies, statements, initiatives, and programs, ranging from the publication of advice literature for mothers to the ratification of international conventions and codes to support of provincial efforts to modify hospital birthing practices. Yet, central to all policy endeavours has been an emphasis on the promotion of breastfeeding through the education of mothers without equal attention paid to the material supports and resources required to do this successfully. Two features of federal health policy on breastfeeding have been more or less constant for the past eighty years: (1) breastfeeding is "the one best way" to feed infants and (2) educating mothers is the main way to increase breastfeeding initiation and duration. While the central message has remained constant, the policy rationale, tone, and intended targets of these two messages have changed over time, as have the specific guidelines regarding duration of breastfeeding and the addition of solid foods and supplements.

In the 1920s, breastfeeding became a moral choice equated with good citizenship and good mothering. Breastfeeding promotion was an imperative for the federal government because it was seen as a key solution to the catastrophically high and intractable infant mortality rates. The strong promotion of mother-centered breastfeeding in the first edition of *The Canadian Mother's Book*, with its insistence on exclusive breastfeeding for nine months as "the one best way" to the exclusion of all other practices, reflected the militancy of the federal health policy experts. This militancy was situated in the context of the post–World War One national crisis over the slowing birth rate and high infant mortality. It also reflected a militant view of women as primarily caretakers of the family with a parallel role as nurturers of the next generation of Canadians.

The tone of this early breastfeeding campaign was singular, dire, patronizing, and imperative. The breastfeeding promotion efforts of the 1920s were targeted almost exclusively at poor and less-educated Canadian women even though they were, in general, much more likely than women of higher social and economic classes to be breastfeeding. These promotion efforts were also based on an idealized conception of mothering and motherhood. MacMurchy and other policy-makers in the 1920s strongly believed that women should remain in the home and therefore provided no practical advice for the large number of poor Canadian women who had no choice but to seek employment outside the home. Breastfeeding promotion efforts of the 1920s can thus be characterized as moralizing in tone, based entirely on the education of mothers, providing no alternatives for women who needed them, and mistargeted as middle class and wealthy women were the ones moving most quickly away from breastfeeding during this time.

In the 1930s, federal breastfeeding promotion efforts waned as, for about half the decade, the federal Division of Child Welfare was closed down. By 1941, while the rhetoric of "the one best way" continued, the actual advice promulgated in *The Canadian Mother's Book* had begun to shift away from an emphasis on exclusive breastfeeding. During the Second World War, formula feeding with evaporated milk was recognized and supported by federal directives which gave new mothers priority access to canned milk. By the late 1940s, advice on formula feeding began to appear in advice literature to mothers, and the duration of exclusive breastfeeding suggested by the federal government began a steady decline over the next twenty years, from nine to three months.

Why did these shifts in breastfeeding promotion policy occur in the 1940s? First, women at this time appear to have been choosing to feed their infants breast milk alternatives instead of breastfeeding for an increasing number of reasons, such as the scientific and modern image associated with formula or the purported ease of formula feeding. Second, infant mortality rates had plummeted by this time in Canada, easing policy-makers' earlier concerns. Notwithstanding the fact that Canada had just come through a second major war, the link between national survival, motherhood, and breastfeeding had been broken. Third, the safety and availability of breast milk alternatives had increased and the cost of these mostly cow's-milk-based alternatives had dropped. Fourth, between 1940 and 1960 childbirth shifted entirely from the home into the hospitals: control over infant feeding advice became firmly entrenched in the hospitals and medical profession. Finally, women giving birth, particularly by the 1950s, represented the daughters of the first generation of mothers in Canadian history who had moved en masse away from breastfeeding. They were, therefore, the first generation who had little, and in some cases, no knowledge of the practical skills required for successful breastfeeding. This loss of knowledge, in conjunction with the medicalization of infant feeding advice and women's own desires to use breast milk alternatives, meant that breastfeeding by the late 1950s was virtually a lost art.

From its nadir in the 1960s, breastfeeding made a spectacular comeback across Canada during the 1970s, although this was not an even return, as its pace differed by class, region, and ethnicity. It is essential to acknowledge the timing of the resurrection of breastfeeding in relation to breastfeeding promotion efforts. The rapid increase in breastfeeding in the 1970s was part of a secular movement of women returning to breastfeeding that *preceded* the rejuvenation of breastfeeding policy initiatives by the federal government in the 1980s. While the breastfeeding promotion efforts of the 1980s were the broadest, best-funded, best-designed, best-programmed, and least dependent on mother's education ever developed by any Canadian federal government, they were promulgated following dramatic increases in breastfeeding rates. As well, during the height of these promotion programs in the mid-1980s, breastfeeding rates remained relatively flat in Canada. While these promotion efforts may have consolidated and helped sustain these increases in breastfeeding practices, they clearly did not cause them.

The breastfeeding promotion efforts in Canada in the 1980s were unique because they involved government promotion of much broader initiatives rather than solely the education of mothers for the first time. The federal government became involved in complex efforts to promote linkages and alliances with women's groups, La Leche League, industry, hospitals and hospital associations, various health professional organizations, and consumers. These efforts were also unique because they occurred within the context of a strong, popular, broadly based, national and international movement against the marketing of infant formula. Education efforts were, for the first time directed at changing the practices of health professionals and, probably most importantly, encouraging hospital practices that valued and supported breastfeeding. Finally, these efforts were universal–that is, they were not targeted at particular "high-risk" groups of mothers–and avoided the moral and patronizing tone of the 1920s.

Federal breastfeeding promotion efforts shifted once again in the mid-1990s, and these coincided with an approximate 10 percent increase, to the 2000s, in breastfeeding initiation rates. But, the efforts of the 1990s were in some ways a retreat from the 1980s. Many initiatives have been only partially or inadequately implemented. While the federal government has been a signatory to international agreements such as the WHO Code, the Innocenti Declaration, and the Convention on the Rights of the Child, these agreements have never been translated into legislation or backed with substantial financial or material resources. Surveys and anecdotal evidence suggest that most health professionals remain woefully ignorant of the benefits of breastfeeding and lack the practical skills to support mothers.

Since the mid-1990s, the formula industry has developed more aggressive and direct marketing campaigns. While Canada has signed on to important international accords promoting breastfeeding, it is not clear that the federal government has followed through on these agreements within Canada. As well, it is unclear how the development of a child-centred research and policy strategy in the mid-1990s has affected breastfeeding promotion. Finally, it appears that the money allocated for breastfeeding promotion over the past decade is significantly less than in the 1980s and that the alliances, activism, and political context of this promotion has drastically shifted.

Since the 1990s, federal breastfeeding policy has become increasingly fragmented. The provincial governments and the non-profit organization known as the Breastfeeding Committee for Canada have taken leadership in promoting breastfeeding across the country. While the federal government has designated the Breastfeeding Committee for Canada as the national authority for the implementation of the Baby-Friendly Initiative, few financial resources are available to further its goals. Instead, the committee works strategically at the provincial/territorial level. Eight years after the launch of the Baby-Friendly campaign in 1998, there are four baby-friendly hospitals and birthing centres in Canada (three in Quebec and one in Ontario) and four baby-friendly community health services (three in Quebec and one in Ontario) (Breastfeeding Committee for Canada 2006). In the absence of federal leadership, several provincial governments have begun to develop and introduce breastfeeding policies, including Quebec (2001), Nova Scotia (2005), and New Brunswick (2006). While several provinces do not have explicit breastfeeding policies, several have provided some funding to support breastfeeding initiatives (e.g., British Columbia, Alberta, Manitoba, and Saskatchewan). While these initiatives are encouraging, they have resulted in a patchwork approach to promoting breastfeeding.

It appears that, in the 2000s, the pendulum has swung back towards earlier promotion strategies. For example, in the 2005 edition of *Baby's Best Chance*, a free perinatal manual for expectant parents produced by the B.C. Ministry of Health, in a somewhat controversial decision, the manual only contains information about breastfeeding. There are two paragraphs under the heading of "Formula Feeding," which state, "It is rare that a woman is unable to or advised not to breastfeed her baby. If you are unsure about breastfeeding or are considering formula feeding, talk first with your health care practitioner or phone the B.C. NurseLine ... They have many ways to help you with breastfeeding" (Province of British Columbia Ministry of Health 2005, 108). Clearly, once again, as in the 1920s and 1930s, all mothers in B.C. in the 2000s are expected to breastfeed. Information on formula feeding is increasingly difficult to obtain from public health sources. Unfortunately, this information is readily available from the formula industry, which often downplays formula's risks. Public health information, on the other hand, often fails to contextualize risk. Knaak comments on the informational biases that appear to be entering educational and promotional literature on breastfeeding, turning it into a "tool for persuasion [rather] than a tool for education." She says, "It is important to uphold the foundational ethics of expert-guided childcare, and to rightly reposition the discourse as a tool for influence via education, not informational manipulation" (Knaak 2006, 412).

Moving Forward: New Directions for Canadian Breastfeeding Policy

One of the consequences of a consistent emphasis on the education of mothers is that women are pressured to make infant feeding decisions that comply with broader social goals without paying attention to their individual circumstances. Rather than equally emphasizing, for example, the importance of industry, the health care system, networks of women, and employers, government policy tends to view mothers as being most responsible for infant health and the social implications of breastfeeding. While individual women do have considerable power to make decisions about whether and for how long to breastfeed, in general, most efforts to promote breastfeeding never consider providing mothers with adequate material and social supports. Overall, breastfeeding policy tends to undermine mothers as it encourages breastfeeding within a context of widespread detrimental hospital practices, the intensification of the direct marketing of infant formula, and hostility to public breastfeeding. Even when appropriate practical supports are available (e.g., knowledgeable health care providers and lactation consultants), they suggest that breastfeeding is a difficult task that requires expert intervention.

There are four principles, garnered from a consideration of the changing history of breastfeeding practices and policy, that we think are important for policy-makers seeking to increase breastfeeding rates in Canada. First, definitions of breastfeeding success (which become the goals of promotion policy) must be made with the full participation of breastfeeding women and, most importantly, with much better knowledge and understanding of their diverse needs. Second, the very real tension between women's productive and reproductive roles and the state's interest and function in supporting these distinct but related roles must be made explicit in the development of breastfeeding policy. The issues connected to women's work have been implicit in past policy-making, and the inability of policy-makers to accurately analyze and understand these issues has historically constrained the design of labour force policies which improve the lives of breastfeeding women and their children. Third, our study indicates that reliance on classical health promotion education methods by themselves does very little to change breastfeeding practices. Fourth, the marketplace must be constrained, as it has historically not been the best place to develop and promote ideas about infant feeding.

1. Redefining Breastfeeding Success

Many industrialized countries, including the United States (2000), Australia (2001), and the United Kingdom (2003), have set targets for national breastfeeding rates. While the Canadian government has not set goals for the number of women initiating and continuing to breastfeed, several provinces have done so. However, at the national level, data on breastfeeding rates continue to be collected and the number of women complying with breastfeeding guidelines continues to be monitored. Breastfeeding success has been defined differently by policy-makers, health professionals, mothers, and researchers from various academic disciplines (Harrison, Morse, and Prowse 1985; Leff, Gagne, and Jefferis 1994). Breastfeeding policy and subsequently developed guidelines for mothers tend to define success by duration and exclusivity of breastfeeding. In practice, historically and currently, health professionals tend to focus on breastfeeding duration, infant growth, and infant mortality. However, as Beske and Garvis (1982) first identified in the early 1980s, research has shown that, for many women, breastfeeding duration is not necessarily an indicator of success.

Studies have highlighted the range of factors that influence women's perceptions of successful breastfeeding, including maternal enjoyment, maternal attitudes towards breastfeeding experiences, the compatibility of breastfeeding with family life, the physiological and health benefits of breastfeeding, the perception of the infant's response to breastfeeding, and the mother's feelings of closeness with her infant. Maternal and infant satisfaction are common indicators of breastfeeding success (Leff, Jefferis, and Gagne 1994; Schmied and Barclay 1999; Ayre-Jaschke 2004; Hauck and Reinbold 1996): "In general, it appears that women will continue to breastfeed if they are satisfied with the experience and if they believe their babies are satisfied. While some women are able to continue breastfeeding despite dissatisfaction with some aspects of the experience, their perception that their infant is satisfied is crucial to continued breastfeeding" (Ayre-Jaschke 2004, 91).

Policy rarely acknowledges that breastfeeding is a central part of women's overall experience of motherhood (Schmied, Sheehan, and Barclay 2001). "A woman's evaluation of her breastfeeding experience may be closely associated with her assessment of her ability as a mother and her level of self-esteem" (Leff, Gagne, and Jefferis 1994, 99). Maternal satisfaction is linked with mothers' meeting their own expectations and personal goals about breastfeeding, and these may greatly diverge from national targets and guidelines (Ayre-Jaschke 2004).

Breastfeeding policies that focus on exclusivity and duration often create a discrepancy between women's experiences and perceptions and policy recommendations. This can lead to comparisons and judgments on the part of mothers themselves, other mothers and family members, and health professionals. In some situations, the incongruity between policy expectations and women's actual experiences may result in women seeing themselves as failures. Successful breastfeeding programs must meet the emotional and developmental needs of both mother and child (Leff, Gagne, and Jefferis 1994). Breastfeeding needs to be promoted in a way that improves the *quality* of women's experiences rather than the *duration* or *exclusivity* of breastfeeding. Ultimately, breastfeeding policy must meet the needs of diverse women, each of whom defines her breastfeeding goals and successes differently.

2. Women's Work: Breastfeeding and Labour Force Policy

Successful breastfeeding policy must consider the relationship between women's reproductive and productive work. At a global level, women's employment and breastfeeding has been a subject of discussion and activism. In Canada, these discussions have been muted, perhaps because of the availability of some form of maternity entitlements since the 1970s. However, both historically (particularly in the 1910s and 1920s) and presently, employment has often been perceived as a barrier to breastfeeding. Currently, a significant proportion of Canadian women are in the workforce, yet research reveals that, for many women, employment is not a barrier to initiating breastfeeding (Millar and Maclean 2005). However, flexible policies that provide women with various ways of combining employment and breastfeeding can influence breastfeeding duration and exclusivity (Greiner 1990; Van Esterik 2002; Van Esterik and Greiner 1981).

While many people assume that paid work outside the home may affect women's decisions to initiate breastfeeding, most studies have shown this is not an important factor in women's decisions to breastfeed. In surveys, only a small proportion of women cite work as a reason for not breastfeeding, for initiating bottle-feeding, or for stopping breastfeeding (Van Esterik and Greiner 1981; Millar and Maclean 2005). Indeed, in some situations, women's employment may even provide conditions favourable to breastfeeding initiation. At a broader level, there is little evidence to support the belief that maternal employment is a contributor to the decline of breastfeeding. In fact, trend data demonstrate that, in the 1970s and 1980s, the proportion of women breastfeeding and the proportion of women in the labour force both increased dramatically. However, while women's employment seems to have little effect on breastfeeding *initiation* at the aggregate level, it does influence the *duration* of breastfeeding. In particular, structural variables such as length of maternity leave and workplace flexibility have been seen to affect breastfeeding duration (McKinley and Hyde 2004).

Currently, in Canada, maternity leave is governed by the provinces, which generally allow fifty-two weeks of leave. However, maternity benefits are provided through the federal Employment Insurance Act. While Canada's policies on maternity leave are generous when compared to those of many other countries, many women, including self-employed, part-time, and contract workers, are ineligible for such benefits. In 1998, only 49 percent of families with newborns qualified for and received maternity benefits: about 30,000 women did not qualify at all. In 2001, the federal government lowered the number of hours required to qualify for benefits. Yet, in 2004, 40 percent of women received no benefits during their maternity leave (Sokoloff 2004). While amendments to the Employment Insurance Act in 2001 have increased accessibility for some women, discrepancies between allowed leave and available benefits, along with difficulties making ends meet on a reduced income, mean that many women are not able to take advantage of the maximum leave allowed. Also, some women who are eligible do not take advantage of available benefits as they believe it may affect their future participation in the labour force. Research shows that the social class of worker and receipt of maternity benefits are important predictors of return to work. For example, of the 367,000 employed women who gave birth in 1993 or 1994, one in five were back at work by the end of the first month after childbirth. Within a year of giving birth, 86 percent of mothers had returned to work, and, within two years, 93 percent had returned to work. The average time off was 6.4 months (Almey et al. 2000). Mothers who did not receive maternity benefits were almost six times more likely to have returned to work by the end of the first month than were those who received benefits. Mothers who were self-employed were almost eight times more likely to have returned to work earlier than were paid employees (Almey et al. 2000).

Research suggests that labour market policies that provide mothers job-protected, paid leave post-birth may be an effective strategy for increasing breastfeeding duration. Mothers with children born before 31 December 2000 were eligible for 15 weeks of maternity leave benefits through Canada's Employment Insurance program. A further 10 weeks could be shared between the mother and father for a total of 25 weeks. Following 31 December 2000, this further 10 weeks was increased to 35 weeks for a total of 50 weeks of entitlement. One study confirmed that increasing the availability of maternity leave increased the period of time before mothers returned to work post-birth: in the first year of life, mothers eligible for maternity entitlements remained out of the workforce for 3 to 3.5 months longer. Further, the duration of breastfeeding in the first year increased by over one month; the duration of *exclusive* breastfeeding increased over one-half month. Overall, the proportion of women attaining six months of exclusive breastfeeding increased by 7.7 and 9.1 percentage points (Baker and Milligan 2008).

Maternity entitlements that provide maximum flexibility are most likely to be conducive to women meeting their breastfeeding goals. Since January 2006, the Quebec government has taken on the responsibility of providing maternity, paternity, parental, and adoption benefits to its residents. This new plan proposes a flexible approach, as it allows individuals to select between longer leave at lower compensation or shorter leave at higher compensation. Quebec's plan may provide a model for other provinces. Ultimately, the availability of combinations of fully paid, partially paid, and unpaid leave can provide opportunities for mothers to adapt breastfeeding to their personal circumstances and employment requirements.

Workplace conditions are also important in determining whether women are able to successfully breastfeed. Flexible hours, part-time or short shifts, and opportunities for breaks throughout the day are conducive to breastfeeding. For older children, the availability of daycare close to the workplace may be relevant. Perhaps as a result of the availability of maternity entitlements, corporate lactation programs have not proliferated in Canada as they have in the United States. Corporate lactation programs often provide women with a "Mother's room" (in which they can express milk) and often provide or subsidize breast pumps and other equipment. In the United States this has resulted in a divide between working mothers who have access to such programs (i.e., primarily white-collar workers) and those who do not. Several states have passed laws protecting women's right to breastfeed in the workplace, although these are primarily symbolic. One of the arguments in support of maternity entitlements is that they support the practice of breastfeeding rather than just the production and provision of breast milk, thereby emphasizing the relationships involved rather than merely the benefits of breast milk for infants.

3. Beyond the Education of Mothers

Historically, breastfeeding promotion has been open to the same critiques as the majority of other health promotion activities; namely, that it is individualistic and victim-blaming. While all mothers are the targets of breastfeeding education, specific groups of mothers receive additional scrutiny. Just as working-class mothers in the 1920s were believed to be at the root of the infant mortality problem, so, over the years, teen mothers, Aboriginal mothers, immigrant and refugee mothers, and mothers from lower socio-economic backgrounds have all received negative attention. Generally, strategies for promoting breastfeeding in these groups involve providing advice that will improve compliance rather than addressing these women's socio-economic circumstances (Zimmerman and Guttman, 2001).

As breastfeeding policy evolves in the twenty-first century, there is a need to expand its scope. Most breastfeeding initiatives target women during the perinatal period. Yet, health promotion officials have long acknowledged that the decision to breastfeed is often made prior to both conception and birth. Further, initiatives to promote breastfeeding rarely differentiate between activities that encourage women to initiate breastfeeding and those that lengthen the duration of breastfeeding (Palda et al. 2004). Greater attention should be given to the development and growth of milk banks across the country. Canada's sole milk bank is hospital-based and attempts to serve women not only across the country but also internationally. As a consequence of limited resources, milk banks remain inaccessible to large numbers of women. This results in a situation in which many women remain convinced of the benefits of breast milk and may be driven to extreme lengths to obtain it.

Over the twentieth century, breastfeeding entered and remained under the purview of health and medicine. Yet, given the complexity of factors that influence breastfeeding, no single group, sector, institution, or intervention can be responsible for increasing breastfeeding success. Mothers have often been left out of discussions on the development of breastfeeding policy, and, unfortunately, breastfeeding still remains a low-priority issue for many women's groups. The promotion of mother-to-mother support groups may provide one alternative to the formal health care system. There has been frequent antagonism between the formula industry and breastfeeding advocates, yet increasing breastfeeding success requires addressing the impact of the formula industry and involving it in policy development so as to ensure that it makes sustained changes to its practices. Breastfeeding policy requires the involvement of numerous areas of government, including Health Canada, Industry Canada, and Human Resources and Social Development Canada. It also requires the ongoing and committed involvement of health institutions and health professionals.

In recent years, the federal government has become less involved in the development and promotion of breastfeeding policy and has made very little movement towards implementing various relevant international codes and conventions. Breastfeeding advocates, in conjunction with several provincial governments, have worked to ensure that breastfeeding remains an important policy goal. As certain areas of health care, including hospitals, are a provincial responsibility, provincial governments have an important role to play in developing and supporting efforts that encourage breastfeeding. However, the federal government must play a leadership role in developing priority areas, coordinating educational materials, and ensuring equitable policies across the country. As well, many policies and initiatives indirectly affect breastfeeding practices. For example, a recent report on barriers to breastfeeding in B.C. hospitals highlighted the role of overall health care system resource constraints on successful breastfeeding initiation. Bed shortages and overworked nurses appeared to be resulting in mothers receiving supplemental formula as a "quick fix" (Roslin 2008). Ultimately,

many changes in breastfeeding practices have been driven by social movements and cultural change both inside and outside Canada. Federal leadership should be able to utilize these movements to create an environment of
dialogue, innovation, and sharing.

4. Constraining Marketing

Since the beginning of the twentieth century, the marketing of breast milk
alternatives, ranging from condensed milk to infant formula, has been recognized as having a detrimental effect on breastfeeding practices. While
marketing practices have changed over time, the messages used to promote
breast milk substitutes have remained remarkably similar. Marketing campaigns have consistently exploited women's uncertainties about their own
ability to breastfeed and their desire to have the healthiest baby possible.
Despite arguments to the contrary, the marketing of breast milk alternatives
is not the same as the marketing of other food or infant products, as the physiological process involved in the production of breast milk is greatly influenced by psychological suggestion and environmental stressors.

In spite of the development of the WHO Code in the early 1980s, the marketing of breast milk substitutes has only intensified in Canada. As the free
distribution of formula samples through hospitals has declined and efforts to
alter other detrimental hospital practices has increased, formula companies
have shifted towards direct marketing to mothers. Mothers receive promo-
tions, discounts, and gifts; are exposed to formula advertisements through
leaflets, direct mailings, in-store coupons, brochures, and magazines; and
can easily gain information through formula company websites and telephone hotlines. Public health services are hard pressed to compete with the
volume of information and strategies used by industry.

In Canada, such marketing practices remain unchecked. While the federal
government has endorsed the WHO Code, it has never translated it into
legislation. Unfortunately, in light of free trade agreements, implementing
the WHO Code no longer appears to be the relatively uncomplicated matter
it might have been two decades ago. In recent years, several countries in
the South, including Mexico and Guatemala, have attempted to introduce
legislation to implement the code. However, they have been forced to retract this
legislation, as the major formula companies have alleged that to implement it
would interfere with free trade agreements. To date, no industrialized nation
has tried to enforce the WHO Code through legislation. If the Canadian
government attempted to do this, it would no doubt face similar challenges.
However, this could result in drawing domestic and international attention
to the issue and could raise issues about national sovereignty with respect to
health and social issues.

Conclusion

Canadian policy has considered breastfeeding to be "the one best way" for over eighty years. Breastfeeding will undoubtedly continue to be the subject of diverse policy areas as its individual and societal benefits continue to be valued in the twenty-first century. Using findings from the past, it is clear that breastfeeding policies should emphasize both education and material resources to ensure that women can breastfeed successfully. Policy for the twenty-first century may need to redefine traditional conceptions of breastfeeding success and focus on increasing the possibility that women will reach their own breastfeeding goals. The fragmentation of breastfeeding policy and programs in the early twenty-first century suggests the need for strong federal leadership that is responsive to the diversity of Canadian women and the changing contexts within which breastfeeding occurs.

The Politics of "Choice"

Breastfeeding has officially been considered "the one best way" for the past 100 years of Canadian history. The "best" way has often been scientifically or politically determined and has shifted from one generation to the next. Women have been encouraged to breastfeed because it was their maternal duty, because it was their patriotic duty, because it was good for their baby, because it was good for them, and/or because it was good for society. The history of breastfeeding raises questions about how to reconcile individual choice with societal benefit, how to balance a desire to promote societal health and well-being and a desire to respect individual autonomy. Canadian policy has often promoted breastfeeding as a way of solving social problems. It has required individual women to make decisions to remedy social problems not of their making. The infant feeding decisions of individual women have been seen as a way of addressing issues ranging from the infant mortality crisis of the 1920s to the obesity epidemic of the 1990s.

For the most part, government and scientific medicine have attempted to influence the infant feeding practices of mothers through education and persuasion. Yet, as we have seen, breastfeeding is clearly more than a matter of individual choice. Breastfeeding is shaped by a woman's socio-cultural context, yet an emphasis on individual choice has resulted in steering us away from examining the social forces that determine that "choice." It has also resulted in scrutinizing the mothering practices of certain groups of people (e.g., mothers of lower socio-economic status) without paying adequate attention to the contexts of their lives. While knowledge and attitudes are important, personal and social context are more important. Acknowledging and investing in changing the structural determinants of women's "choices" reframes breastfeeding as a societal rather than an individual responsibility.

At the turn of the twenty-first century, the decision to breastfeed has become a somewhat moralistic one, bearing some resemblance to the imperatives of the early breastfeeding campaigns of the 1920s. "Pressure," "guilt," "bullied," and "coercion" are words now often associated with breastfeeding promotion (Battersby 2000). Anecdotes and media discussions abound with stories of women who wanted to breastfeed but could not; feelings of shame, guilt, and isolation related to infant feeding choices; incidents of lying to public health nurses; fears of attitudes of other mothers; and the great lengths to which women will go to breastfeed (Van Esterik 2002; Reed 1999). For many women, breastfeeding has become associated with being a "good mother" (Murphy 1999; Schmied, Sheehan, and Barclay 2001).

Policies and programs based on the idea that there is "one best way" often end in a breastfeeding zeal that can result in judgment and socially induced guilt and grief. This is by no means to suggest that breastfeeding should not be promoted at an individual level or be a societal goal. However, it does suggest that we need to acknowledge that breastfeeding is an emotional issue that is often tied to a woman's sense of worth as a mother. It requires acknowledging the feelings of grief, sorrow, and sense of failure that some women feel when their breastfeeding expectations are not met. Further, individual attitudes towards breastfeeding are shaped by personal experience. Over the past 100 years, women have demonstrated ambivalence and resistance to infant feeding advice. Regardless of the time period, what happens to the mother whose personal feelings about an infant feeding method conflict with the advice of experts or others? Ultimately, women who have negative experiences of breastfeeding do not become advocates for it and may well perceive breastfeeding policies to be oppressive and judgmental.

At the turn of the twenty-first century, Canadian women do not have to breastfeed out of need or because of tradition. And, while breastfeeding is and should remain an important societal goal, it is not currently a real "choice" for many women. Wong Wah, at the launch of the Canadian Baby-Friendly Initiative in 1998, commented on working with mothers who decide not to breastfeed. He suggested that another step be added to the "Ten Steps for Successful Breastfeeding": "Thou (we) shall not judge the bottle-feeding mom, But shall love and support her as we do the breastfeeding mom" (Wah 2000, 10). Current breastfeeding rates and practices have been shaped by a long history. In the wake of this legacy, it may behoove us all to view individual breastfeeding decisions with respect and compassion.

Appendices
Notes
References
Index

Appendix A: Timeline of Infant Feeding in Canada
Timeline of infant feeding in Canada

1851	Population of Canada: 2.5 million.
	80 percent of Canadians live in rural areas.
1867	Canadian confederation. The British colonies of New Brunswick, Nova Scotia, Quebec, and Ontario form a new country: the Dominion of Canada.
	25 percent of Canadians live in urban centres.
1887	Nestlé canned, condensed milk is imported from Europe and is available in Canada.
1888	Thomas Rotch develops percentage feeding.
1891	The first Walker-Gordon milk laboratory is opened in the U.S.A.; by 1903, there are laboratories in Montreal, Ottawa, and Toronto.
1900	40 percent of Canadians live in urban centres.
1901	16 percent of women aged 15 and older are in the paid labour force.
1910	Helen MacMurchy publishes the first of her three reports on infant mortality for the Ontario government.
1915	A survey in six Canadian cities finds that 44.4 percent of infant deaths are caused by gastrointestinal problems.
	Approximately 80 percent of mothers in Toronto initiate breastfeeding.
1919	The Federal Department of Health is formed.
1921	The first edition of *The Canadian Mother's Book* is published.
	102.1 infant deaths per 1000 live births.
	50 percent of Canadians live in urban centres.
	Population of Canada: 9 million.
1922	The Canadian Society for the Study of Disease of Children is formed (later to become the Canadian Paediatric Society).
1930	Alan Brown, Frederick Tisdall, and Theodore Drake create Pablum, the first precooked cereal for infants, at Toronto's Hospital for Sick Children.
1934	The Dionne quintuplets are born in Callander, Ontario, on May 28. Their survival is attributed to donations of breast milk; they later became the celebrity face of Carnation Milk.
1936	The first human milk bank in Canada is established in Montreal.
1940	The first edition of *The Canadian Mother and Child* is published.
1941	50 percent of babies are born in hospital.
1944	55 infant deaths per 1000 live births.
1950	Approximately 25–50 percent of mothers initiate breastfeeding.
1960	28 percent of women aged 15 and older are in the paid labour force.
1961	97 percent of babies are born in hospital.
1965	There are five La Leche League groups in Quebec, Ontario, and Alberta.
	According to the national Nutrition Canada survey, approximately 25 percent of mothers initiate breastfeeding between 1965 and 1971.

Appendix A continues

Appendix A: Timeline of Infant Feeding in Canada, *continued*
Timeline of infant feeding in Canada

1968	Dr. Derrick Jelliffe coins the phrase "commerciogenic malnutrition."
1971	Maternity benefits are added to Canada's Employment Insurance Program.
1975	55 percent of women aged 15 and older are in the paid labour force.
1976	La Leche League has 140 groups and 325 leaders in Canada.
1978	The Nestlé Boycott begins in Canada.
	The Canadian Paediatric Society publish a position paper entitled "Breastfeeding: What Is Left besides the Poetry?"
1979	The federal government launches a national campaign to promote breastfeeding.
1981	WHO/UNICEF Code of Marketing of Breast-Milk Substitutes is endorsed by the federal government.
1982	Approximately 70 percent of mothers initiate breastfeeding.
1984	The Nestlé Boycott ends.
1988	The Nestlé Boycott is reinstated.
1993	Over 80 percent of Canadian hospitals have exclusive contracts with infant formula manufacturers.
	In the early 1990s, La Leche League has 300 groups and 640 leaders.
1994	The federal government initiates the "Breastfeeding Anytime, Anywhere" campaign to promote breastfeeding.
	73 percent of mothers in Canada initiate breastfeeding.
1995	B.C. Women's Hospital is the first facility to refuse free supplies of infant formula.
1996	The Breastfeeding Committee of Canada is formed.
1997	The decision by the B.C. Human Rights Tribunal in the case of *Poirier v. British Columbia* is the first legal decision on breastfeeding issues in Canada.
1998	The Baby-Friendly Initiative is launched in Canada.
	49 percent of families with newborns qualify for and receive maternity benefits.
2000	60 percent of women aged 15 and older are in the paid labour force.
2002	There are 1,191 lactation consultants in Canada.
2003	Approximately 85 percent of mothers in Canada initiate breastfeeding.
2004	La Leche League Canada has 188 groups and 466 leaders.

Appendix B: Infant Mortality in Canada
Infant mortality in Canada, 1926–44

Year	Number	Deaths under one year of age per 1000 live births
1926	23,692	102
1927	22,101	94
1928	21,195	90
1929	21,674	92
1930	21,742	89
1931	21,360	85
1932	17,263	73
1933	16,284	73
1934	15,870	72
1935	15,730	71
1936	14,574	66
1937	16,693	76
1938	14,517	63
1939	13,939	62
1940	13,783	56
1941	15,236	60
1942	14,651	54
1943	15,217	54
1944	15,539	55

Source: 1946 Annual Report, Department of National Health and Welfare.

Appendix C: *The Canadian Mother's Book*
Eleven editions of *The Canadian Mother's Book* were published between 1921 and 1991. These advice manuals for mothers reflect changing federal government advice and policy on breastfeeding (Lewis and Watson, 1991/92)

Title	Edition	Author/editor	Distribution
The Canadian Mother's Book	1921, 1923, 1927, 1932	Helen MacMurchy (author)	800,000 copies, 1 for every 4 live births between 1921 and 1932
The Canadian Mother's Book	1934	Canadian Council on Child and Family Welfare (editor)	
The Canadian Mother and Child	1940	Ernest Couture (author)	2 million copies; reprinted 12 times between 1940 and 1953
The Canadian Mother and Child	1953, 1957	Jean Webb (editor)	13 printings
The Canadian Mother and Child	1967	Jean Webb and Anne Burns (editors)	Reprinted in 1968, 1969, 1970, 1975
The Canadian Mother and Child	1979	Anne Burns (editor)	
You and Your Baby	1991		

Appendix D: Percentage of Births Occurring in Hospital, 1926–74

Year	Percentage
1926	17.8
1927	19.3
1928	21.5
1929	24.5
1930	26.6
1931	26.8
1932	27.5
1933	28.5
1934	30.0
1935	32.3
1936	34.5
1937	36.4
1938	39.4
1939	41.7
1940	45.3
1941	48.9
1942	53.7
1943	54.7
1944	61.0
1945	63.2
1946	67.6
1947	71.0
1948	72.3
1949	74.3
1950	76.0
1951	79.1
1952	81.4
1953	83.4
1954	84.6
1955	86.5
1956	88.4
1957	90.2
1958	91.7
1959	93.1
1960	94.6
1961	96.9
1962	97.8
1963	98.3
1964	98.7
1965	99.0
1966	99.2
1967	99.4
1968	99.5
1969	99.5
1970	99.6
1971	99.6
1972	99.6
1973	99.6
1974	99.7

Source: Statistics Canada, "Historical Statistics of Canada," http://www.statcan.gc.ca/pub/11-516-x/
sectionb/4147437-eng.htm, Table B1-14: Live Births, Crude Birth Rate, Age-Specific Fertility Rates, Gross
Reproduction Rate and Percentage of Births in Hospital, Canada, 1921–1974. Excludes Newfoundland;
excludes Yukon and NWT, 1926–49.

Appendix E: National Surveys of Breastfeeding Practices

All surveys of breastfeeding practices have relied on self-reported information. The federal government has collected national data on breastfeeding since the 1970s.

Year of data collection	Sample	Data collected	Source
1963–82	Nine cross-sectional studies – mail-out questionnaire sent to mothers with infants under 6 months of age	Initiation and duration of breastfeeding up to 6 months	McNally, Hendricks, and Horowitz 1985
	1963–79 – mothers selected from women answering ads in a popular baby magazine (readership = 10% of total births)	Measured types of milk fed to baby at the hospital and at each month during the first six months: breast-milk, commercial infant formula, cow's milk (skim, 2%, whole)	
	1980–82 – mothers who applied for a baby gift through a retail outlet (represent 30% of yearly births)	Years: 1963, 1973, 1976, 1977, 1978, 1979, 1980, 1981, 1982	
	Response Rate 54–88%; weighted sample		
1965–71	Retrospective data for 1965–1971, collected during the Nutrition Canada Survey (1970–72)	1965–71	Myres 1979a
		Was/is the child breastfed?	
	1965–71: Mothers with children under the age of six	Age at which breastfeeding was discontinued?	
		Was/is the child bottle-fed?	
	1970–1972: Infants under the age of one	Age at which bottle-feeding started?	
		Age at which bottle-feeding discontinued	
		Age at which non-milk foods were started	
		1970–72	
		Food consumption of infants under the age of 1 – 24 h dietary recall – type and quantity of milk, use of vitamin/mineral supplements	

Appendix E continues

Appendix E: National Surveys of Breastfeeding Practices, *continued*

Year of data collection	Sample	Data collected	Source
1982	Questionnaire mailed to 18,000 nationally representative households: sample of all mothers with children under the age of two; results weighted according to StatsCan estimates	Percentage of mothers starting breastfeeding Duration of breastfeeding Milk and formula supplementation for breastfed babies Duration of formula feeding and supplementation type	Health and Welfare Canada 1985
1983	Longitudinal data of Aboriginal people across Canada (including the territories and excluding Quebec) All Aboriginal infants born in 1983 and receiving services from Medical Services Branch (data also includes entire population in NWT and Yukon, as they receive medical care from MSB) Response rate: 75%	Infant feeding from birth to six months – breastfeeding, supplementary bottles, formula	Stewart and Steckle 1987
1994/95	National Population Health Survey (NPHS) – surveyed mothers with one or more children under the age of 5 – results for youngest child only National Longitudinal Study on Children and Youth (NLSCY) – children aged 0–23 months at time of survey	BF Initiation = proportion of women who report breastfeeding their child (not necessarily exclusively), regardless of duration. Based on women who were currently breastfeeding or had done so at the time of the survey BF Duration = total length of time the infant was breastfed (not necessarily exclusively). Based on women who had completed bf at the time of the survey.	Health Canada 1998d

Appendix E: National Surveys of Breastfeeding Practices, *continued*

Year of data collection	Sample	Data collected	Source
1994–99	NLSCY Biennial – 2-year intervals (1994–95, 1996–97, 1998–99)	Breastfeeding Initiation= percentage of children under 2 years of age whose mother chose to breastfeed Breastfeeding duration= percentage of children over 2 years of age whose mother reported breastfeeding 3 months or more	Dzakpasu 2003 Statistics Canada 2001a
2003	Canadian Community Health Survey (CCHS) National sample of 7,266 women aged 15–55 who had a baby in the previous five years (weighted to represent 1.4 million women in 10 provinces)	Breastfeeding initiation= "Did you breastfeed or try to breastfeed your baby, even if only for a short time?" Breastfeeding duration= "For how long did you breastfeed?" Duration of exclusive breast-feeding = length of time before the introduction of solid foods or other liquids	Millar and Maclean 2005

Appendix F: Evolution of Canadian Infant Feeding Guidelines, 1923–2004

Infant feeding advice from *The Canadian Mother's Book*[1] (MacMurchy 1923, 1928); *The Canadian Mother and Child*[2] (Couture 1940, 1949, 1953, 1965); *The Canadian Mother and Child*[3] (Canadian Department of National Health and Welfare 1975, 1979); *Feeding Babies: A Counselling Guide on Practical Solutions to Common Infant Feeding Questions* (Health and Welfare Canada and the Canadian Paediatric Society 1986); *You and Your Baby* (Nonesuch 1991); *Nutrition for Healthy Term Infants* (Canadian Pediatric Society, Dieticians of Canada, Health Canada 1998, 2004)

Year	Breastfeeding and alternative methods	Supplements	Introduction of other foods
1923	Breastfeeding for 9 months Baby must feed regularly, according to a timetable. No advice on artificial feeding. Baby should be fed according to a timetable, every 3 hours.	Boiled cooled water – from birth – 2 or 3 little teaspoonfuls about 3 times a day, between nursings (preparation for weaning). Fruit Juice – at 1 month – strained orange, apple, or prune juice, diluted with water. Begin with a few drops at 1 month and increase to a teaspoon at 3 months; a dessert spoon at 6 months; a tablespoon 2 or 3 a day at 12 months; at 6 months, other strained juice or tomato juice. Give between nursings (for health reasons). Chicken bone or crust of bread – at 6 months (exercises teeth, jaws, and facial muscles).	Milk – from 9 to 24 months – 2 pints a day (enables proper growth) Milk must be pasteurized; during weaning, mix milk with water and sugar. Summer care: Don't leave milk in the sun and feed less when the weather is hot. Solids – at 10 months – barley, cereal, and oat jelly; from 11 to 24 months – gradually introduce cereals, bread and butter, apple and potatoes, purée of green vegetables, eggs, stewed fruit, pieces of beef or chicken, simple desserts, and fruit jellies. By age 2, child should be fed half milk and half other foods.
1928	Breastfeeding for 9 months No advice on artificial feeding. Baby should be fed according to a timetable, every 3 hours.	Cod-liver oil – at 2 weeks · 2–3 drops (increase to teaspoon at 3 months, a dessert spoon at 6 months, and a tablespoon 2 or 3 times per day at 12 months); give between nursings; in the summer, cod-liver oil may be eliminated. Sunshine (UV rays) is necessary to growth and development. Fruit Juice – at 2 weeks – strained orange, apple or	·Milk – from 9 to 24 months · 2 pints a day (enables proper growth) During weaning, mix milk with water and sugar. Do not wean in hot weather. Keep milk cool and pure. Solids – at 10 months – barley, cereal, and oat jelly; from 11 to 24 months – gradually introduce cereals, bread and butter, apple and potatoes, purée of green

1. *The Canadian Mother's Book* was published in both French and English. The 1921, 1923, 1927, and 1932 editions were all edited and revised by Helen MacMurchy.
2. *The Canadian Mother and Child*, written by Ernest Couture, replaced *The Canadian Mother's Book* (first edition 1940 [twelve printings]; second edition 1953 [thirteen printings]; third edition 1967 [ten printings]; fourth edition [1979]).
3. Revised edition of *The Canadian Mother and Child*, co-published by Douglas and McIntyre and Health and Welfare Canada.

Appendix F: Evolution of Canadian Infant Feeding Guidelines, 1923–2004, *continued*

Year	Breastfeeding and alternative methods	Supplements	Introduction of other foods
1928, continued		prune juice, diluted with water (begin with a few drops at 2 weeks and increase to a teaspoon at 3 months; a dessert spoon at 6 months; a tablespoon 2 or 3 times a day at 12 months); at 6 months, other strained juice or tomato juice. Give between nursings (for health reasons). Chicken bone or crust of bread – at 6 months (exercises teeth, jaws and facial muscles).	vegetables, eggs, stewed fruit, pieces of beef or chicken, simple desserts, and fruit jellies.

Summary of evolution of guidelines from 1923 to 1928

Changes: None.

Additions: Introduction of cod-liver oil at 2 weeks (unnecessary during summer); discussion of importance of sunshine to growth.

Deletions: No information on supplementing breast milk with water.

Year	Breastfeeding and alternative methods	Supplements	Introduction of other foods
1940	If mother does not have enough milk, supplement with a mixture of cow's milk (boiled), sugar, and water. Wean gradually through addition of foods. Artificial feeding – from birth if mother cannot nurse her baby successfully – use fresh, evaporated, or powdered cow's milk mixed with sugar and water. "For the first 3 months the baby needs 50 calories per pound of body weight in 24 hours." Feedings should be every 3 or 4 hours.	Boiled water (unsweetened or mildly sweetened) – from birth – 3–5 times per day (particularly important in the summer). Cod-liver oil – second week, 5 drops twice a day, gradually increasing to 1 teaspoon twice a day at 3 months (to prevent rickets and tetany – required even during the summer months). Orange juice or tomato juice – beginning of second month 15 drops of orange juice or 30 drops of tomato juice; gradually increase to 2 tablespoons and 4 tablespoons, respectively (to prevent scurvy). Iron – at 3 months, begin food containing iron (as milk does not contain).	Solids – 2½–9 months – introduce cooked cereal or sieved vegetables; gradually introduce eggs, whole wheat toast and butter; cow's milk at 6 months, fruit, green vegetables (iron). "Baby foods" should not be used, as they lack many nutrients.

Appendix F continues

Appendix F: Evolution of Canadian Infant Feeding Guidelines, 1923–2004, *continued*

Summary of evolution of guidelines from 1928 to 1940

Changes: (1) Duration of exclusive breastfeeding reduced from 9 to 6 months. (2) Babies should be fed according to a timetable—a 3-hour and a 4-hour interval are acceptable. (4) Age of introduction of cod-liver oil remains at 2 weeks; however, begin with 5 drops instead of 2. Supplements should be given all year, not just in the winter months. Rationale for cod-liver oil is given (prevention of rickets and scurvy). (4) Age of introduction of solids changes from 10 months to 2 and a half months.

Additions: (1) Information on artificial feeding provided for the first time. Combination of breastfeeding and artificial feeding is discussed. (2) If mother does not have enough breast milk, can supplement with a cow's-milk formula. (3) Boiled, sweetened, or unsweetened, water should be offered to infants, especially in the summer months. (4) At 2 months, infants should receive daily doses of orange or tomato juice, to prevent scurvy. (5) At 3 months, infants should receive food containing iron. (6) First mention of the importance of iron-containing solid foods.

Deletions: None.

Year	Breastfeeding and alternative methods	Supplements	Introduction of other foods
1949	Breastfeeding for 6 months If mother does not have enough milk, supplement with a mixture of cow's milk (boiled), sugar, and water. Wean gradually through addition of foods. Artificial feeding – from birth if mother cannot nurse her baby successfully – use fresh, evaporated or powdered cow's milk mixed with sugar and water. Milk must be boiled. By 6 months, baby should be getting whole, undiluted milk. "For the first 3 months the baby needs 50 calories per pound of body weight in 24 hours." 3-hour or 4-hour schedule; or self-demand feedings.	Boiled water (unsweetened or mildly sweetened) – from birth – 3–5 times per day (particularly important in the summer). Cod-liver oil – second week, 5 drops twice a day, gradually increasing to 1 teaspoon twice a day at 3 months. Fruit juice – at 4 weeks, orange juice, vitaminized apple juice or tomato juice, gradually increasing dosage to 1 oz. orange juice, 1 oz. apple juice, or 2 oz. tomato juice at 1 year.	Solid foods – at 10–12 weeks, cereal mixtures (to augment breast or artificial feeding with desirable minerals and vitamin B_1 and to train the infant to accept solids); also give solid foods containing iron. From 4 to 8 months – gradually introduce sieved vegetables, egg yolks, stewed puréed fruits, scrapings of meat, bread (early introduction of solids allows baby to learn about variety of foods).

Summary of evolution of guidelines from 1940 to 1949

Changes: (1) Artificial feeding – at birth, formula should be diluted cow's milk; by 6 months, infant should receive whole, undiluted milk. (2) As in 1940, feeding intervals should be every 3 or 4 hours; as well, self-demand feedings are acceptable.

Additions: (1) In addition to orange and tomato juice, vitaminized apple juice is another fruit juice option to prevent scurvy. (2) Rationale for introduction of cereals at 2 and a half months provided (to augment breast- or artificial feeding with desirable minerals and vitamin B_1 and to train the infant to accept solids).

Deletions: None.

Appendix F: Evolution of Canadian Infant Feeding Guidelines, 1923–2004, *continued*

Year	Breastfeeding and alternative methods	Supplements	Introduction of other foods
1953	Breastfeeding for 6 months At 3 months, replace 1 breastfeeding with 1 bottle-feeding (accustoms baby to bottle); at 6 months, start a second bottle-feeding. Supplement with formula if necessary. *Breastfeeding provides infant with maternal attention. Artificial feeding – if impossible to breastfeed, use fresh pasteurized cow's milk, evaporated milk, or powdered milk mixed with water and sugar: 2 oz. of whole milk and 1 oz. of water for every pound of body weight. *Artificial feeding allows father to interact with infant. Self-demand feeding (allow infant to establish his or her own schedule).	Vitamin D – at 1 week, pure fish-liver oil or concentrates; at second week, 200 IU per day, increasing to 800 IU per day at 4 weeks (winter and summer). Vitamin C – at 2 weeks, 1 teaspoon diluted orange juice or undiluted tomato juice; gradually increase to 2 oz. orange juice or 4 oz. tomato juice at 2 months; or use 25–50 mg of ascorbic acid liquid or tablets each day.	Solids – 2½–9 months – introduce prepared, pre-cooked cereal, fruit, strained vegetables (canned or homemade), canned meats, egg yolks, whole egg, baby biscuits or hard crust (to chew on at 5 months), toast.

Summary of evolution of guidelines from 1949 to 1953

Changes: (1) Self-demand feeding is considered the best way to feed a baby. (2) Age of introduction of vitamin D/fish concentrates decreases from 2 weeks to 1 week. (3) Age of introduction of vitamin C/fruit juice decreases from 4 weeks to 2 weeks.

Additions: (1) First discussion of importance of maternal attention (breastfeeding) and paternal attention (artificial feeding). (2) Ascorbic acid liquid or tablets can be used instead of fruit juice.

Deletions: (1) Boiled water no longer recommended as a supplement.

Year	Breastfeeding and aternative methods	Supplements	Introduction of other foods
1965	Breastfeeding for 6 months Combined breast- and artificial feeding Ensure baby is receiving enough milk – Weigh baby before and after feedings – should take in 2 oz. of milk for every pound of body weight; supplement with formula, if necessary. At 3 months, replace 1 breastfeeding with 1	Vitamin D – at 1 week, 200 IU of pure fish-liver oil or concentrates; increase to 800 IU at 4 weeks. Vitamin C – at 2 weeks, diluted orange juice or undiluted tomato juice or another source of vitamin C (i.e., ascorbic liquid or tablets).	Do not wean during summer; don't give more than 30 oz. milk or 40 oz. formula per day, as he will be receiving solids and will not need this amount. Milk – by 6 months, whole milk daily. Solids – at 2½ months, pre-pared, precooked cereals mixed with warm milk or formula at 10 a.m.

Appendix F continues

Appendix F: Evolution of Canadian Infant Feeding Guidelines, 1923–2004, *continued*

Year	Breastfeeding and alternative methods	Supplements	Introduction of other foods
1965, continued	bottle-feeding (preparation for weaning) Artificial Feeding – when breastfeeding is not possible, use mixture of fresh pasteurized cow's milk, evaporated milk (which is more digestible than ordinary milk), or powdered milk, water, and sugar. 2 oz. milk and 1 oz. water for every pound of body weight (1 oz. evaporated milk and 2 oz. water); 1 tablespoon powdered milk and 3 oz. water for every pound of body weight. After 10 lbs., gradually reduce water and sugar; by 6 months, use whole milk Self-demand feeding (however, objective is always to establish a regular 3–4 hour schedule; infant will have developed a regular schedule by the end of the first few weeks)		and 6 p.m. feedings; at 3–4 months, fruit at 2 p.m. feeding – strained canned baby foods or strained fruits at home such as applesauce and apricots (do not add sugar) or ripe mashed bananas; at 4 months, raw, hard-boiled or sieved egg yolk; at 5–6 months, introduce strained vegetables at noon feeding; at 5 months, hard crust or baby biscuits (for teeth); gradually introduce canned meats, egg white (scrambled, poached, soft-boiled, or hard-boiled), toast, pudding, bacon, jelly.

Summary of evolution of guidelines from 1953 to 1965

Changes: None.

Additions: None.

Deletions: None.

Year	Breastfeeding and alternative methods	Supplements	Introduction of other foods
1975	Breastfeeding for 6 months If baby is not getting enough to eat, supplement with formula (but not too much or will lose breast milk). Once breastfeeding is established, substitute with 1 bottle-feeding (chance to go out or rest). Artificial feeding – mixture of water, sugar, and cow's milk. – fresh cow's milk, canned	Vitamin C – at 3 weeks, 1 teaspoon diluted orange juice; or tomato juice or vitaminized apple juice, gradually increasing to 2 oz. by 2 months. Vitamin D – at 2 weeks, concentrate drops or liquid, gradually increasing to 400 IU.	Solids – no one pattern of introducing solid foods – solids meet vitamin needs, introduce new textures and flavours; infants physiologically ready after 3 months Generally: at 2½–3 months, baby cereals and fruit (e.g., applesauce or banana); at 4 months, vegetables (coloured vegetables have vitamin A); at 5–7 months, egg yolk and meats (source of protein); at 8–9 months, whole egg.

Appendix F: Evolution of Canadian Infant Feeding Guidelines, 1923–2004, *continued*

Year	Breastfeeding and alternative methods	Supplements	Introduction of other foods
1975, continued	evaporated whole or half skimmed milk or powdered whole milk (powdered skimmed milk not recommended; half skimmed evaporated milk most easily digested) – granulated sugar or corn syrup – 1 oz. evaporated milk to 2 oz. fresh whole milk for every pound of body weight – can increase formula if infant is hungry – reduce amount of water and sugar gradually Self-demand feeding (infant will soon develop a schedule).		

Summary of evolution of guidelines from 1965 to 1975

Changes: (1) Age of introduction of vitamin C increases from 2 to 3 weeks. (2) Age of introduction of vitamin D increases from 1 to 2 weeks. (3) Greater flexibility in the order of solid foods introduced.

Additions: None.

Deletions: None.

Year	Breastfeeding and alternative methods	Supplements	Introduction of other foods
1979	Breastfeeding – exclusive for 4–6 months; breastfeed for 9–12 months or more. If infant is hungry and milk supply cannot be increased after 1–2 days, supplement with small amount of artificial milk. Artificial feeding – wean from bottle to cup between 5 and 12 months – use commercial milk products such as ready-to-feed formulas, concentrated formulas that require addition of water, powdered formulas that require water and mixing; or homemade formulas from evaporated milk or whole cow's milk mixed with	Vitamin C – at least 20 mg/day at 3 weeks; if using homemade cow- or goat-milk formula, supplement with orange, apple, or tomato juice diluted with water (evaporated milk and commercial formula are fortified). Vitamin D – at least 400 IU/day – supplement if breastfeeding or using goat's milk (cow's milk and commercial formula are fortified). Iron – at least 7 mg/day – baby's iron stores last for 3 months – supplement at 4 months if breastfeeding or using homemade formula; after 4 months, infant	Solids – age at which solids are introduced is more important than the other foods. At 3-4 months, introduce cereal; at 5 months, vegetables; at 6 months, fruits; at 7 months, cooked meat. Do not add sugar or seasonings (e.g., salt) to baby's food. Use home prepared or commercially prepared infant foods.

Appendix F continues

Appendix F: Evolution of Canadian Infant Feeding Guidelines, 1923–2004, *continued*

Year	Breastfeeding and alternative methods	Supplements	Introduction of other foods
1979, continued	water and sugar (no skim or 2% milk). Self-demand feeding (unless less than 2½–3 hours). If upset, do not feed. Comfort infant with cool, unsweetened boiled water.	receives iron through commercial formula, iron-enriched cereals, and introduced solids Fluoride – if water supply is not fluoridated; do not allow infant to suck at bottles of sweetened liquid for long periods of time.	

Summary of evolution of guidelines from 1975 to 1979

Changes: (1) Distinction between exclusive breastfeeding and combination breastfeeding. Exclusive feeding recommended for 4–6 months. Breastfeed for 9–12 months. (2) Vitamin C supplements required only for infants receiving homemade cow or goat formula. (3) Vitamin D supplements required only for breastfed infants and infants receiving goat's milk. (4) Age of introduction of solids emphasized; order of foods not important. Commercially prepared foods are accepted.

Additions: (1) Commercial milk products (as opposed to homemade formulas) mentioned for the first time. (2) Goat's-milk formula mentioned for the first time. (3) Mention of cool boiled water to supplement feedings. (4) Iron supplementation described for the first time. (5) Fluoride mentioned for the first time.

Deletions: None.

Year	Breastfeeding and alternative methods	Supplements	Introduction of other foods
1986	Breastfeeding From birth to 6 months. Breastfeeding may continue beyond 6 months; however, a commercially prepared formula, cow's milk, or evaporated milk substitute may be used as a replacement by 9 months. Supplements should be avoided; do not attempt before 8 weeks. Artificial Feeding Commercially prepared formulas are the most acceptable substitute (milk-based, soy-based, or casein hydrolysate-based formula provides 68 kcal/100 mL) – average daily intake of 180 mL/kg; evaporated whole milk should be used only when economic resources do not permit purchase of formula (dilute 1 part	Vitamin D – until 24 months, infants require a daily supplement of vitamin D (400 IU/day); infants receiving commercially prepared or evaporated whole milk formula do not require vitamin supplements; all breastfed infants should receive a daily vitamin D supplement. Iron – from 4 to 12 months, 7 mg/day (exclusively breastfed infants do not require supplement until 6 months). Iron sources include fortified infant cereal, liquid ferrous sulfate or iron-fortified infant formula. Vitamin B_{12} – from one week, breastfed infants of strict vegetarian or vegan mothers should receive a vitamin B_{12} supplement (during lactation,	Milk – at 6–9 months – Unmodified, pasteurized cow's milk may be introduced if infant has begun eating solids; 2% and skim milk should not be introduced before 12 months; goat's milk should not be introduced before six months and must be supplemented with vitamin D, C, and folic acid. Solids – at 4–6 months; no rigorous order to introduction; recommended sequence: iron-fortified infant cereals, vegetables and fruits, meat and protein alternates (e.g., legumes, tofu, cheese), fruit juice. Egg yolks introduced at same time as meat; egg white introduced at end of first year to minimize allergic manifestations.

Appendix F: Evolution of Canadian Infant Feeding Guidelines, 1923–2004, *continued*

Year	Breastfeeding and alternative methods	Supplements	Introduction of other foods
1986 continued	evaporated milk with 2 parts water plus powdered carbohydrate such as dextrose or sucrose). Self-demand feeding – strict timetable is not appropriate – longer intervals as infant grows older (at birth, nurse every hour or 2; at 2–3 weeks, every 3 hours; at 3 months, every 4 hours). Increased demands may be noted at second week, 5–6 weeks, and around 12 weeks of age.	2.5 µg/day; from birth – 24 months, 0.3 µg/day). Vitamin A – recommended intake is 1400 IU/day – easily attained without supplementation. Fluoride – at birth, supplementation remains controversial; 6 months–2 years, infants should receive 0.25 mg/day if water supply contains less than 0.3 ppm of fluoride. Water – breastfed infants do not require a water supplement, as breast milk meets their fluid needs (may offer in 2–3 months to accustom infant to the bottle); formula-fed infants may require additional water during very hot weather; infants eating cow's-milk formula and high solute foods may require extra water. Vitamin C – from birth to 24 months, 20 mg/day; no supplement required (800 mL breast milk contains 33 mg; 800 mL formula contains 44 mg).	Honey and corn syrup should not be offered before 12 months. Commercially prepared or home prepared foods.

Summary of evolution of guidelines from 1979 to 1986

Changes: (1) Explicit warning not to supplement breastfeeding with formula feeding before 8 weeks. (2) Commercially prepared formulas favoured over homemade formulas. (3) Age of iron supplementation for breastfed infants increases from 4 to 6 months. (4) More detailed instructions on fluoride supplementation. (5) No vitamin C supplement required for all infants.

Additions: (1) Vitamin B_{12} supplement recommended for infants of vegetarian/vegan infants. (2) Statement regarding vitamin A requirements. (3) Water supplementation for artificially fed infants permitted. (4) Skim milk, 2% milk, and goat's milk should not be used with newborns. (5) Specific instructions for goat's milk supplementation.

Deletions: None.

Appendix F continues

Appendix F: Evolution of Canadian Infant Feeding Guidelines, 1923–2004, *continued*

Year	Breastfeeding and alternative methods	Supplements	Introduction of other foods
1991	Breastfeeding – no explicit time frame provided – "from a number of weeks up to 12 months or longer" Artificial Feeding – from birth to 4–6 months, use ready-to-serve concentrated liquid or powdered formula. Self-demand feeding (every 2–3 hours at first).	Water – from 0 to 3 months, boiled water from tap or bottle; do not use water from lake, mineral water, or from water softener (infants may require water during hot weather or if they have a fever or diarrhea – some will accept, others will not). Formula-fed infants do not need any vitamin or mineral supplements. If infant is breastfed: Vitamin D – recommended by some doctors, especially if child infant doesn't receive ample sunshine. Vitamin B_{12} – if mother is a strict vegetarian, breast milk may not contain enough B_{12}. Iron – breastfed infants need iron after 6 months (e.g., use fortified baby cereal). Fluoride – if water supply is not fluorinated, use a supplement at 6 months.	Whole cow's milk – at 9–12 months (do not use skim or 2%). Solids – beginning at 4–6 months, gradually introduce iron-fortified infant cereals, vegetable purées, fruit purées, meat and alternatives (meat, fish, poultry, egg yolks, cheese, yogurt, tofu, well-cooked legumes) – solids can be commercially prepared or homemade. Suggestions for vegetarian babies: soy formula, iron-fortified cereal, whole-wheat bread, puréed vegetables, peanut butter, tahini. Fruit juice – when infant can drink from a cup (about 10 months), 2 oz. fruit juice.

Summary of evolution of guidelines from 1986 to 1991

Changes: (1) No explicit time frame given for breastfeeding. (2) Formula-fed infants do not require any supplements. (3) Vitamin D supplementation is permitted but not required. (3) Age of introduction of whole milk increases from 6–9 months to 9–12 months.

Additions: (1) Suggested solids for vegetarian infants.

Deletions: None.

Year	Breastfeeding and alternative methods	Supplements	Introduction of other foods
1998	Breastfeeding – Exclusive breastfeeding for 4 months; continuation of breastfeeding with complementary foods until 2 years and beyond. Artificial feeding – if infant is not breastfed, or only partially, use commercial formulas; from birth	Vitamin D – breastfed infants should receive extra vitamin D supplements; infant formula and milk are fortified with vitamin D. Fluids – water is generally suitable for infants (boil for 2 minutes for infants below 4 months); limit fruit juice to avoid interfering with the	Milk –from 9–12 months to 2 years, use pasteurized whole cow's milk (partly skimmed milk not recommended; skim milk and soy or rice beverages are not appropriate). Solids – at 4–6 months, introduce solids – infants are physiologically and

Appendix F: Evolution of Canadian Infant Feeding Guidelines, 1923–2004, *continued*

Year	Breastfeeding and alternative methods	Supplements	Introduction of other foods
1998 continued	to 9–12 months, use cow's-milk-based, iron-fortified formulas; from 6 months to 9–12 months, iron-fortified follow-up formulas are preferred to cow's milk; soy formulas for infants who cannot take dairy-based products for health or cultural reasons. Frequent feedings are encouraged.	intake of nutrient-contained foods; herbal teas and other beverages may be harmful. Iron – for breastfed infants, introduce iron-containing foods at 4–6 months.	developmentally ready for new foods, textures, and modes of feeding. Iron-containing foods, such as iron-fortified cereals, are recommended first foods. Do not use honey (prevents infant botulism) and cook all eggs well (prevents salmonella). Vegetarian diets – can meet nutritional needs; get professional advice for limited diets.

Summary of evolution of guidelines from 1991 to 1998

Changes: (1) Explicit statement regarding exclusive breastfeeding for 4 months; breastfeeding may be continued for 2 years or more. (2) Vitamin D supplements for breastfed infants recommended. (3) Fruit juice not recommended for infants. (4) Vitamin B$_{12}$ supplementation no longer advised for vegetarian/vegan infants.

Additions: Soy formula and soy and rice beverages mentioned.

Deletions: None.

Year	Breastfeeding and alternative methods	Supplements	Introduction of other foods
2004	Breastfeeding – exclusive breastfeeding for 6 months; breastfeeding should continue till 2 years.	Vitamin D – at birth, breastfed infants should receive 400 IU/day until child's diet includes at least 200 IU from other dietary sources.	Solids – at 6 months, introduction to iron-rich solid foods.

Summary of evolution of guidelines from 1998 to 2004

Changes: (1) Exclusive breastfeeding increases from 4 to 6 months. (2) Solids should be introduced at 6 months instead of 4.

Additions: None.

Deletions: None.

Notes

Notes to Chapter 1

1 Breastfeeding for long periods of time often has a contraceptive effect, thereby increasing the spacing between children and affecting the total birth rate. Prentice et al. (1988) suggest that Aboriginal women on average had three or four children, which may have been helpful in groups that were highly mobile.
2 "The nursing bottle is the real cause of excess mortality of newborns in summer. The real remedy, the only remedy, is breastfeeding" (Lachapelle, quoted in Thornton and Olson 2001).

Notes to Chapter 3

1 MacMurchy attributed this phrase to the Right Honorable John Burns, who made this statement at the first conference on infant mortality in London.
2 Birth registration was vital to child welfare efforts: if births were not registered promptly, babies might not be seen until it was too late to help with any health problems the baby (or mother) had.

Notes to Chapter 4

1 The Division of Child Welfare was formed in 1919 and was closed in 1934. In 1937, the Division of Child and Maternal Hygiene was formed (Lewis and Watson 1991/92).
2 The term "infant soldier" is found in the 1923 edition of *The Canadian Mother's Book*, page 68.
3 The department included both in-patient and outpatient services. Among other things, it comprised a pasteurizing plant and milk-modifying laboratory, which produced 150 milk modifications per day.

Notes to Chapter 5

1 "Pablum" is a corruption of the Latin *pabulum*, which means "food" or "nourishment."
2 *Chatelaine* was first published in 1928 and has enjoyed a wide readership throughout its history. It was distributed to 12,270 individuals in 1920. In 1939 it was distributed to 22,285 in British Columbia alone (N.L. Lewis 1982–83).

Notes to Chapter 6

1 The 1953 *The Canadian Mother and Child* was slightly more conservative, suggesting the gradual introduction of solids at ten weeks.
2 Between 1945 and 1958, the average circulation for *Chatelaine* ranged from 250,000 to 450,000.

Notes to Chapter 7

1 From a taped recording of the conference session "Affirming Our Beliefs: Differences in Leaders' Perceptions of La Leche League Philosophy," National Conference, La Leche League of Canada, Ottawa, June 1986.
2 This group had formed in 1955 to study infant malnutrition in less industrialized nations.
3 Note that these surveys were conducted at slightly different times, used different methods, and focused on different regions, which may explain the range in initiation rates observed.

Notes to Chapter 9

1 Infant formula manufacturers acknowledged that breastfeeding was superior to formula but used its nutritional and immunological benefits to argue for the acceptability of infant formula.
2 Enfalac had 39 percent of the $175-million market share, while Similac had 37 percent (Canadian Press Newswire 1996).

References

Abeele, Cynthia Commachio. 1988. The mothers of the land must suffer: Child and maternal welfare in rural and outpost Ontario, 1918–1940. *Ontario History* 75 (3): 183–205.

Agnew, Theresa, Joanne Gilmore, and Pattie Sullivan. 1997. *A multicultural perspective on breastfeeding in Canada.* Ottawa: Health Canada.

Agriculture and Agri-Food Canada. 1998. *Canada's action plan for food security: A response to the World Food Summit.* Ottawa: Agriculture and Agri-Food Canada.

——. 1999. *Canada's progress report to the Committee on World Food Security in implementing the World Food Summit Plan of Action.* Ottawa.

——. 2006. *Canada's action plan for food security: A response to the World Food Summit.* Agriculture and Agri-Food Canada 2003. http://www4.agr.gc.ca/AAFC-AAC/display-afficher.do?id=1196888128319&lang=e.

Almey, Maria, Josée Normand, Colin Lindsay, Jennifer Chard, Sandra Besserer, Valerie Pottie Bunge, Heather Tait, Marcia Almey, and Nancy Zukewich. 2000. *Women in Canada 2000: A gender-based statistical report.* Ottawa: Statistics Canada.

Ames, Herbert Brown. 1897. *The city below the hill: A sociological study of a portion of the city of Montreal, Canada.* Repr. The social history of Canada. Toronto: University of Toronto Press, 1972.

Anderson, M. Doris. 1954. Establishing good lactation. *Canadian Nurse* 50 (7): 895–96.

Anonymous. 1884. Infant mortality in Ottawa. *Canada Lancet* 16 (5): 156.

——. 1912. Child Welfare Exhibition, Montreal. *Dominion Medical Monthly* 39 (1): 210.

——. 1913. Domestic: Baby clinics. *Public Health Journal* 4 (2): 94.

——. 1933. Far better for babies—and better for cooking, too. *Chatelaine* 6, 3.

——. 1936. A Sikh well-baby clinic in British Columbia. *Canadian Child Welfare News* 11 (6): 17–19.

——. 1938. Does bottle bother baby? *Chatelaine*, 10, 59.

——. 1951. Milk survey. *Canadian Nurse* 47 (10): 714.

——. 1982a. Canada: 10% Toronto residents actively boycott Nestlé. *INFACT Update*, cited in Chetley 1986, 54.

——. 1982b. Keeping the lid on the babymilk menace. *New Internationalist,* April, 110.

——. 1993. Hospital sold its soul for $1-million grant, critics charge: Infant formula contract raises howls of protest, but some say such deals are inevitable. *Gazette,* 6 March, A14.

——. 2000. On the uddered breast. *Public Culture* 12 (1): 173–75.

——. 2004. News review: Nestlé USA adds Martek's oils to infant formula. *Lipid Technology* 16 (1): 2.

——. 2005. Broke? Your body's worth more than you think. *Dose* vol. 061.

Apple, Rima D. 1980. "To be used only under the direction of a physician": Commercial infant feeding and medical practice, 1870–1940. *Bulletin of the History of Medicine* 54 (3): 402–17.

——. 1987. *Mothers and medicine: A social history of infant feeding, 1890–1950.* Wisconsin Publications in the History of Science and Medicine. Madison: University of Wisconsin Press.

——. 1995. Constructing mothers: Scientific motherhood in the nineteenth and twentieth Centuries. *Social History of Medicine* 8 (2): 161–78.

——. 2006. *Perfect motherhood: Science and childrearing in America.* New Brunswick, NJ: Rutgers University Press.

Applebaum, Richard M. 1970. The modern management of successful breastfeeding. *Child and Family* 9 (1): 61–86.

Armstrong, David. 1986. The invention of infant mortality. *Sociology of Health and Illness* 8 (3): 211–32.

Arneil, Barbara. 2000. The politics of the breast. *Canadian Journal of Women and Law* 345: 345–70.

Arnup, Katherine. 1994. *Education for motherhood: Advice for mothers in twentieth-century Canada.* Toronto: University of Toronto Press.

——. 1994–1995. Raising the Dionne quintuplets: Lessons for modern mothers. *Journal of Canadian Studies* 29 (4): 65–81.

Arnup, K., A. Levesque, and R. Pierson, eds. 1990. *Delivering motherhood: Maternal ideologies and practices in the 19th and 20th centuries.* London: Routledge.

Associated Press. 1964. Poor imitate well-off, refuse to nurse: MD. *Globe and Mail,* 12 December, 15.

——. 1976. Formulas for babies adequate, panel says. *Globe and Mail,* 3 March, 11.

Atkinson, William B. 1889. The infant food problem. *Canada Lancet* 11 (5): 137–40.

Audy, Fiona. 2004. The Year of the group: History of LLL Canada. *LEAVEN* 40 (4): 82–83.

Austin, Marsha. 2006. Sides clash over putting price on mothers' milk. *Denver Post,* 26 March, A1.

Ayre-Jaschke, Leslie E. 2004. Preparing for breastfeeding: Mothers' perspectives on learning from unsuccessful and successful experiences. MA thesis. Faculty of Graduate Studies and Research, University of Alberta, Edmonton.

Baby Milk Action. 1993. Baby milk manufacturer offered to pay Canadian hospitals for exclusive distribution of their baby milk. *Baby Milk Action,* 11 July, 1.

The bad news in babyland. 1972. *Dun's Review* 100: 104.

Baillargeon, Denyse. 1996. Fréquenter les gouttes de lait: L'expérience des mères montréalaises 1910–1965. *Revue d'histoire de l'Amérique francaise* 50 (1): 29–68.

——. 1998. Gouttes de lait et soif de pouvoir: Les dessous de la lutte contre la mortalité infantile à Montréal, 1910–1953. *Canadian Bulletin of Medical History* 15 (1): 27–57.

——. 2002. Entre la "Revanche" et la "Veillée" des Berceaux: Les médecins québécois francophones, la mortalité infantile et la question nationale, 1910–1940. *Canadian Bulletin of Medical History* 19 (1): 113–37.

Baker, Michael, and Kevin Milligan. 2008. Maternal employment, breastfeeding, and health: Evidence from maternity leave mandates. *Journal of Health Economics* 27 (4): 871–87.

Ball, Helen L. 2003. Breastfeeding, bed-sharing, and infant sleep. *Birth* 30 (3): 181.

Ball, T.M., and A.L. Wright. 1999. Health care costs of formula-feeding in the first year of life. *Pediatrics* 103 (4 Pt 2): 870–76.

Barber, C.M., T. Abernathy, B. Steinmetz, and J. Charlebois. 1997. Using a breastfeeding prevalence survey to identify a population for targeted programs. *Canadian Journal of Public Health* 88 (4): 242–45.

Battersby, Sue. 2000. Breastfeeding and bullying: Who's putting the pressure on? *Practicing Midwife* 3 (8): 36–38.

Baumslag, N., and D.L. Michels. 1995. *Milk, money, and madness: The culture and politics of breastfeeding.* Westport, CT: Bergin & Garvey.

Beaudry, M., and L. Aucoin-Larade. 1989. Who breastfeeds in New Brunswick, when and why? *Canadian Journal of Public Health* 80 (3): 166–76.

Beaudry, Micheline, Renée Dufour, and Sylvie Marcoux. 1995. Relation between infant feeding and infections during the first six months of life. *Journal of Pediatrics* 126: 191–97.

Bell, Patricia. 1979. Hospitals loosening maternity rules. *Globe and Mail*, 15 March, T3.

Bergevin, Yves. 1983. Infant feeding: Do infant formula samples shorten the duration of breast-feeding? *Lancet* 8334 (1): 1148–51.

Bernhard, Blythe. 2005. Breast-milk clinic confronts criticisms. *Orange County Register*, 5 August.

Bertin, Oliver. 2000. Gauge could cost Nestlé millions. *Globe and Mail*, 22 March, B7.

Berton, Pierre. 1977. *The Dionne years: A thirties melodrama.* Toronto: McClelland and Stewart.

Beske, E. Jean, and Marlene S. Garvis. 1982. Important Factors in Breast-Feeding Success. *American Journal of Maternal Child Nursing* 7: 174–79.

Bideau, A., B. Desjardins, and H.P. Brignoli, eds. 1997. *Infant and child mortality in the past.* Oxford: Clarendon Press.

Black, Naomi. 1993. The Canadian women's movement: The second wave. In Burt, Code, and Dorney 1993.

Blatz, William Emet. 1938. *The five sisters: A study of child psychology.* Toronto: McClelland and Stewart.

Bourgoin, G.L., N.R. Lahaie, B.A. Rheaume, M.G. Berger, C.V. Dovigi, L.M. Picard, and V.F. Sahai. 1997. Factors influencing the duration of breastfeeding in the Sudbury region. *Canadian Journal of Public Health* 88 (4): 238–41.

Bourne, Hilary B. 1950. Breast feeding. *Canadian Nurse* 46 (12): 969–71.

Bowman, Bonnie. 2005. Quebec's specialists await mat leave delivery. *National Review of Medicine* 2 (5). http://www.nationalreviewofmedicine.com/issue/2005/03_15/2_contents_05.html.

Braungart, Susan. 1990. Breastfeeding creates ruckus. *Calgary Herald*, 5 August, B1.

Breastfeeding Committee for Canada. 2002a. The baby friendly initiative in community health services: A Canadian implementation guide. Toronto: Breastfeeding Committee for Canada.

——. 2002b. The implementation and evaluation of the baby-friendly initiative in Canada: Final project report 1999–2002. Toronto: Breastfeeding Committee for Canada.

——. 2006. Breastfeeding Canada newsletter, issue 1. Toronto: Breastfeeding Committee for Canada.

Brosco, Jeffrey P. 2002. Weight charts and well child care: When the pediatrician became the expert in child health. In *Formative years: Children's health in the United States: 1880–2000*, ed. A.M. Stern and H. Markel. Ann Arbor: University of Michigan Press.

Brown, Alan. 1917a. The ability of mothers to nurse their infants. *Canadian Medical Association Journal* 7: 241–49.

——. 1917b. The deficiency diseases of infancy and childhood. *Canadian Medical Association Journal* 7: 911–24.

——. 1918a. Infant and child welfare work. *Public Health Journal* 9 (4): 145–62.

——. 1918b. Problems of the rural mother in the feeding of her children. *Public Health Journal* 9 (7): 297–301.

——. 1919a. Protein milk powder. *Canadian Medical Association Journal* 9: 528–37.

——. 1919b. The relation of the pediatrician to the community. *Public Health Journal* 10 (2): 49–55.

——. 1920. Toronto as a pediatric centre. *Canadian Medical Monthly* 5 (6): 204–10.

——. 1923. *The normal child: Its care and feeding*. New York: Century Co.

——. 1933. The prevention of neonatal mortality. *Canadian Medical Association Journal* 29: 264–68.

——. 1938. Some factors concerning the care of the new-born. *Canadian Public Health Journal* 29: 337–44.

——. 1940. A decade of paediatric progress. 4th Blackader Lecture. *Canadian Medical Association Journal* 43 (4): 305–13.

——. 1948. Scientific construction of the normal child's diet. *Lancet* 2 (6536): 877–81.

Brown, Alan, Howard Spohn, and Ida MacLachlan. 1918. Protein milk—its composition, preparation and application in the treatment of digestive disturbances. *Canadian Medical Association Journal* 8: 510–22.

Brown, Alan, and Frederick F. Tisdall. 1932. *Common procedures in the practice of paediatrics: Being a detailed description of diagnostic, therapeutic and dietetic methods employed at the Hospital for Sick Children, Toronto*. 2nd ed. Toronto: McClelland and Stewart.

——. 1939. *Common procedures in the practice of paediatrics: Being a detailed description of diagnostic, therapeutic, and dietetic methods employed at the Hospital for Sick Children, Toronto*. 3rd ed. Toronto: McClelland and Stewart.

Buckley, Suzann. 1977. Efforts to reduce infant maternity mortality in Canada between the two World Wars. *Atlantis* 2 (Part 2): 76–84.

——. 1979. Ladies or midwives? Efforts to reduce infant and maternal mortality. In *A not unreasonable claim: Women and reform in Canada, 1880s–1920s*, ed. L. Kealey. Toronto: Women's Press.

Bueckert, Dennis. 2006. Pediatric society likely to soften stance against moms, infants sharing bed. *Vancouver Sun*, 14 February, A5.

Burglehaus, Maria J., and Sam B. Sheps. 1997. Physicians and breastfeeding: Beliefs, knowledge, self-efficacy, and counselling practices. *Canadian Journal of Public Health* 88 (6): 383–87.

Burns, Anne Y. 1967. The Child and Maternal Health Division of the Department of National Health and Welfare. *Medical Services Journal* April 1967: 678–702.

Burt, S., L. Code, and L. Dorney, eds. 1993. *Changing patterns: Women in Canada*. 2nd ed. Toronto: McClelland and Stewart.

Callen, Jennifer, and Janet Pinelli. 2004. Incidence and duration of breastfeeding for term infants in Canada, United States, Europe, and Australia: A literature review. *Birth* 31 (4): 285–92.

Canada. Department of National Health and Welfare. 1967. *The Canadian mother and child*. Ottawa: Department of National Health and Welfare.

——. 1979. *The Canadian mother and child*. Hull, QC: Health Services and Promotion Branch, Canadian Government Publishing Centre.

Canada NewsWire. 2000. Nestlé voluntarily recalls liquid concentrate infant formula. Ottawa: Canada NewsWire.

Canadian Council on Child Welfare. 1929. Development of breast-fed and artificially fed children. *Child Welfare News* 5 (2): 40–41.

——. 1930. Breast feeding continues to decline. *Canadian Child Welfare News* 6 (1): 29–30.

Canadian Food Inspection Agency. (2006). Health Hazard Advisory. 18 August. http://www.inspection.gc.ca/english/corpaffr/recarapp/2006/20060818be.shtml.

Canadian Heritage. 2007. *Human rights* program 2007. http://www.pch.gc.ca/progs/pdp-hrp/docs/crc/intro_e.cfm (accessed 31 January 2007).

Canadian Home Economics Association. 1997. CHEA position paper on breastfeeding. *Canadian Home Economics Journal* 47 (4): 170–76.

Canadian Institute for Health Information. 2004a. *Improving the health of Canadians*. Ottawa: Canadian Institute for Health Information.

——. 2004b. *Giving birth in Canada: Providers of maternity and infant care*. Ottawa: CIHI.

Canadian Institute of Child Health. 1996. *National breastfeeding guidelines for health care providers*. Ottawa: Canadian Institute of Child Health.

Canadian Paediatric Society. 1978. Breast-feeding: What is left besides the poetry? *Canadian Journal of Public Health* 69 (January/February): 13–19.

——. 1979. Infant feeding. *Canadian Journal of Public Health* 70 (November/December): 376–85.

——. 1996. Human milk banking and storage. *Paediatrics & Child Health* 1 (3): 141–45.

Canadian Paediatric Society Nutrition Committee and American Academy of Pediatrics Committee on Nutrition. 1978. Breast-feeding: A commentary in celebration of the International Year of the Child, 1979. *Pediatrics* 62 (4): 591–601.

Canadian Press. 1943. Canned milk is rationed in some areas. *Globe and Mail*, 29 November, 15.

——. 1980. Churches get behind boycott. *Globe and Mail*, 11 January, 13.

——. 1994a. Breast-feeding moms furious with formula pushers. *Canadian Press NewsWire*, 4 August.

——. 1994b. It's OK to nurse in public, theme of new ad campaign. *Edmonton Journal*, 25 August, A1.

——. 1996. Formula producer told to scrap ads. *Canadian Press NewsWire*, 6 November.

——. 2004. Type of powder Enfalac recalled; incorrect scoop may cause overconcentration. Toronto: Canadian Press NewsWire.

Chandler, A.B. 1929. Breast feeding in health centres. *Canadian Nurse* 25 (11): 665–70.

Cherry, Zena. 1977. 35,000 diapers herald La Leche group. *Globe and Mail*, 14 July, F2.

Chetley, Andrew. 1986. *The politics of baby foods: Successful challenges to an international marketing strategy.* New York: St. Martin's Press.

Child and Maternal Health Division. 1968. *Recommended standards for maternity and newborn care.* Ottawa: Department of National Health and Welfare.

Clio Collective, Micheline Dumont, Michele Jean, Marie Lavigne, and Jennifer Stoddart. 1987. *Quebec women: A history.* Trans. R. Gannon and R. Gill. Toronto: Women's Press.

Cochrane, W.A. 1959. Nutritional excess in infancy and childhood. *Canadian Medical Association Journal* 81: 454–56.

Cody, W.L. 1915. The scope and function of the medical staff of the babies' dispensary, Hamilton. *Public Health Journal* 6 (11): 545–47.

Cohen, Elizabeth. 2006. *Not your mother's breast milk.* Cable News Network. http://web.lexis-nexis.com (accessed 13 April 2006).

Colon, A.R. 1999. *Nurturing children: A history of pediatrics.* Westport, CT: Greenwood Press.

Comacchio, Cynthia R. 1993. *"Nations are built of babies": Saving Ontario's mothers and children 1900–1940.* Montreal: McGill-Queen's University Press.

Committee on the Evaluation of the Addition of Ingredients New to Infant Formula. 2004. *Infant formula: Evaluating the safety of new ingredients.* Washington, DC: National Academies Press.

Cooke, Ethel R. 1955. Nutrition of Infants. *The Canadian Nurse* 51 (5): 381–82.

Copp, Terry. 1981. Public health in Montreal, 1870–1930. In Shortt 1981.

Cosh, Colby. 2000. Lactation nation: Canada's last human milk bank may be forced to close by budget cuts. *Report Newsmagazine*, 14 August, 47.

Coutts, Jane. 1997. Obstetrics journal chided for infant formula advertisements. *Globe and Mail*, 14 October, A6.

Couture, Ernest. 1940. *The Canadian mother and child.* Ottawa: Department of National Health and Welfare.

——. 1949. *The Canadian mother and child.* Ottawa: Department of National Health and Welfare.

Cox, Wendy. 1997. B.C. woman seeks tribunal ruling breastfeeding at office. *Globe and Mail*, 18 March, A8.

Cross, D. Suzanne. 1977. The neglected majority: The changing role of women in 19th century Montreal. In Trofimenkoff and Prentice 1977.

Dafoe, Allan Roy. 1936. Further history of the care and feeding of the Dionne quintuplets. *Canadian Medical Association Journal* 34: 26–32.

Davin, Anna. 1978. Imperialism and motherhood. *History Workshop Journal* 5 (1): 9–66.

De Kiriline, Louise. 1936. *The quintuplets' first year.* Toronto: Macmillan.

Department of National Health and Welfare. 1946. *Annual Report.* Ottawa, Ont.: Department of National Health and Welfare & Government of Canada.

Department of National Health and Welfare. 1952. *Annual Report.* Ottawa: Department of National Health and Welfare & Government of Canada.

Desjardins, Bertrand. 1997. Family formation and infant mortality in New France. In Bideau, Desjardins, and Brignoli 1997.

Dodd, Dianne. 1991. Advice to parents: The blue books, Helen MacMurchy, MD, and the federal Department of Health, 1920–34. *Canadian Bulletin of Medical History* 8: 203–30.

Dodgson, Joan E., and Roxanne Struthers. 2003. Traditional breastfeeding practices of the Ojibwe of northern Minnesota. *Health Care for Women International* 24: 49–61.

Doran, L., and S. Evers. 1997. Energy and nutrient inadequacies in the diets of low income breastfeeding women. *Journal of the American Dietetic Association* 97: 1283–87.

Dormandy, T. 2000. *The white death: A history of tuberculosis.* New York: New York University Press.

Dunlop, Marilyn. 1995. Few Canadian hospitals qualify for "baby-friendly" designation by promoting breast-feeding: Survey. *Canadian Medical Association Journal* 152 (1): 87–89.

Dwork, Deborah. 1987. The milk option: An aspect of the history of the infant welfare movement in England 1898–1908. *Medical History* 31: 51–69.

Dzakpasu, Susie. 2003. *Canadian perinatal health report.* Ottawa: Public Health Agency of Canada.

Ensor, Deborah. 2006. Land of milk and money: Breast-milk enterprise raises concerns among those who view collection and distribution as a philanthropic endeavor. *San Diego Union-Tribune,* 12 February, B1.

Ermann, M. David, and William H. Clements II. 1984. The Interfaith Center on Corporate Responsibility and its campaign against marketing infant formula in the Third World. *Social Problems* 32 (2): 185–96.

Euromonitor International. 2006. Baby foods in Canada. Global Market Information database. University of British Columbia Library, David Lam Branch.

Everitt, Joanna. 1998. Public opinion and social movements: The women's movement and the gender gap in Canada. *Canadian Journal of Political Science* 31 (4): 743–65.

Expert Working Group on Breastfeeding. 1993. *Report of the Expert Working Group on Breastfeeding.* Ottawa: Expert Working Group on Breastfeeding.

Farnsworth, Clyde H. 1994. Quebec bets on subsidized milk, mother's kind. *New York Times,* A4.

Fildes, Valerie. 1988. Wet nursing in colonial America. In *Wet nursing: A history from antiquity to the present.* Oxford: Basil Blackwell.

Finlayson, Judith. 1982. Between the sexes. New winner in the battle of the bottle. *Globe and Mail,* 23 January, F8.

Fomon, Samuel J. 1991. Infant feeding. In Nichols, Ballabriga, and Kretchmer 1991.

Food Controller for Canada. 1917. *Report of the milk committee appointed by the Food Controller for Canada, to investigate milk supplies for urban municipalities: Including a plan for the re-organisation of milk distribution*. Ottawa: Food Controller for Canada.

Friel, James K. 1997. Evaluation of full-term infants fed an evaporated milk formula. *Acta Pediatrica* 86: 448–53.

Fylyshtan, Alassandra. 1994. Shameful treatment. *Ottawa Citizen*, 18 October, A8.

Gazette. 1993. Hospital sold its soul for $1-million grant, critics charge: Infant formula contract raises howls of protest, but some say such deals are inevitable. 6 March, A14.

Gerrard, John W. 1975. Breast-feeding: Should it be recommended? *Canadian Medical Association Journal* 113: 138.

Globe. 1900. Dentonia Dairy.19 May, 4.

——. 1912a. The bottle-fed infant. 28 May, 11.

——. 1912b. Best babies in Toronto are found in Earlscourt. 27 April, 8.

——. 1917. Maternal nursing shirked in Canada. 29 September, 21.

——. 1919. Infant mortality.22 April, 6.

Globe and Mail. 1937. Death rate cut by human milk. 22 April, 10.

——. 1943. Mothers get all the condensed milk needed. 8 January, 1.

——. 1964. Doctors, fashion, status vary attitudes of breast-feeding in Canada. 27 August, W3.

——. 1969. Breastfeeding decline under way in 1920s. 9 October, W3.

——. 1980. NWT babies are bouncing back. 12 May, 5.

——. 1981. Timbrell won't ban formula giveaways. 25 May, 5.

Goldbloom, Alton. 1924. Modern tendencies in infant feeding. *Canadian Medical Association Journal* 14 (8): 709–12.

——. 1930. Special feeding methods for infants. *Canadian Medical Association Journal* 23: 807–10.

——. 1945. A twenty-five year retrospective of infant feeding. *Canadian Nurse* 41 (4): 279–84.

——. 1959. *Small Patients: The Autobiography of a Children's Doctor*. Toronto: Longmans, Green, and Company.

Golden, Janet L. 1996. *A social history of wet nursing in America: From breast to bottle*. Cambridge: Cambridge University Press.

Gorham, Deborah, and Florence Keller Andrews. 1990. The La Leche League: A feminist perspective. In Arnup, Levesque, and Pierson 1990.

Gough, W.M.F. 1953. A new approach to infant feeding. *Canadian Medical Association Journal* 68: 544–45.

Government of Canada. 2002. *National report–Canada: Ten-year review of the World Summit for Children*. Ottawa: Government of Canada.

Grant, Dorothy Metie. 1968. Breast feeding may be a dying "art." *Canadian Nurse* 64: 45–47.

Greene-Finestone, L., W. Feldman, H. Heick, and B. Luke. 1989. Infant feeding practices and socio-demographic factors in Ottawa-Carleton. *Canadian Journal of Public Health* 80 (3): 173–76.

Greer, Frank R. 1991. Physicians, formula companies, and advertising. *American Journal of Diseases of Children* 145 (3): 282–86.

Greiner, Ted. 1990. Breastfeeding and working women: Thinking strategically. Paper read at Work, Women, and Breastfeeding, at Brasilia.

Grewar, David. 1958. Infantile scurvy in Manitoba. *Canadian Medical Association Journal* 78: 675–80.

——. 1959. Breast feeding. *Canadian Medical Association Journal* 81: 844–45.

Grier, Stella. 1929. The baby's routine and management. *Chatelaine* 19, 53.

Habib, Marlene. 1997. Human milk banks are controversial wet nurses [International seminar organized by Toronto's Infant Feeding Action Coalition]. *Canadian Press NewsWire*, 5 June.

——. 1999. Vitamin D campaign sucks: Breast-feeding group. *Gazette*, 29 April, A12.

——. 2002. New survey shows which baby foods contain genetically modified ingredients. *Canadian Press NewsWire*, 9 October.

Haley, Lynn. 2001. B.C. breastfeeding challenge raises awareness, acceptance. *Medical Post* 37 (6).

Hankins, Gerald W. 2000. *Sunrise over Pangnirtung: The story of Otto Schaefer, M.D.* Komatik Series. Calgary: Arctic Institute of North America.

Hanvey, Louise, and Shirley Post. 1986. Changing patterns in maternity care. *Canadian Nurse* 82 (8): 28–34.

Harrison, Harold E. 1991. Rickets. In Nichols, Ballabriga, and Kretchmer 1991.

Harrison, M.J., J.M. Morse, and M. Prowse. 1985. Successful breastfeeding: The mother's dilemma. *Journal of Advanced Nursing* 19: 261–69.

Hauck, Y., and J. Reinbold. 1996. Criteria for successful breastfeeding: Mother's perceptions. *Australian College of Midwives Incorporated Journal* 9: 21–27.

Hausman, Bernice L. 2003. *Mother's milk: Breastfeeding controversies in American culture.* New York: Routledge.

Health and Welfare Canada. 1975. *Recommended standards for maternity and newborn care.* Ottawa: Information Canada.

——. 1985. *Canadian infant feeding patterns: Results of a national survey, 1982.* Ottawa: Minister of Supply and Services Canada.

——. 1987. *Family-centred maternity and newborn care: National guidelines.* Ottawa.

——. 1990. *Present patterns and trends in infant feeding in Canada.* Ottawa: Minister of Supply and Services Canada.

Health Canada. 1997. *Breastfeeding: A selected bibliography and resource guide.* Ottawa: Minister of Public Works and Government Services Canada.

——. 1998a. *10 great reasons to breastfeed.* Ottawa: Minister of Public Works and Government Services Canada.

——. 1998b. *10 valuable tips for successful breastfeeding.* Ottawa: Minister of Public Works and Government Services Canada.

——. 1998c. *Breastfeeding in Canada: A review and update.* Ottawa: Minister of Public Works and Government Services Canada.

——. 1998d. *Canadian perinatal surveillance system–breastfeeding.* Ottawa: Health Canada.

——. 2000. *Family-centred maternity and newborn care: National guidelines.* Ottawa: Health Canada.

——. 2006. *Information update: Health Canada raises concerns about the sale and distribution of human milk.* http://www.hc-sc.gc.ca/ahc-asc/media/advisories-avis/2006/2006_56_e.html (accessed 11 September 2006).

Health Programs Branch. 1975. *The Canadian mother and child.* Ottawa: National Health and Welfare.

Heinrich, Jeff. 1996. New infant formula a "non-event," breast-feeding advocates say. *Gazette*, 16 June, A4.

Henripin, J. 1954. La fécondité des ménages canadiens au début du XVIIIe siècle. *Population* (French ed.) 9e Année (1): 61–84.

Hill, Lee Forrest. 1967. Infant feeding: Historical and current. *Pediatric Clinics of North America* 14 (1): 255–68.

Hogan, Denys. 1979a. Churches fight formula promotion: Nestlé smarting from boycott. *Globe and Mail*, 15 December, 15.

——. 1979b. Risk to native infants. *Globe and Mail*, 15 December, 15.

Hollingsworth, J.B. 1925. Milk and dairy inspection. *Public Health Journal* 15: 223–26.

Hollobon, Joan. 1975. Doctors urged to end neutrality, back breast feeding of babies. *Globe and Mail*, 12 November, 12.

Holmes, Oliver W. 1911. Scholastic and bedside teaching. In *Medical essays*. Boston: Houghton Mifflin. Quoted in Pearson, Howard A. 1991. Pediatrics in the United States. In Nichols, Ballabriga, and Kretchmer 1991, 60.

Holt, L. Emmett. 1907. *The care and feeding of children: A catechism for the use of mothers and children's nurses.* 4th ed. New York: D. Appleton and Company. *Project Gutenberg's The care and feeding of children, by L. Emmett Holt.* http://www.gutenberg.net.

Howes, Helen Claire. 1949. Newborn babies "room in." *Saturday Night*, May, 24.

——. 1950. Cheapest baby food ... and the best. *Saturday Night*, November, 46–47.

Huetis, Archibald M. 1918. Mother's pensions vs. provincial aid for children. *Public Health Journal* 9 (4): 163–70.

Immigrants coming to Canada. 1908. *Canada Lancet* 42 (2): 139–40.

INFACT Canada. 1995. BC Women's Hospital takes lead on rejecting free formula–a step to being baby friendly. *INFACT Canada Newsletter*, Fall.

——. 1996. Women on the frontlines: Breastfeeding and human rights. *INFACT Canada Newsletter*. http://www.infactcanada.ca/br_bf_frontlines.htm.

——. 1997. Michelle Poirier versus the BC Ministry of Municipal Affairs. *INFACT Canada Newsletter*, Winter.

——. 2000. Women's breastfeeding rights chart. *INFACT Canada Newsletter*, Spring.

——. 2001. The WHO International Code in Canada: Twenty years later. *INFACT Canada Newsletter*, Spring.

——. 2002a. Warning: Filling out coupons may hook you into artificial promotion machine. *INFACT Canada Newsletter*, Summer/Fall.

——. 2002b. Health protection and health care in Canada: Protecting the health of Canadians and the health care system in Canada: A submission to the Commission on the Future of Health Care in Canada. http://www.infactcanada.ca/news_releases_Soy_Formula.htm.

——. *INFACT Canada fact sheet: Environment: Working together for a toxic-free future.* http://www.infactcanada.ca/Environment,%20Working%20Together%20for%20a%20Toxic-Free%20Future.pdf.

International Baby Food Action Network (IBFAN). 2001. *Mead Johnson–breaking the rules.* http://www.ibfan.org/english/codewatch/btro1/MEADJ-en.html (accessed 12 May 2005).

International Women's Rights Watch. 1994. Government of Quebec increased public assistance to women who breastfeed and has ceased payment for infant formulas. *Women's Watch* 8 (3): 6.

Jasen, Patricia. 2002. Race, culture, and the colonization of childbirth in northern Canada. In *Rethinking Canada: The promise of women's history*, ed. V. Strong-Boag, M.L. Gleason, and A. Perry. Oxford: Oxford University Press.

Jones, Debbie. 1980. Inuit babies die at 5 times national rate, study shows. *Globe and Mail*, 1 February, 8.

Jones, Frances. 2003. History of North American donor milk banking: One hundred years of progress. *Journal of Human Lactation* 19 (3): 313–18.

——. 2006. From the Chair. *MNBANA Matter* 3: 3.

Jones, Frances, and Marina Green. 1996. The B.C. Baby-Friendly Initiative. *Nursing BC* 28 (5): 7–8.

Kealey, G. 1980. *Toronto workers respond to industrial capitalism, 1867–1892.* Toronto: University of Toronto Press.

Kingsmill, A.B. 1995. *Dr. Alan Brown–portrait of a tyrant.* Canadian Medical Lives, ed. T. Morley. Markham, ON: Fitzhenry & Whiteside.

Kintner, Hallie J. 1985. Trends and regional differences in breastfeeding in Germany from 1871 to 1937. *Journal of Family History* 10 (2): 163–79.

Kirkey, Sharon. 2005. Mamas, don't let your babies grow up to be chunky ds. Don Mills, ON: CanWest News Service.

Knaak, Stephanie J. 2006. The problem with breastfeeding discourse. *Canadian Journal of Public Health* 97 (5): 412.

Kome, Penney. 1981. Formula-feeding is hurting native infants' health: MD. *Globe and Mail*, 16 July, T2.

Kopun, Francine. 2006. Investing in motherhood. *Toronto Star*, 19 February, D3.

Krahn, Harvey J., and Graham S. Lowe. 2002. Women's employment. In *Work, industry and Canadian society.* Scarborough, ON: Thomson Nelson.

Kroeger, Mary. 2004. *Impact of birthing practices on breastfeeding: Protecting the mother and baby continuum.* Sudbury, MA: Jones and Bartlett Publishers.

Kryhul, Angela. 2000. Bringing up baby: Sampling, coupons and baby clubs are key tools for infant care marketers. *Marketing Magazine* 105 (28): 13.

La Leche League International. 1981. *The womanly art of breastfeeding.* 3rd ed. Franklin Park, IL: La Leche League International.

Lachapelle, Séverin. 1888. *La mère et l'enfant.* Vol. 5, Bk. 10. Quoted in Thornton and Olson 2001, 118.

Lalou, Richard. 1997. Endogenous mortality in New France: At the crossroads of natural and social selection. In Bideau, Desjardins, and Brignoli 1997.

Langford, Nanci. 2000. Childbirth on the Canadian prairies, 1880–1930. In *Telling tales: Essays in western women's history*, ed. C.A. Cavanaugh and R.R. Warne. Vancouver: University of British Columbia Press.

Laurie, C.N. 1913. Sanitary work among the foreign population. *Public Health Journal* 4 (8): 455–57.

Law, Jules. 2000. The politics of breastfeeding: Assessing risk, dividing labour. *Journal of Women in Culture and Society* 25 (2): 407–50.

Ledogar, Robert J. 1975. Formula for malnutrition. In *Hungry for profits: U.S. food and drug multinationals in Latin America.* New York: IDOC.

Leff, Ellen W., Margaret P. Gagne, and Sandra C. Jefferis. 1994. Maternal perceptions of successful breastfeeding. *Journal of Human Lactation* 10 (2): 99–104.

Leff, Ellen W., Sandra C. Jefferis, and Margaret P. Gagne. 1994. The development of the maternal breastfeeding evaluation scale. *Journal of Human Lactation* 10 (2): 105–11.

Lent, Barbara, Susan P. Phillips, Beverley Richardson, and Donna Stewart. 2000. Promoting parental leave for female and male physicians. *Canadian Medical Association Journal* 162 (11): 1575–76.

Levinson, Abraham. 1943. *Pioneers of pediatrics.* New York: Froben Press.

Levitt, Cheryl. 1995. Canada urged to ban free infant-formula samples. *Canadian Medical Association Journal* 152 (10): 1587.

Levitt, C.A., J. Kaczorowski, L. Hanvey, D. Avard, and G. Chance. 1996. Breast-feeding policies and practices in Canadian hospitals providing maternity care. *Canadian Medical Association Journal* 155 (2): 181–88.

Lewis, Milton. 1980. The problem of infant feeding: The Australian experience from the mid-nineteenth century to the 1920s. *Journal of the History of Medicine and Applied Sciences* 35 (2): 174–87.

Lewis, Norah Lillian. 1980. Advising the parents: Child rearing in British Columbia during the inter-war years. PhD diss., University of British Columbia, Vancouver. In Arnup 1994.

——. 1982–83. Creating the little machine: Child rearing in British Columbia, 1919–1939. *BC Studies* 56: 44–60.

Lewis, Norah, and Judy Watson. 1991/92. *The Canadian mother and child*: A time-honoured tradition. *Health Promotion* (Winter): 10–13.

Light, Beth, and Joy Parr, eds. 1983. *Canadian women on the move 1867–1920.* Vol. 2 of *Documents in Canadian women's history.* Toronto: New Hogtown Press and Ontario Institute for Studies in Education.

Light, Beth, and Ruth Roach Pierson, eds. 1990. *No easy road: Women in Canada 1920s to 1960s.* Vol. 3 of *Documents in Canadian women's history.* Toronto: New Hogtown Press.

Lowry, Lynda. 2004. Breast milk substitutes–an update. *In-Touch* 21 (2): 1–4.

Macdougall, Chas S. 1923. Malnutrition in children of school age. *Public Health Journal* 14: 25–35.

MacDougall, Heather. 1990. *Activists and advocates: Toronto's Health Department, 1883–1983.* Toronto: Dundurn Press.

MacGregor, R.R. 1923. Supplemental feeding in gastro-intestinal disturbances of the breast fed infant. *Canadian Medical Association Journal* 13 (3): 179–80.

Maclean, Heather. 1990. *Women's experiences of breast feeding.* Toronto: University of Toronto Press.

——. 1998. Breastfeeding in Canada: A demographic and experiential perspective. *Journal of the Canadian Dietetic Association* 59 (1): 15–23.

MacMurchy, Helen. 1910. *Infant mortality: Special report.* Toronto: Legislative Assembly of Ontario.

——. 1911. *Infant mortality: Second special report.* Toronto: Legislative Assembly of Ontario.

——. 1912. *Infant mortality: Third report.* Toronto: Legislative Assembly of Ontario.

——. 1918. The baby's father. *Public Health Journal* 9 (7): 315–19.

——. 1923. *The Canadian mother's book.* The Little Blue Books: Mothers' Series no. 1. Ottawa: Department of Health (F.A. Acland).

——. 1928a. *Maternal mortality in Canada: Report of an enquiry made by the Department of Health Division of Child Welfare.* Ottawa: Department of Health.

——. 1928b. *The Canadian mother's book.* Ottawa: Department of Health (F.A. Acland).

MacMurchy, Helen, and Canada. Department of Health. 1923. *The Canadian mother's book.* Ottawa: F.A. Acland.

——. 1928. *The Canadian mother's book.* Ottawa.

MacMurchy, Helen, and Canada. Division of Child Welfare. 1929. *Rickets: Prevention and cure.* National Health Publication no. 43. Ottawa: F.A. Acland.

Makin, Kirk. 1981. Quick to back code on infant formula, Canada slow to act. *Globe and Mail,* 9 July, 5.

Martyn, Tessa. 2003. Artificial baby milks: How safe is soya? *Midwives: The Official Journal of the Royal College of Midwives* 6 (5): 212–15.

McCaulay, Ann C., Nancy Hanusaik, and Janet E. Beauvais. 1989. Breastfeeding in the Mohawk community of Kahnawake: Revisited and redefined. *Canadian Journal of Public Health* 80: 177–81.

McConnachie, Kathleen. 1983. Methodology in the study of women in history: A case study of Helen MacMurchy, M.D. *Ontario History* 75 (1): 61–70.

McCullough, John W.S. 1933a. Chatelaine's baby clinic, no. 4: Artificial feeding. *Chatelaine* 6: 66–67.

——. 1933b. Chatelaine's baby clinic, no. 6: The nursing mother. *Chatelaine* 6: 64–65.

——. 1936. Milk for holiday children. *Chatelaine* 9: 42.

McGinnis, Janice P. Dickin. 1981. The impact of epidemic influenza: Canada, 1918–1919. In Shortt 1981.

McInnis, Marvin. 1997. Infant mortality in late nineteenth-century Canada. In Bideau, Desjardins, and Brignoli 1997.

McKendry, J.B.J., and J.D. Bailey. 1990. *Paediatrics in Canada.* Ottawa: Canadian Paediatric Society.

McKenna, James, Sarah Mosko, and Christopher Richard. 1997. Bedsharing promotes breastfeeding. *Pediatrics* 100 (2): 214–19.

McKim, E., M. Laryea, S. Banoub-Baddour, K. Matthews, and K. Webber. 1998. Infant feeding practices in coastal Labrador. *Journal of the Canadian Dietetic Association* 59 (1): 35–42.

McKinley, Nita Mary, and Janet Shibley Hyde. 2004. Personal attitudes or structural factors? A contextual analysis of breastfeeding duration. *Psychology of Women Quarterly* 28: 388–99.

McLaren, Angus. 1981. Birth control and abortion in Canada, 1870–1920. In Shortt 1981.

——. 1990. *Our own master race: Eugenics in Canada, 1885–1945.* Toronto: McClelland and Stewart.

McNally, E., S. Hendricks, and I. Horowitz. 1985. A look at breast-feeding trends in Canada (1963–1982). *Canadian Journal of Public Health* 76 (March/April): 101–7.

Mercier, Michael E., and Christopher G. Boone. 2002. Infant mortality in Ottawa, Canada, 1901: Assessing cultural, economic and environmental factors. *Journal of Historical Geography* 4: 486.

Millar, Wayne J., and Heather Maclean. 2005. Breastfeeding practices. *Health Reports* 16 (2): 23–31.

Millard, Ann V. 1990. The place of the clock in pediatric advice: Rationales, cultural themes, and impediments to breastfeeding. *Social Science and Medicine* 31 (2): 211–21.

Mitchinson, Wendy. 1993. The medical treatment of women. In Burt, Code, and Dorney 1993.

Montreal Health Bureau. 1914. How to take care of babies during hot weather: No other milk, no other food, not even a wet nurse, can take the place of milk from the child's own mother. Montreal: Montreal Health Bureau.

Moore, Michael. 1978. Baby bottle, not just a liquor bottle, hurting way of life, Indian says. *Globe and Mail*, 12 January, F4.

Morrow, Marina. 2007. "Our Bodies Our Selves" in context: Reflections on the women's health movement in Canada. In *Women's health in Canada: Critical perspectives on theory and policy*, ed. M. Morrow, O. Hankivsky, and C. Varcoe. Toronto: University of Toronto Press.

Morse, Janice M. 1989. "Euch, those are for your husband!" Examination of cultural values and assumptions associated with breast-feeding. *Health Care for Women International* 11 (2): 223–32.

Morse, Janice M., and Margaret Harrison. 1987. Social coercion for weaning. *Journal of Nurse-Midwifery* 32 (4): 205–10.

Moxley, Susan, Nicki Sims-Jones, Agnes Vargha, and Marie Chamberlain. 1997. Breastfeeding: A course for health professionals. *Canadian Nurse* 93 (9): 35–38.

Mullen, Heurner. 1915. History of the organization of the Babies' Dispensary Guild, Hamilton. *Public Health Journal* 6 (11): 542–44.

Murphy, Elizabeth. 1999. "Breast is best": Infant feeding decisions and maternal deviance. *Sociology of Health and Illness* 21 (2): 187–208.

Myres, A.W. 1979a. A retrospective look at infant feeding practices in Canada: 1965–1978. *Journal of the Canadian Dietetic Association* 40 (3): 200–211.

——. 1979b. Every baby deserves the breast. *Canadian Consumer*, February, 12–14.

——. 1980. Recent developments in nutrition and infant feeding. *Canadian Pharmaceutical Journal* 113: 11–15.

——. 1981. Breast-feeding–a national priority for infant health. *Journal of the Canadian Dietetic Association* 42 (2): 130–41.

——. 1983. The national breast-feeding promotion program. Part 2: Public information phase–a note on its development, distribution and impact. *Canadian Journal of Public Health* 74 (November/December): 404–8.

——. 1988. National initiatives to promote breastfeeding: Canada, 1979–85. In *Programmes to promote breastfeeding*, ed. D. Jelliffe and E. Jelliffe. Oxford: Oxford University Press.

Myres, A.W., J. Watson, and C. Harrison. 1981. The national breast-feeding promotion program. Part 1: Professional phase–a note on its development, distribution and impact. *Canadian Journal of Public Health* 72 (September/October): 307–11.

Nault, Francois, Bertrand Desjardins, and Jacques Legare. 1990. Effects of reproductive behaviour on infant mortality of French-Canadians during the seventeenth and eighteenth centuries. *Population Studies* 44: 273–85.

Naylor, Audrey J. 2001. Baby Friendly Hospital Initiative: Protecting, promoting, and supporting breastfeeding in the twenty first century. *Pediatric Clinics of North America* 48 (2): 475–83.

Neander, Wendy L., and Janice M. Morse. 1989. Tradition and change in the northern Alberta Woodlands Cree: Implications for infant feeding practices. *Canadian Journal of Public Health* 80: 190–94.

Nestlé Canada. 2005. *Milestones 2005.* http://www.nestle.ca (accessed 20 May 2005).

Netscribes. 2005. *Market trends: Baby/toddler food and beverage products.* Ed. D. Montuori, *Packaged Facts.* New York: MarketResearch.com.

Newton, Lisa H. 1999. Truth is the daughter of time: The real story of the Nestle case. *Business and Society Review* 104 (4): 367–95.

Newton, Michael, and Niles Newton. 1970. The Normal Course and Management of Lactation. *Child and Family* 9 (2): 102–20.

Nichols, B.L., A. Ballabriga, and N. Kretchmer, eds. 1991. *History of pediatrics 1850–1950.* New York: Raven Press.

Nicholson, Patricia. 2005. Inside Canada's breast milk bank. *Medical Post,* 9 August, 1–2.

Nolan, Liana, and Vivek Goel. 1995. Sociodemographic factors related to breastfeeding in Ontario: Results from the Ontario Health Survey. *Canadian Journal of Public Health* 86 (5): 309–12.

Nonesuch, Kate, and Health and Welfare Canada Health Services Promotion Branch. 1991. *You and your baby.* Vancouver/Toronto: Douglas & McIntyre.

Nutrition Canada, Bureau of Nutritional Sciences. 1976. *Food consumption patterns report.* Ottawa: Department of National Health and Welfare.

Office of the United Nations High Commissioner for Human Rights. 1990. *Convention on the rights of the child.* http://www.unhchr.ch/html/menu3/b/k2crc.htm (accessed 4 December 2008).

O'Neil, John, and Patricia A. Kaufert. 1996. The politics of obstetric care: The Inuit experience. In *Canadian women: A reader,* ed. W. Mitchinson, P. Bourne, A. Prentice, G. Guthbert Brandt, B. Light, and N. Black. Toronto: Harcourt Brace & Company Canada.

Ostry, Aleck. 1994. Public health and the Canadian state: The formative years, 1880 to 1920. *Canadian Journal of Public Health* 85 (5): 293–94.

——. 1995a. Prelude to medicare: Institutional change and continuity in Saskatchewan, 1944–1962. *Prairie Forum* (Spring): 87–105.

——. 1995b. Theories of disease causation and their impact on public health in 19th century Canada. *Canadian Journal of Public Health* 85 (6): 368–69.

——. 2006. *Change and continuity in the Canadian health care system.* Ottawa: Canadian Healthcare Association.

Palda, Valerie A., Jeanne-Marie Guise, C. Nadine Wathen, and Canadian Task Force on Preventive Care. 2004. Interventions to promote breast-feeding: Applying the evidence in clinical practice. *Canadian Medical Association Journal* 170 (6): 976–78.

Payne, Elizabeth. 2005. Breast is best: When Katrina hit, many bottle-fed infants were at high risk. *Ottawa Citizen,* 17 September, I2.

Pearce, Tralee. 2007. Breast friends. *Globe and Mail,* 1 May, L1.

Phillipp, Barbara L., and Anne Merewood. 2004. The baby-friendly way: The breastfeeding start. *Pediatric Clinics of North America* 51 (3).

Philipp, Barbara L., Anne Merewood, Lisa W. Miller, Neetu Chawla, Melissa Murphy-Smith, Jenifer S. Gomes, Sabrina Cimo, and John T. Cook. 2001. Baby-Friendly Hospital Initiative improves breastfeeding initiation rates in a US hospital setting. *Pediatrics* 108 (3): 677–81.

Picard, Andre. 2005. Take it to the bank, breast milk is best. *Globe and Mail*, 25 August, A13.

Pierson, Ruth. 1977. Women's emancipation and the recruitment of women into the labour force in World War II. In Trofimenkoff and Prentice 1977.

Poirier v. British Columbia (Ministry of Municipal Affairs, Recreation and Housing). 1997. In *Canadian Human Rights Reporter.* British Columbia Human Rights Tribunal.

Post, Shirley. 1981. Family-centered maternity care: The Canadian picture. *Dimensions in Health Service* (June): 26–31.

Potter, Beth, Judy Sheeshka, and Ruta Valaitis. 2000. Content analysis of infant feeding messages in a Canadian women's magazine, 1945 to 1995. *Journal of Nutrition Education* 32 (4): 196–203.

Prentice, Alison, Gail Cuthbert Bourne, Beth Light, Wendy Mitchinson, and Naomi Black. 1988. *Canadian women: A history.* Toronto: Harcourt Brace Jovanovich.

Priest, Alicia. 1990. "Breast is best." That's the well-worn adage ... *Vancouver Sun*, 10 November, 1.

Province of British Columbia, Ministry of Health. 2005. *Baby's best chance: Parents' handbook of pregnancy and baby care.* 6th ed. Victoria, BC: Open School BC.

Reed, Pauline. 1999. When the milk doesn't come in: A first-time mother feels guilt and shame for bottlefeeding her baby. *Province*, 31 October, B4.

Reid, Anthony J. 1996. Adopting the WHO International Code of Marketing of Breast-milk Substitutes. *Canadian Family Physician* 42: 1639–41.

Rollet, Catherine. 1997. The fight against infant mortality in the past: An international comparison. In Bideau, Desjardins, and Brignoli 1997.

Rorke, Robert. 1916. Infant feeding. *Canadian Nurse* 12 (2): 67–70.

Roslin, Alex. 2008. Breast-feeding gets cold shoulder in B.C. hospitals. *Straight*, 3 July. http://www.straight.com/article-151971/breastfeeding-gets-cold-shoulder-hospitals.

Royer, Albert. 1962. Problems in infant feeding. *Canadian Nurse* 58 (11): 991–92.

Rozee, Emily. 1976. New concepts in infant nutrition. *Canadian Nurse* 72: 18–21.

Rudolf, Robert D. 1912. Low percentages in infant feeding. *Canadian Medical Association Journal* 2 (3): 173–80.

Ryan, Kathleen M., and Victoria M. Grace. 2001. Medicalization and women's knowledge: The construction of understanding of infant feeding experiences in post WWII New Zealand. *Health Care for Women International* 22: 483–500.

Sallot, Jeff. 1979. Insurance against ear infections: Breastfeeding urged on native mothers. *Globe and Mail*, 13 September, T8.

Samuel, Jean. 1997. Breastfeeding and the empowerment of women. *Canadian Nurse* 93 (2): 47–48.

Sandelowski, Margarete. 1984. *Pain, pleasure, and American childbirth: From the twilight sleep to the Read method, 1914–1960.* Westport, CT: Greenwood Press.

Sauve, R., K. Buchan, A. Clyne, and D. McIntosh. 1984. Mothers' milk banking: Microbiological aspects. *Canadian Journal of Public Health* 75: 133–36.

Schaefer, Otto, and Donald W. Spady. 1982. Changing trends in infant feeding patterns in the Northwest Territories 1973–1979. *Canadian Journal of Public Health* 73 (September/October): 304–9.

Schmied, V., and L. Barclay. 1999. Connection and pleasure, disruption and distress: Women's experiences of breastfeeding. *Journal of Human Lactation* 15 (4): 325–34.

Schmied, Virginia, Athena Sheehan, and Lesley Barclay. 2001. Contemporary breast-feeding policy and practice: Implications for midwives. *Midwifery* 17: 44–54.

Sharkey, Ann. 1952. Starting baby off. *Canadian Nurse* 48 (3): 188–89.

Shortt, S.E.D., ed. 1981. *Medicine in Canadian society: Historical perspectives.* Montreal: McGill-Queen's University Press.

Sibbald, Barbara. 2000. Canada's only human milk bank may close. *Canadian Medical Association Journal* 163 (3): 319.

Siegel, Linda S. 1984. Child health and development in English Canada, 1790–1850. In *Health, disease and medicine: Essays in Canadian history*, ed. C.G. Roland. Toronto: Hannah Institute for the History of Medicine.

Smith, Julie P. 1999. Human milk supply in Australia. *Food Policy* 24: 71–91.

Smith, Julie P., and Lindy H. Ingham. 2005. Mothers' milk and measures of economic output. *Feminist Economics* 11 (1): 41–62.

Sokoloff, Heather. 2004. 40% get nothing for maternity leave. The myth of maternity leave [series]. *National Post*, 15 March, A1. Fro.

Sommer, Allison Kaplan. 2005. Israeli study: Probiotics in baby formula can prevent illness and infection. Canada-Israel Committee. http://www. Israel21c.org.

Sorg, Marcella H., and Beatrice C. Craig. 1983. Patterns of infant mortality in the Upper St. John Valley French population: 1791–1838. *Human Biology* 55 (1): 100–113.

Spohn, Howard. 1920. Infant feeding. *Canadian Medical Monthly* 5 (9): 363–73.

Statistics Canada. 2001a. *Breastfeeding practices.* http://www.statcan.ca/english/freepub/82-221-XIE/01201/high/breast.htm (accessed 11 September 2006).

——. 2001b. 2001 Aboriginal peoples survey. Catalogue no. 89M0021XCB. Ottawa: Statistics Canada.

Statistics Canada. 1983. Historical Statistics of Canada. Table B1-14: Live births, cude birth rate, age-specific fertility rates, gross reproduction rate and percentage of births in hospital, Canada, 1921–1974. http://www .statcan.gc.ca/pub/11-516-x/sectionb/4147437-eng.htm.

Sterken, Elisabeth. 2002. *Out of the mouths of babes: How Canada's infant foods industry defies World Health Organization rules and puts infant health at risk.* Toronto: INFACT Canada.

——. 2004. Edmonton works to re-open human milk bank. *INFACT Canada Newsletter* (Fall): 10.

Stewart, Paula J., and Jean Steckle. 1987. Breastfeeding among Canadian Indians on-reserve and women in the Yukon and N.W.T. *Canadian Journal of Public Health* 78: 255–61.

Strong-Boag, Veronica. 1977. "Setting the stage": National organization and the women's movement in the late 19th century. In Trofimenkoff and Prentice 1977.

——. 1982. Intruders in the nursery: Childcare professionals reshape the years one to five, 1920–1940. In *Childhood and family in Canadian history*, ed. J. Parr. Toronto: McClelland and Stewart.

——. 1994. *"Janey Canuck": Women in Canada, 1919–1939*. Historical Booklet no. 53. Ottawa: Canadian Historical Society.

Strong-Boag, Veronica, and Kathryn McPherson. 1990. The confinement of women: Childbirth and hospitalization in Vancouver, 1919–1939. In Arnup, Levesque, and Pierson 1990.

Struthers, R.R. 1925. Comparison and interpretation on a caloric basis of the milk mixtures used in infant feeding. *Canadian Medical Association Journal* 15 (12): 1276–77.

Sussman, George D. 1982. *Selling mother's milk: The wet-nursing business in France, 1715–1914*. Urbana: University of Illinois Press.

Taggart, Marie-Elizabeth. 1976. A practical guide to successful breast feeding. *Canadian Nurse* 72: 25–35.

Thompson, Elizabeth. 1968. Group aims to teach art of breastfeeding. *Globe and Mail*, 18 July, W4.

Thornton, Patricia, and Sherry Olson. 1991. Family contexts of fertility and infant survival in nineteenth-century Montreal. *Journal of Family History* 16 (4): 401–17.

——. 1997. Infant vulnerability in three cultural settings in Montreal, 1880. In Bideau, Desjardins, and Brignoli 1997.

——. 2001. A deadly discrimination among Montreal infants, 1860–1900. *Continuity and Change* 16 (1): 95–135.

Tinkiss, Ruby. 1948. Mothers' milk services in Saskatchewan. *Canada's Health and Welfare* 3 (5): 6–7.

Tisdall, Frederick F. 1942. *The home care of the infant and child*. New York: New Home Library.

Tomes, Nancy. 1999. Spreading the germ theory: Sanitary science and home economics, 1880–1930. In *Women and health in America: Historical readings*, ed. J.W. Leavitt. Madison: University of Wisconsin Press.

Trofimenkoff, S.M., and A. Prentice, eds. 1977. *The neglected majority: Essays in Canadian women's history*. Toronto: McClelland and Stewart.

Tseng, Marilyn. 2006. Editorial. Breastfeeding–part of the slow food movement? *Public Health Journal* 9 (6): 667–68.

Tully, Mary Rose, Laraine Lockhart-Borman, and Kim Updegrove. 2004. Stories of success: The use of donor milk is increasing in North America. *Journal of Human Lactation* 20 (1): 75–77.

Tyson, Holliday. 1991. Outcomes of 1001 midwife-attended home births in Toronto, 1983–1988. *Birth* 18 (1): 14–19.

Ursel, Jane. 1992. *Private lives, public policy: 100 years of state intervention in the family*. Toronto: Women's Press.

Van Esterik, Penny. 1989. *Beyond the breast-bottle controversy*. New Brunswick, NJ: Rutgers University Press.

——. 1994. Breastfeeding and feminism. *International Journal of Gynecology and Obstetrics* 47: s41–s54.

——. 1997. The politics of breastfeeding: An advocacy perspective. In *Food and culture: A reader*, ed. C. Counihan and P. Van Esterik. New York: Routledge.

——. 2000. Nurturing cycles. Paper read at The Gender of Genetic Futures: The Canadian Biotechnology Strategy, Women and Health, at York University.

——. 2002. Contemporary trends in infant feeding research. *Annual Review of Anthropology* 31: 257–78.

Van Esterik, P., and T. Greiner. 1981. Breastfeeding and women's work: Constraints and opportunities. *Studies in Family Planning* 12 (4): 184–97.

Vipond, Mary. 1977. The image of women in mass circulation magazines in the 1920s. In Trofimenkoff and Prentice 1977.

Wah, Wong. 2000. Advanced breastfeeding: WHO and UNICEF's existing Ten Steps to Successful Breastfeeding should be extended to 12 steps. *Canadian Nurse* 96 (7): 10.

Wall, G. 2001. Moral constructions of motherhood in breastfeeding discourse. *Gender & Society* 15 (4): 592–610.

Wall, R.J., D.E. Kerr, and K.R. Bondioli. 1997. Transgenic dairy cattle: Genetic engineering on a large scale. *Journal of Dairy Science* 80: 2213–24.

Wallace, Anne. 1980. Nursing mothers then and now. *Canadian Nurse* (October): 44–47. .

Ward, W.P., and P.C. Ward. 1984. Infant birth weight and nutrition in industrializing Montreal. *American Historical Review* 89 (2): 324–45.

Weaver, John D. 1974. *Carnation: The first 75 years.* Los Angeles: Anderson, Ritchie & Simon.

Webb, Jean. 1953. *The Canadian mother and child.* Ottawa: Department of National Health and Welfare.

Weekend Magazine. 1978. *The Globe and Mail,* 13 May, 01.

Weiner, Lynn. 1994. Reconstructing motherhood: The La Leche League in postwar America. *Journal of American History* 80 (4): 1357–81.

Williams, P.L., S.M. Innis, and A.M.P. Vogel. 1996. Breastfeeding and weaning practices in Vancouver. *Canadian Journal of Public Health* 87 (4): 231–36.

WHO. *See* World Health Organization.

Wolf, Jacqueline H. 2001. *Don't kill your baby: Public health and the decline of breastfeeding in the nineteenth and twentieth century.* Women and health: Cultural and social perspectives. Columbus: Ohio State University Press.

Woodard, Joe. 1997. Let it all hang out: Swiss Chalet strikes a blow for natural nursing in public. *Alberta Report,* 27 October, 43.

World Health Organization (WHO) and United Nations Children's Fund (UNICEF). 1989. *Protecting, promoting and supporting breast-feeding: The special role of maternity services.* Geneva: WHO.

——. 1990. Protecting, promoting and supporting breastfeeding: The special role of maternity services. *International Journal of Gynecology and Obstetrics* 31 (Suppl. 1): 171–83.

——. 2006. *Innocenti declaration: On the protection, promotion and support of breastfeeding.* WHO/UNICEF 1990. http://www.unicef.org/programme/breastfeeding/innocenti.htm (accessed 6 September 2006).

Yalom, Marilyn. 1997. *A history of the breast.* New York: Alfred A. Knopf.

Yeung, D.L., M. Pennell, M. Leung, and J. Hall. 1981. Breastfeeding: Prevalence and influencing factors. *Canadian Journal of Public Health* 72 (September/October): 323–30.

Zimmerman, Deena R., and Nurit Guttman. 2001. "Breast is best": Knowledge among low income mothers is not enough. *Journal of Human Lactation* 17 (1): 14–19.

Index

Books in the Studies in Childhood and Family in Canada Series
Published by Wilfrid Laurier University Press

Making Do: Women, Family, and Home in Montreal during the Great Depression by Denyse Baillargeon, translated by Yvonne Klein • 1999 / xii + 232 pp. / ISBN: 0-88920-326-1 / ISBN-13: 978-0-88920-326-6

Children in English-Canadian Society: Framing the Twentieth-Century Consensus by Neil Sutherland with a new foreword by Cynthia Comacchio • 2000 / xxiv + 336 pp. / illus. / ISBN: 0-88920-351-2 / ISBN-13: 978-0-88920-351-8

Love Strong as Death: Lucy Peel's Canadian Journal, 1833–1836 edited by J.I. Little • 2001 / x + 229 pp. / illus. / ISBN: 0-88920-389-X / ISBN-13: 978-0-88920-389-230-X

The Challenge of Children's Rights for Canada by Katherine Covell and R. Brian Howe • 2001 / viii + 244 pp. / ISBN: 0-88920-380-6 / ISBN-13: 978-0-88920-380-8

NFB Kids: Portrayals of Children by the National Film Board of Canada, 1939–1989 by Brian J. Low • 2002 / vi + 288 pp. / illus. / ISBN: 0-88920-386-5 / ISBN-13: 978-0-88920-386-0

Something to Cry About: An Argument against Corporal Punishment of Children in Canada by Susan M. Turner • 2002 / xx + 317 pp. / ISBN: 0-88920-382-2 / ISBN-13: 978-0-88920-382-2

Freedom to Play: We Made Our Own Fun edited by Norah L. Lewis • 2002 / xiv + 210 pp. / ISBN: 0-88920-406-3 / ISBN-13: 978-0-88920-406-5

The Dominion of Youth: Adolescence and the Making of Modern Canada, 1920–1950 by Cynthia Comacchio • 2006 / x + 302 pp. / illus. / ISBN: 0-88920-488-8 / ISBN-13: 978-0-88920-488-1

Evangelical Balance Sheet: Character, Family, and Business in Mid-Victorian Nova Scotia by B. Anne Wood • 2006 / xxx + 198 pp. / illus. / ISBN: 0-88920-500-0 / ISBN-13: 978-0-88920-500-0

A Question of Commitment: Children's Rights in Canada edited by R. Brian Howe and Katherine Covell • 2007 / xiv + 442 pp. / ISBN: 978-1-55458-003-3

Taking Responsibility for Children edited by Samantha Brennan and Robert Noggle • 2007 / xxii + 188 pp. / ISBN: 978-1-55458-015-6

Home Words: Discourses of Children's Literature in Canada edited by Mavis Reimer • 2008 / xx + 280 pp. / illus. / ISBN: 978-1-55458-016-3

Depicting Canada's Children edited by Loren Lerner • 2009 / xxvi + 442 pp. / illus. / ISBN: 978-1-55458-050-7

The One Best Way? Breastfeeding History, Politics, and Policy in Canada by Tasnim Nathoo and Aleck Ostry • 2009 / xvi + 266 pp. / illus. / ISBN: 978-1-55458-147-4